Assessment and Treatment of Infant Sleep

Assessment and Treatment of Infant Sleep

Medical and Behavioral Sleep Disorders From Birth to 24 Months

IGNACIO E. TAPIA, MD, MS

Professor
Department of Pediatrics
Chief
Division of Pediatric Pulmonology and Sleep
Medicine
Department of Pediatrics
University of Miami
Miami, Florida

LIAT TIKOTZKY, PhD

Associate Professor
Department of Psychology
Ben-Gurion University of the Negev
Beer-Sheva, Israel

CHRISTOPHER M. CIELO, DO, MS

Assistant Professor of Pediatrics
Division of Pulmonary and Sleep Medicine
Children's Hospital of Philadelphia
Philadelphia, Pennsylvania

ELSEVIER

Elsevier
1600 John F. Kennedy Blvd.
Ste 1800
Philadelphia, PA 19103-2899

Notice

Content Strategist: Mary Hegeler
Content Development Specialist: Ranjana Sharma
Publishing Services Manager: Shereen Jameel
Project Manager: Nandhini Thanga Alagu
Design Direction: Bridget Hoette

Printed in India

Last digit is the print number: 9 8 7 6 5 4 3 2 1

Working together
to grow libraries in
developing countries

www.elsevier.com • www.bookaid.org

CONTRIBUTORS

Olufunke Afolabi-Brown, MD
Attending Physician
Division of Pediatric Pulmonology and Sleep
    Medicine
Department of Pediatrics
Children's Hospital of Philadelphia
Philadelphia, Pennsylvania

Chun Ting Au, PhD
Adjunct Assistant Professor
Department of Paediatrics
The Chinese University of Hong Kong
Sha Tin, Hong Kong
Research Fellow
Department of Translational Medicine
The Hospital for Sick Children
Toronto, Ontario, Canada

**Kate C. Chan, MBChB, MRCPCH, FHKAM (Paed),
FHKC (Paed)**
Associate Professor
Division of Paediatrics
The Chinese University of Hong Kong
Sha Tin, Hong Kong

Ambika Gnanam Chidambaram, MBBS, MS
Assistant Professor
Division of Pediatric Pulmonology
Department of Pediatrics
University of California
Davis, California

Yeilim Cho, MD
Advanced Fellow
Department of Sleep Medicine
VISN 20 Mental Illness Research
Education and Clinical Center
Sleep Physician
Department of Psychiatry and Behavioral
    Sciences
University of Washington School of Medicine
Seattle, Washington

Christopher M. Cielo, DO, MS
Assistant Professor of Pediatrics
Division of Pulmonary and Sleep Medicine
Children's Hospital of Philadelphia
Philadelphia, Pennsylvania

Kelsey D. Csumitta, MS
Doctoral Candidate
Department of Psychological and Brain
    Sciences
Drexel University
Philadelphia, Pennsylvania

Majalisa Dunnewald, MS
MS Student
Department of Psychology
Saint Joseph's University
Philadelphia, Pennsylvania

Zarmina Ehsan, MD
Associate Professor
Department of Pediatrics
University of Missouri Kansas City
Kansas City, Missouri

Lance Feld, MD
Physician
Departments of Pediatric Pulmonary and
    Sleep Medicine
Children's Hospital of Philadelphia
Philadelphia, Pennsylvania

Alisha George, MD
Assistant Professor
Department of Pediatrics
Cincinnati Children's Hospital Medical
    Center
Cincinnati, Ohio

Jennifer Gingrasfield, BFA, RN, MSN, PNP-BC
Pediatric Nurse Practitioner
Sleep Center
Boston Children's Hospital
Boston, Massachusetts

Madeleine M. Grigg-Damberger, MS
Professor
Department of Neurology
University of New Mexico School of
  Medicine
Medical Director
Pediatric Sleep Medicine Services
University of New Mexico Sleep Center
University of New Mexico
Associate Medical Director
Clinical Neurodiagnostic Laboratory
University of New Mexico Medical Center
Vice Chair, Faculty Development
Department of Neurology
Univerrsity of New Mexico
Albuquerque, New Mexico

Wendy A. Hall, RN, BN, MSN, PhD
Professor Emeritus
School of Nursing
University of British Columbia
Vancouver, British Columbia, Canada

Courtney R.J. Kaar, MD
Assistant Professor
Department of Pediatrics
Washington University School of Medicine
St. Louis, Missouri

Michal Kahn, PhD
Assistant Professor
School of Psychological Sciences
Tel Aviv University
Tel Aviv, Israel

Thomas G. Keens, MD
Professor of Pediatrics
Departments of Physiology and Neuroscience
Keck School of Medicine
University of Southern California
Pediatric Pulmonologist
Division of Pediatric Pulmonology and Sleep
  Medicine
Children's Hospital Los Angeles
Los Angeles, California

James S. Kemp, MD
Professor
Department of Pediatrics
Washington University School of Medicine
University City, Missouri

Francesca Lupini, BS, MS
Doctoral Student
Department of Psychology
University of South Carolina
Columbia, South Carolina

Joanna E. MacLean, MD, PhD, FRCPC
Associate Professor
Department of Pediatrics
University of Alberta
Medical Director
Pediatric Sleep Laboratory
Stollery Children's Hospital
Edmonton, Alberta, Canada

Katarina N. A. McKenzie, MSc
Doctoral Student
Department of Psychology
The University of Western Ontario
London, Ontario, Canada

Michael E. McLeland, PhD
Director of Research
Sleep Medicine and Research Center
St. Luke's Hospital
Chesterfield, Missouri

Maile A. Moore, MSN, CPNP-PC
Pediatric Nurse Practitioner
Department of Sleep Medicine
Boston Children's Hospital
Boston, Massachusetts

Melisa E. Moore, PhD, DBSM
Licensed Clinical Psychologist
Los Angeles, California

Judith A. Owens, MD, MPH
Sleep Center Senior Faculty
Department of Neurology
Boston Children's Hospital
Professor
Department of Neurology
Harvard Medical School
Boston, Massachusetts

Graham J. Reid, PhD
Associate Professor
Department of Psychology
The University of Western Ontario
Scientist
Children's Health Research Institute
London, Ontario, Canada

Robert Clinton Stowe, MD
Instructor
Division of Epilepsy and Clinical
    Neurophysiology
Boston Children's Hospital
Boston, Massachusetts

Ignacio E. Tapia, MD, MS
Professor
Department of Pediatrics
Chief
Division of Pediatric Pulmonology and Sleep
    Medicine
Department of Pediatrics
University of Miami
Miami, Florida

Liat Tikotzky, PhD
Associate Professor
Department of Psychology
Ben-Gurion University of the Negev
Beer-Sheva, Israel

Sally L. Davidson Ward, MD
Professor of Clinical Pediatrics
Department of Pediatrics
Children's Hospital Los Angeles
Keck School of Medicine
University of Southern California
Los Angeles, California

Hannah Whittall, PhD
College of Education, Psychology and Social
Work
Flinders University
Bedford Park, South Australia, Australia

Ariel A. Williamson, PhD, DBSM
Licensed Psychologist
Assistant Professor of Child Behavioral
    Health
The Ballmer Institute for Children's
    Behavioral Health
Department of Psychology (clinical area)
University of Oregon
Portland, Oregon

Kathy M. Wolfe, MD, MS
Assistant Professor
Department of Neurology
University of New Mexico School of
    Medicine
Albuquerque, New Mexico

The first 2 years of life in humans are critical for the development of functions and skills that can determine a lifelong trajectory of well-being. Infants experience significant growth and maturation during this period, which requires a nurturing environment, adequate energy intake, and healthy sleep. The latter is affected by sleep duration and timing, sleep consolidation, and regulation, as well as medical conditions affecting sleep or those related to breathing, movements, or other factors. Disrupted sleep health has been associated with delayed developmental milestones, failure to thrive, overall poor physical and mental health, impaired family functioning and parental quality of life, and more—all of which emphasize the utmost importance of this subject.

As clinicians and clinical researchers specializing in pediatric sleep and working in academic settings, we have had the privilege of meeting many colleagues during their training and at conferences and had numerous discussions about the lack of resources available for this age group. Importantly, these discussions led to the realization that a book including an integrative view on medical, developmental, and behavioral topics on sleep during early childhood was needed. With this text, we hope to fill that gap by offering a comprehensive, evidence-based resource that includes the latest research and clinical knowledge about important topics in infant sleep for trainees, researchers, and clinicians.

The first section of the book provides information about normal physiological and behavioral milestones that are relevant to infant sleep; the second section describes the unique evaluation and management of medical sleep disorders specific to infants; and the third section discusses the etiology, assessment, and treatment of behavioral sleep problems in infancy.

We hope that readers will enjoy this work and be as excited as we are about pediatric sleep health.

Ignacio E. Tapia
Christopher M. Cielo
Liat Tikotzky

CONTENTS

Developmental Aspects of Sleep

Developmental Changes in EEG and Sleep Architecture From Prematurity Through Infancy

Robert Clinton Stowe

Introduction

Since the first human electroencephalography (EEG) recordings in the 1920s,[1] researchers have sought to best understand the significance of these tracings as they relate to the generators (e.g., cortical versus thalamic) of these rhythms and how these may provide insight into brain activity and function in different states (e.g., pathological versus normal and wakefulness versus sleep versus coma). At its core, the voltage fields recorded by the scalp EEG electrodes are the summation of excitatory and inhibitory postsynaptic potentials from pyramidal neurons in the most superficial cortex. The frequencies recorded via scalp EEG that can be visually interpreted (without the assistance of advanced automated software) are limited to a band of frequencies under 30 Hz due to attenuation of recorded signals by skull and interceding tissue layers.[2]

The adult EEG tends to be quite predictable. In polysomnograms (PSGs) there may be mild differences observed in voltages with increasing age, changing distributions of sleep stages, and lower thresholds for arousals, but generally speaking there is not much differentiating the EEG of a 24-year-old from that of a 70-year-old. In stark contrast, there are well-described maturational changes in the EEG in pediatrics; the differences between the EEGs of a full-term newborn and a 6-month-old are profound. The predictable electrographic evolution from the *tracé discontinú* pattern of an extremely premature neonate to the expected appearance of vertex waves and sleep spindles in infancy reflects the progressive, continued development of the brain from the simplified and smooth gyral pattern of premature neonates to that of a more mature postnatal brain.

This chapter will seek to review the maturational changes of the sleep EEG from prematurity (i.e., <37 weeks gestational age) to term (i.e., 37–42 weeks gestational age) and through infancy and early childhood to the second year of life. To effectively address the stark evolution of the sleep EEG of the extremely premature neonate and a 2-year-old, a broad review of both wake and sleep EEG features is necessary. This will entail a description of core concepts defining the maturing EEG background such as synchrony/asynchrony, continuity/discontinuity, symmetry/asymmetry, and neonatal *graphoelements*. In this review, key clinical and research correlates to the developmental sleep EEG will be highlighted.

Defining Ages and Conceptional Age

Based on the American Academy of Pediatrics recommendations on age terminology, newborns are considered premature if less than 37 weeks of gestation have been completed, term if 37 to 42 weeks of gestation have been completed, and postterm if they are born after 42 weeks.[3] The term "neonate" refers to a child during the first 28 days after birth and "infant" refers to a child aged 1 to 12 months.

One core concept of neonatal EEG interpretation is establishing the corrected age (CA, sometimes referred to as correct gestational age (GA), conceptional age, postconceptional age, postmenstrual age, or adjusted age). The CA is the estimated GA at birth plus the chronological, actual age (i.e., the number of days and weeks postpartum). The GA is the time elapsed between the first day of the mother's last menstrual period and day of the neonate's birth, expressed in completed weeks. Beyond timing of menstrual cycles, fetal ultrasounds and the baby's postnatal physical examination can be used to modify the GA. A 7-week-old born at 33 weeks' gestation has a CA of 40 weeks for the purposes of EEG interpretation. Determining the accurate CA is crucial for interpretation of the EEG in neonates as the brain and EEG are expected to develop and mature at a similar rate whether the baby is *in utero* or *ex utero*.[2,4-7] For example, the neonate born at 41 weeks' gestation is expected to share the same EEG features as the 10-week-old neonate born at 31 weeks' gestation. This example holds true under the assumption that both of these hypothetical neonates are otherwise neurologically normal; there are of course various pathological processes that may negatively influence orderly EEG maturation and development, such as cerebral dysgenesis disorders, hypoxic-ischemic injury, and metabolic and genetic disorders, among others.

Most professionals working with premature infants will continue to use these aforementioned concepts including CA until the chronological age of the child is somewhere around 2 to 2.5 years old, which is luckily within the scope of this chapter. At this age, it is generally felt that most (healthy) premature babies have had an opportunity to "catch up" to age-matched term peers.[8,9] Some developmental specialists have estimated a rule of thumb needed to correct the developmental gap from prematurity by multiplying the number of prematurity weeks by 10. For example, a premature infant born at 34 weeks' gestation (6 weeks early) would be estimated to require 60 weeks (1 year and 2 months) to prospectively catch up to age-matched term-delivered peers.

PRACTICAL CONSIDERATIONS

Of note, different institutions may utilize different EEG electrode recording montages for the recording of newborns. There are varying opinions on the utility of a full 10–20 EEG montage versus a reduced ("double-distance") montage for neonatal recordings (Fig. 1.1). The American Society of Clinical Neurophysiology position statement on neonatal EEG recording recommends at least the double distance montage but does not go so far to recommend one montage over the other.[7] The primary argument for the reduced montage relies upon the perspective that the smaller cranial vault is effectively recorded by a reduced complement of electrodes. The contrary concern is that the reduced montage is more likely to miss seizures or be less apt to confidently delineate artifact from ictal recording, which has been borne out in some studies.[10] In institutions that do utilize the double-distance montage, once an infant reaches a CA of approximately 48 weeks, then the standard 10–20 EEG montage is implemented. The double-distance neonatal montage still utilizes a greater array of electrodes than the typical EEG montage recommended by the American Academy of Sleep Medicine (AASM) Manual for the Scoring of Sleep and Associated Events for PSG in children and infants.[4] It is noteworthy that many academic pediatric sleep centers utilize a higher number of electrodes during their PSG recordings, such as midline derivations, than those explicitly recommended by the AASM. Regardless of montage, newborn EEGs have traditionally been recorded and interpreted at "half paper speed" (15 mm/second, or approximately 25–30 seconds per page), that is, a compressed EEG view more similar to what sleep physicians typically review and score on PSG. Once an infant reaches a CA of 48 weeks (i.e., 2 months old), the AASM recommends scoring PSGs based on typical NREM and REM sleep stages.

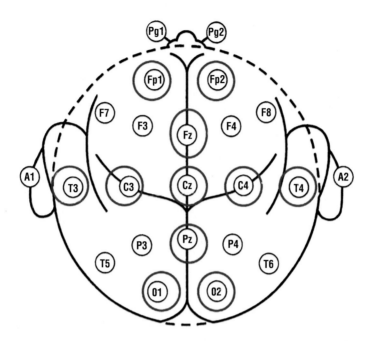

Fig. 1.1 The International 10–20 System for electrode placement, modified for neonates. Electrode positions circled in red are included in the "double distance" neonatal montage. Note that some laboratories use an alternate location for the position of the frontal polar electrodes.

Premature EEGs (23 Weeks to <37 Weeks)

It is worthwhile to mention some of the nuances and challenges (both historical and present-day) inherent to the interpretation of premature neonatal EEGs. From a technical perspective, EEG recording is challenging and potentially inadvisable in the extremely premature neonates (i.e., <28 weeks' gestation) who may have exceptionally fragile and underkeratinized epidermis; the application of EEG electrodes puts these neonates at risk of skin tears and breakdown as well as possibly infection. Thankfully the general indications for EEG monitoring in children at this age are sparse, as seizures are considered generally rare and the baseline biobehavioral states can demonstrate poor reactivity to stimulus. An exceptionally challenging perspective is defining true "normal" in the premature neonate, both in terms of neurological function and EEG activity. Typically neonates who receive any sort of EEG recording have some clinical indication for neurophysiological monitoring, which inherently suggests there is a higher likelihood of neurological abnormality. We have the benefit of more than 50 years of research supporting normative patterns.[2,5,6] There are several conceptual approaches that may help best understand the early sleep EEG recording: a review of the major background patterns, in particular the expected progression from discontinuity to continuity, and neonatal graphoelements will lay the groundwork to approach our patients' EEGs based on CA.

CONTINUITY VERSUS DISCONTINUITY AND SYNCHRONY VERSUS ASYNCHRONY

There are two essential electrical patterns to recognize in neonatal EEG. Continuity refers to uninterrupted electrical activity with less than 2 seconds of relative voltage attenuation less than 25 μV. Discontinuity is defined by bursts of high-voltage electrical activity separated by interburst intervals (IBIs) of relative voltage attenuation less than 25 to 50 μV for a period of at least 2 seconds.[2,6,7,11] Discontinuity and IBI are a function of age and are best defined in background tracings of *tracé discontinú* and *tracé alternant*. Discontinuity may be most easily described as sections of the recording with "on" and "off" periods.

Tracé discontinú (French for "discontinuous tracing") is a pattern of early prematurity seen up to 30 weeks CA. It is defined by high-voltage (50–300 μV) polymorphic bursts of variable frequencies, often containing spiky or sharply contoured waveforms, separated by dramatically attenuated voltages (<25 μV) in IBIs up to 20 seconds or longer in length (Fig. 1.2). From 30 weeks CA to about 34 weeks CA, *tracé discontinú* may remain as a marker of quiet sleep.

Tracé alternant (French for "alternating tracing") is a normal discontinuous EEG pattern in full-term infants representative of quiet (or "N") sleep. This is characterized by at least three alternating runs of bilateral, symmetrical, synchronous high-voltage (50–150 μV) bursts of 1 to 3 Hz delta activity of 3 to 8 seconds alternating with IBIs of 25 to 50 μV, 4 to 7 Hz, theta activity (Fig. 1.3). Bursts often have polyfrequencies beyond just delta activity. Generally, bursts and IBIs are of similar duration. This pattern becomes apparent around 30 weeks CA, slowly replacing the *tracé discontinú* pattern. As the CA progresses, this pattern undergoes a transient period of

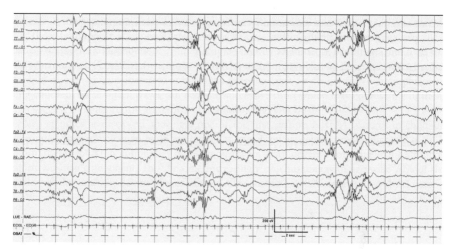

Fig. 1.2 *Tracé discontinú.*

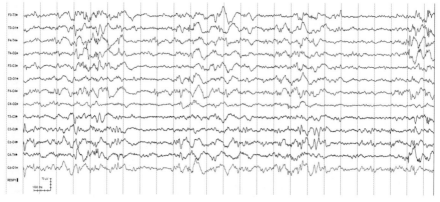

Fig. 1.3 *Tracé alternant.*

asynchrony between 30 weeks CA and term while IBIs shorten and interburst voltages increase. This pattern persists as a marker of quiet sleep up until about 42 to 44 weeks CA.[2,4,6,7,11-13]

There are normative values regarding IBI voltages and durations[7,6] which help to define an appropriately discontinuous from the excessively discontinuous and dysmature EEG (Table 1.1). While discontinuity is a normal feature (if not the prevailing background) of early neonatal EEGs, EEGs should never be discontinuous beyond 2 months of age (46–48 weeks CA); this would be suggestive of diffuse cerebral dysfunction of nonspecific etiology or, possibly, an inaccurate CA.

There is an important caveat regarding discontinuity in that it is expected to be spontaneous and unrelated to specific interventions. It is normal for neonates to have relative voltage attenuation, which may produce a discontinuous-appearing recording during an arousal from sleep or movement and this may best be defined by the concomitant presence of abrupt muscle artifact (Fig. 1.4).

In the extreme perspective of discontinuity is burst suppression. Burst suppression is a markedly abnormal EEG finding of excessively discontinuous background with suppressed (<5 μV) interburst voltages and prolonged IBIs. Burst suppression is invariant, devoid of expected age-appropriate EEG features, absent association to a particular biobehavioral state, and lacking variability and reactivity. The bursts of activity typically contain sharply contoured and spikey-appearing epileptiform discharges. This EEG pattern is associated with severe encephalopathy of nonspecific etiology (e.g., epileptic encephalopathy such as Ohtahara syndrome, severe hypoxic-ischemic encephalopathy) and almost uniformly portends very poor prognosis.[14,15]

The premature neonatal EEG demonstrates a peculiar pattern regarding synchronization of bilateral hemispheric electrical activity. Asynchronous bursts are defined as interhemispheric bursts that are separated by more than 1.5 to 2 seconds of each other. Very early neonatal EEGs

TABLE 1.1 ■ Normal IBI Durations and Amplitudes

Corrected Gestational Age (Weeks)	Typical Interburst Interval (Seconds)	Maximum Interburst Interval (Seconds)	Voltage of Interburst (μV)
<30	6–12	35	<25
30–33	5–8	20	<25
34–36	4–6	10	~25
37–40	2–4	6	>25 (typically 50–75)
41–44	2–4	2–4	>50 (typically 75–100)

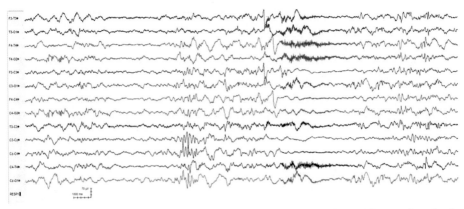

Fig. 1.4 Neonatal arousal demonstrating voltage attenuation in association with overriding muscle artifact in the second half of the record.

(<30 weeks) demonstrate entirely synchronous (often called "hypersynchronous") bursts in their *tracé discontinú* background.[2,6,7,11] Around 30 weeks CA the EEG bursts become notably asynchronous. These asynchronous bursts become progressively more synchronous again such that approximately 70% of bursts are synchronous by 34 weeks' gestation and up to 100% of bursts are synchronous at 40 weeks' gestation. Some very mild asynchrony may persist in normal neonates until the pattern completes abates to the more continuous sleep backgrounds. While this will be discussed in greater detail later, it is important to note that certain developmental sleep features in infancy through early childhood, such as sleep spindles and vertex waves, are expected to be initially asynchronous and eventually become more synchronous.[6]

Normal Continuous Background Patterns of Neonates and Defining Biobehavioral States

In contrast to the discontinuous tracings of early neonates, an increasingly continuous background develops as neonates approach term. A continuous EEG tracing has no recognizable pauses in activity and there are three primary patterns defined in neonates[2,4-7,11-13]:

1. Low voltage irregular (LVI): The LVI pattern is defined by continuous low voltage (~15–35 μV) predominantly theta > delta frequencies. This is observed in active ("R") sleep and wakefulness. See Fig. 1.5 for the LVI pattern observed in active sleep.
2. High-voltage slow (HVS): The HVS pattern is defined by continuous, synchronous, and symmetrical high-voltage (~50–150 μV) delta activity. This activity may be highest amplitude in occipital or central regions. This pattern is observed predominantly in quiet ("N") sleep, although it may rarely occur in active sleep. The *tracé alternant* evolves into the HVS pattern as it becomes less discontinuous/more continuous. This pattern is sometimes referred to as a continuous slow wave sleep (CSWS) pattern and is the predecessor of the more mature slow-wave/stage 3 NREM sleep. See Fig. 1.6 for the HVS pattern.
3. Mixed (M): The M pattern is an intermingling of high-voltage delta (albeit of lower-voltage than the true HVS pattern) and lower-voltage polyfrequencies. This pattern may be observed in any biobehavioral state, although it is most frequently representative of wakefulness and active sleep. This pattern is often still referred to by many EEG readers to its French terminology—*activité moyenne* ("average activity"). See Fig. 1.7 for mixed frequency EEG in active sleep.

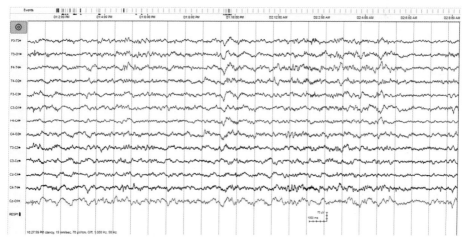

Fig. 1.5 Low voltage irregular pattern observed in active sleep.

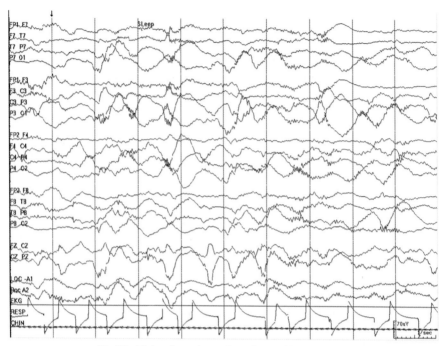

Fig. 1.6   High-voltage slow pattern observed in quiet sleep.

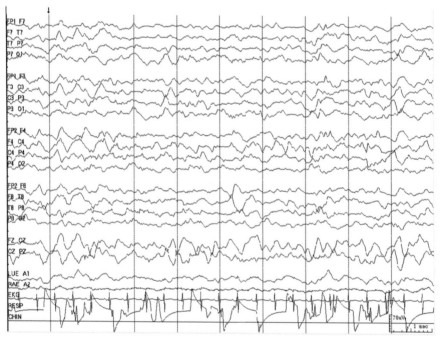

Fig. 1.7   Mixed frequency EEG in active sleep.

TABLE 1.2 ■ Summary of Biobehavioral State Characteristics

Stage	EEG Patterns	Behavior	Respiration	EOG	Chin EMG
Wake	LVI or M	Eyes open, crying, feeding	Irregular, rapid, shallow	Blinks, rapid or scanning eye movements	Present
Quiet Sleep/N	Tracé alternant, HVS, rarely M	Eyes closed, very few movements, some periodic sucking	Deep and regular	No eye movements	Present or may be lower than wake
Active Sleep/R	LVI or M	Eyes closed, random small movements (e.g., squirm, grimace)	Irregular, occasional pauses	Rapid eye movements or no eye movements	Low with brief transient phasic EMG bursts

As is rather apparent in their definitions, these are somewhat nonspecific EEG patterns to state (compared to the expected biobehavioral state of an infant with sleep spindles). It is essential to combine multiple observations to fully assess state as some of these electrophysiological recordings are not standard on every EEG recording (although may be available dependent on the institution). These are the inherent features of a good PSG recording, including visual behavioral assessment, respiratory patterns, EEG, electrooculogram (EOG), and chin electromyogram (EMG). Table 1.2 shows a summary of state characteristics for scoring infants less than 37 weeks CA on PSG[4]:

To add to the confusion of summating multiple parameters to assess sleep state in neonates and infants, there exist definitions of transitional ("T") and indeterminate sleep. Transitional sleep is, intuitively, a period of transition from one sleep state to another and includes elements of both active and quiet sleep (i.e., a combination of either 2 N and 3 R features or 2 R and 3 N features). Indeterminate sleep is defined by the American Clinical Neurophysiology Society (ACNS) as a state of sleep in which the behavioral state is supportive of sleep (i.e., eye closure) but there is a lack of anticipated features to assign a specific sleep state.[7] The AASM does not recommend scoring of indeterminate sleep and encourages assigning a specific stage of N, R, or T.[4,12,13] Typical sleep cycling in newborns occurs in approximate 60-minute cycles with initial sleep entry into the active/REM sleep state up through the first 2 to 3 months of life. Newborns tend to have an equal distribution of active and quiet sleep, although the active/REM sleep component slowly decreases with age such that by age 5 years, children have the general composition of sleep architecture and REM distribution of adults.

NEONATAL GRAPHOELEMENTS

This overview of neonatal graphoelements is helpful in the identification of normal and abnormal EEG features as well as concepts that may provide clues to a wake/sleep EEG epoch. This will not, however, represent an exhaustive review of all neonatal graphoelements. The reader is referred to various pediatric and neonatal EEG atlases for discussion on non–state-defined developmental graphoelements such as temporal sawtooth waves, rhythmic occipital theta activity, and centrotemporal delta activity.[2,6,5]

Delta Brushes ("Ripples of Prematurity" or "Beta-Delta Complexes") and Monorhythmic Occipital Delta

Delta brushes are composed of a combination of a delta frequency transient with superimposed 8 to 22 Hz, typically beta, frequency activity. These tend to be symmetrically represented between

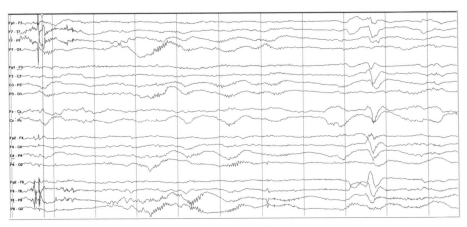

Fig. 1.8   Delta brushes.

the two hemispheres and appear in awake and sleeping infants. These are primarily observed in posterior brain regions and rarely frontally (Fig. 1.8). These first appear in the central/rolandic regions at 26 to 28 weeks CA and peak at 32 to 34 weeks, at which point they are most prominent in occipital electrodes.

Delta brushes may occur in synchronous bilateral hemispheric runs of monorhythmic occipital delta activity (MROD). This is another neonatal graphoelement defined by stereotyped runs of monomorphic high-amplitude 0.5 to 1 Hz delta waves in the occipital regions lasting 2 to 60 seconds. This MROD element appears as early at 23 to 24 weeks, peaks between 31 and 33 weeks, and should entirely abate by 35 weeks. After 34 weeks CA, the delta brushes become a prominent pattern in *tracé alternant* (i.e., quiet sleep) and are rarely observed in active sleep or wakefulness. Delta brushes are rare by term gestation and should be absent by 44 weeks CA.

Anterior Dysrhythmia and Encoches Frontales

Anterior, or frontal, dysrhythmia is a paroxysm of frontally dominant 50 to 150 μV semirhythmic delta (usually 2–4 Hz) activity which may have some subtle evolution over several (generally <6) seconds to acquire a frontal sharp transient morphology. Although the term "dysrhythmia" may appear to suggest abnormality, this is a normal neonatal graphoelement that arises symmetrically and synchronously between frontal regions in any behavioral state but is most obvious in transition from active to quiet sleep. This tends to appear at 32 weeks CA and persists until about 40 to 44 weeks CA.

Encoches frontales are high amplitude (>150 μV) frontal sharp wave transients with biphasic morphology (negative to positive) best observed in the frontopolar electrodes in symmetric, bilateral, synchronous solitary bursts or admixed in runs of anterior dysrhythmia, again showing a predilection toward the transition from active to quiet sleep and occurring most often in quiet sleep (Fig. 1.9). These may appear as early as 26 weeks but may be asynchronous at inception. They are maximal between 34 and 35 weeks and tend to abate after about 44 to 48 weeks CA.

A Word on Sharp Transients

Beyond the normal sharp transients of *encoches frontales*, neonates have frequent sharply contoured waveforms, which may be multifocal, of negative polarity, and are entirely normal. It is

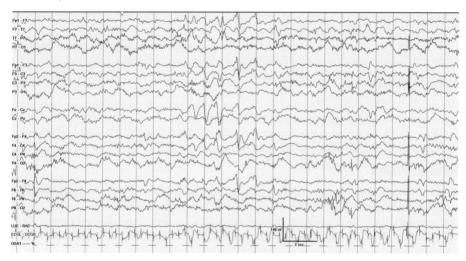

Fig. 1.9 Anterior dysrhythmia and encoches frontales.

important to not consider sharply contoured waveforms occurring within the bursts of *tracé discontinú* and *tracé alternant as potentially abnormal*, but rather those that occur during the IBIs. Normal sharp transients may be considered as the sporadic popping of popcorn at low heat; it should not be of high volume and it should be unpredictable in terms of location.

Certain features of sharp transients may portend an increased risk of seizures. One metric is termed "excessive" sharp transients, which is generally defined as greater than one sharp transient per minute. Features that would support a likely abnormal include sharp transients with very high voltage ($>$150 μV), asymmetry (e.g., persistent occurrence only in left hemisphere), polyphasic or complex morphology, repetitive or persistent focus (e.g., occurring with high frequency in the right frontal region), positive polarity (which may suggest subcortical white matter injury as seen in hypoxic-ischemic encephalopathy, intraventricular hemorrhage, and periventricular leukomalacia), and midline (Cz) location.[2,6,7,11]

Sleep EEGs by Preterm Age Groups

24 to 29 Weeks

Neuronal electrical activity is present overlying a hypersynchronous, *tracé discontinú* background observed in both wakefulness and sleep without any definite EEG features that help differentiate the states. Normative values regarding maximal permissible IBI are not well established; some authors and textbooks suggest a cut-off of 35 seconds, while others suggest IBI durations as long as 60 seconds are permissible in the extremely premature neonate.[2,6,7] IBI voltages are very low ($<$25 μV). Sporadic sharp transients are normal and common. Between 24 and 30 weeks CA, there is a tendency for the attenuated IBI periods to become shorter and the amount of activity during the interburst to increase. Delta brushes are centrally located between 26 and 28 weeks and MROD is a prominent graphoelement.

30 to 32 Weeks

We are now able to differentiate quiet sleep as a unique EEG feature; however, we are unable to differentiate wakefulness from active sleep based on EEG review alone. We observe variable but longer periods of continuity and decreasing IBIs. There is increasing continuous activity as LVI and/or M patterns may be seen during active sleep.

Discontinuous activity pattern continues and the *tracé discontinú* pattern begins to be replaced by the *tracé alternant* pattern as the IBI voltages slowly increase with age.

33 to 34 Weeks

We are able to start distinguishing active and quiet sleep. Awake and active sleep are more continuous with fewer IBIs of 4 to 6 seconds duration. MROD activity begins to dissipate and there are more occipitally-occurring delta brushes in awake and active sleep than quiet sleep. *Encoches frontales* pattern becomes prominent in conjunction with anterior dysrhythmia.

35 to 36 Weeks

These neonates demonstrate increasing continuity and the continuous M *(activité moyenne)* pattern in wakefulness and active sleep. Delta brushes become less common. Quiet sleep is still discontinuous but IBI voltages are increasing above 25 μV and the *tracé alternant* pattern is expected to fully replace the *tracé discontinú* pattern. Persistence of very low IBI voltages consistently less than 25 μV suggests excessive discontinuity for age.

Term Neonates (37–44 Weeks CA)

We have finally made it to term and we will observe an increasingly continuous pattern.

Weeks 37 to 40

Tracé alternant pattern of discontinuous quiet sleep activity continues, but the relatively quiescent intervals and slow-wave bursts are persistently shortened and may begin to become a more continuous HVS pattern of uninterrupted delta activity. A second pattern consists of continuous irregular waves in the theta-delta frequencies appearing during wakefulness and active sleep. The delta brushes tend to disappear and/or only occur in the context of *tracé alternant*. A pattern of diffuse, irregular slow waves with an amplitude of less than 50 μV is an alternative to the previous pattern defining wakefulness and active sleep. Active sleep may be defined by the LVI pattern with *encoches frontales* or the M pattern.[2,4,6,12,13]

Weeks 41 to 44

Delta brushes disappear by 42 to 44 weeks and *encoches frontales* abate by 44 to 46 weeks.

CSWS/HVS consistently has replaced *tracé alternant* pattern, except possibly at the initial onset of quiet sleep.

Weeks 45 to 48

By this time, there should essentially be no further evidence of a discontinuous background. Very brief fragments of relative voltage attenuation may be observed, but frank persistence of the *tracé alternant* pattern and discontinuity beyond 46 to 48 weeks may be suggestive of a dysmature brain, or an incorrectly calculated CA.

Rudimentary sleep spindles (discussed in greater detail below) begin to appear in the sleep EEG sometime between 6 and 8 weeks of life (46–48 weeks CA) and rudimentary vertex weeks may also begin around 48 weeks CA. Rudimentary sleep spindle waveforms may occur slightly sooner at the vertex (Cz) region and may be slightly slower at a frequency of 12 to 14 Hz and not show the full breadth of faster frequencies observed in adulthood (11–16 Hz). These early spindles also have a predilection toward being quite long in duration (up to 10–15 seconds) compared to the typical duration of approximately 1 second in adulthood (Fig. 1.10). These are typically asynchronous and occur independently over each hemisphere. Sleep spindles become progressively

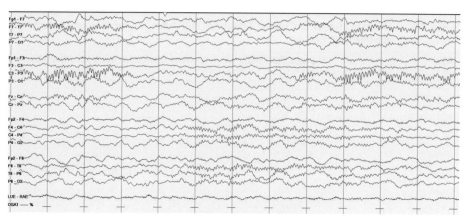

Fig. 1.10 Asynchronous sleep spindles.

more synchronous over the first 2 years of life and asynchrony of sleep spindles should not be considered abnormal prior to 2 years of age.[16]

Infancy and Early Childhood (48 Weeks CA to 2 Years)

As we move into infancy (>48 weeks CA or 2 months) and have more identifiable sleep architecture of mature adults beginning to form, the AASM recommends scoring PSGs based on the pediatric scoring criteria as the continuous infant EEG patterns are replaced with more easily discernible, distinct, and mature organized EEG backgrounds.[4] We will transition to broader perspective of typical wakeful and sleep architecture in their development. The CA principle is still important and valid; however, the following age groups will be defined in terms of chronological age from a term gestation birth.

NORMAL WAKING BACKGROUND

While it may seem nonessential to discuss some features of the developing normal waking background of early childhood, knowledge of these features will help the clinician have a better sense of the normal EEG background and the appropriate transitions into sleep (particularly the subtle dropout of the normal background rhythms and the onset of slow-rolling eye movements of stage 1 NREM sleep) and some of the peculiar, but benign features that may be encountered in the liminal states of drowsiness and arousals from sleep.

Between 3 and 4 months, infants will begin to develop a posterior dominant rhythm (PDR) with a nascent anterior-posterior (AP) gradient.[5,6] The PDR is a posteriorly located sinusoidal rhythm responsive to eye opening (enhanced in relaxed wakeful states with eye closure and diminish with eye opening). The AP gradient is defined by lower amplitude and higher-frequency rhythms in the more anterior brain regions and higher amplitude and slower-frequency rhythms in the more posterior brain regions. There are many descriptions in the literature about expected average, and lowest acceptable, PDR values per age through childhood and into adulthood (Table 1.3). It is worthwhile to know that much of this historic data was derived from a homogeneous Scandinavian population and has not been replicated due to the cost and labor-intensive

TABLE 1.3 ■ **Expected Average, and Lowest Acceptable, PDR Values per Age Through Childhood and Into Adulthood**

Age	Average PDR (Hz)	Lower Limit of Acceptable PDR (Hz)
3–4 months	3–4	
6 months	5	
12 months	6	5
24 months	7	6
3 years	8	7
8 years	9	8
9 years	9	8
15 years	10	8
Adults	8–13 (Alpha)	

nature of such research; these data may not fully capture the diversity of normal PDR development in more heterogeneous populations.[6]

The infantile PDR is the predecessor of the adult "alpha" rhythm and the PDR is sometimes colloquially called the alpha rhythm in spite of it not achieving the expected alpha range frequencies. Many children have a mild voltage asymmetry in their PDR—98% of those children with a PDR voltage asymmetry show higher voltages in the right hemisphere, with the right-sided PDR potentially being up to 50% higher voltage than the left.[6] Asymmetries greater than a 2:1 ratio are abnormal. Although uncommon in children under 2 years of age, posterior slow waves of youth may be observed as random or rhythmic moderate amplitude delta waves with the superimposed alpha rhythm/PDR overlying it. This is a normal phenomenon of unclear significance and does not warrant further investigation but caution is urged in defining such segments as a pathologically slow background.

Drowsy and Arousal EEG Patterns

Hypnagogic hypersynchrony is the abrupt onset of diffuse high-voltage (typically 75–350 μV, but can be higher) sinusoidal delta-theta (predominantly 3 to 4.5 Hz) frequencies maximal in the parasagittal EEG derivations occurring in the drowsy state as children are about to fall asleep. It is first observed in 3 to 4 months of life in about one-third of infants and is observed in approximately 95% of children by 6 months.[6,12] It may be slightly asymmetric particularly prior to 12 months of life and at times have a notched appearance due to overriding faster frequencies (Fig. 1.11). Higher voltage and slightly slower delta rhythms may be observed more posteriorly compared to slow theta-range (4 to 5 Hz) rhythms more anteriorly.

A postarousal hypersynchrony pattern (sometimes referred to as hypnopompic hypersynchrony) may be encountered in similar age groups and with similar morphology, frequencies, and EEG distribution. As the child arouses, a high-voltage run of slow (2.5 to 4 Hz) monomorphic frontally predominant rhythm appears and can persist for several minutes before subsiding back into the prearousal sleep pattern or become admixed with faster frequencies and potentially lead to an awakening.

Normal Sleep Activity and Development

Vertex waves are one of the hallmarks of stage 1 NREM sleep, although they are not essential for scoring of stage 1 sleep.[4] Vertex waves are high-voltage bilateral, synchronous biphasic sharp-wave

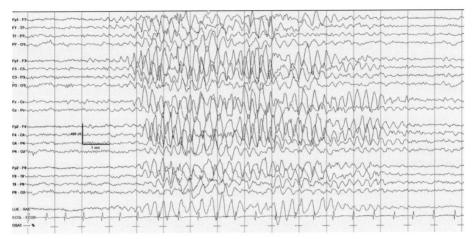

Fig. 1.11 Hypnagogic hypersynchrony.

transients in the parasagittal central electrodes, often with maximal negativity at Cz (i.e., the "vertex"). These first appear at approximately 48 weeks CA, and in young children they may have a broader frontocentral distribution.[6,13] They may be slightly asymmetric in voltages, but tend to be quite synchronous. Persistent asynchrony or development of asynchrony in vertex waves has been described in scenarios of increased intracranial pressure such as obstructive hydrocephalus.[6] In young children, these vertex waves can occur in successive runs, which may confuse the untrained eye to suggest an epileptiform waveform appearance (Fig. 1.12).

Sleep spindles as discussed above are one of the first mature NREM features in childhood, appearing at approximately 46 to 48 weeks CA as asynchronous central predominant 12 to 14 Hz fusiform rhythms.[4] At inception they may demonstrate a sharp negative component and a rounded, arciform positive component. They become increasingly synchronous with age with 70% of sleep spindles synchronized by 12 months of life and they should be 100% synchronous by 2 years old

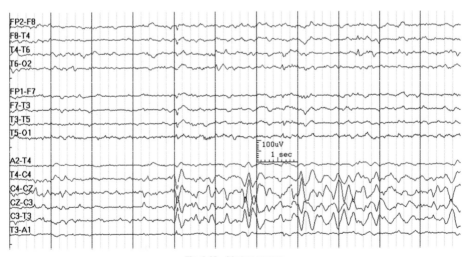

Fig. 1.12 Vertex waves.

and include higher frequencies up to 16 Hz.[6,16] The spindle-specific frequency bands overlap both alpha and beta frequency ranges and have been provided the "sigma" moniker, classically 12 to 16 Hz. Depending upon the publication, however, researchers may use a rather broad frequency band between 10 and 18 Hz to define sigma and spindle-related activity. Central EEG leads tend to have the highest voltages, although up to 5% of children may have frontally predominant sleep spindles.[6,16,17] Children may have both frontal- and central-predominant spindles and these curiously have slightly discordant frequencies at 12 to 14 Hz and 14 to 16 Hz, respectively.

Sleep spindles are generated by the thalamoreticular nucleus. The absence of sleep spindles after 50 weeks CA (and with adequate sleep EEG recording) has been described as a nonspecific EEG abnormality possibly of dysmaturity and portending risk of developmental delays.[6] More importantly, the persistence of asymmetric sleep spindles (e.g., presence only in right hemisphere or unilaterally slow spindle frequency) beyond 3 months of life OR the persistence of asynchronous sleep spindles beyond 2 years of life are both worrisome for intracranial pathology (e.g., thalamic abnormalities, agenesis of corpus callosum). There are historic descriptions of children with "constant spindling" and "extreme" or "exaggerated" spindles often with severe intellectual and developmental disabilities. There are additional descriptions of sleep-based waveforms of a typical fusiform morphology as observed in sleep spindles but slower than the expected sigma range frequency (e.g., 9–10 Hz) in patients with neurodevelopmental disorders such as trisomy 21.[18,19]

K-complexes are a peculiar waveform of some EEG lore; these are often described as an auditory stimulus arousal pattern typically observed in stage 2 NREM sleep. The origin of the "K" is derived from how this EEG waveform was first described in sleep after a Knock on the door of the EEG recording room. These may first arise in infants aged 3 to 6 months old as well-delineated negative sharp wave and immediately followed by a positive component lasting at least 0.5 seconds of maximal voltage in frontal and prefrontal EEG electrodes.[4,12] These may often become intermingled with, or are followed by, a sleep spindle (Fig. 1.13).

Fast activity of low-voltage beta frequencies in the early sleep stages begins around months 5 or 6 of life similar to K-complexes (Fig. 1.14). These frequencies may be most pronounced

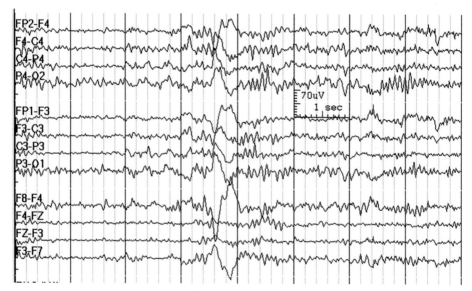

Fig. 1.13   K-complex.

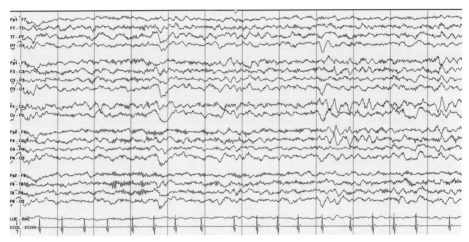

Fig. 1.14 Fast activity of early sleep defined by low-voltage beta frequency waveforms.

in the central regions and become maximal in amplitude around 12 to 18 months old.[6,12] This pattern tends to abate after about 3 years of life. It is worthwhile to consider subtle asymmetries (i.e., depression or absence focally or unilaterally) as abnormal as fast frequencies of cortical origin are quite susceptible to intracranial perturbations, such as ischemia.

Slow wave activity of 0.5 to 2 Hz and 100 to 400 μV amplitudes as measured in the frontal EEG derivations may first develop as early as 2 to 3 months of life. It is typically present by 4 to 5 months and thus clear epochs of stage 3 NREM sleep may be scored. As such, the ability to score stage 3 NREM sleep is typically achievable around 4 to 5 months of life.[4,12] This delta frequency may be first recorded in more occipital regions in younger infants and slowly evolves to include more frontal regions; this is a function of cortical development progressing in a caudal-to-rostral fashion.[20,21]

REM Sleep

As our NREM markers become more obvious, active sleep also develops a more mature REM sleep pattern. The maturing REM background is defined by a desynchronized low voltage mixed frequency pattern reminiscent of the waking background. Low-voltage irregular delta waves intermixed with theta activity are expected around 4 to 4.5 months. At 6 months the average voltage is approximately 100 μV and includes delta, theta, and beta frequencies. Around 5 to 6 months of life sawtooth waves develop. These begin as 4 to 5 Hz bursts in centrotemporal distribution, which tend to develop into faster theta rhythms (5–7 Hz) with an occasional notched morphology between 1 and 5 years of life. Notably, sleep spindles may be present in REM in early childhood (usually before age 2 years) and do not preclude a determination of a REM epoch.[4,12]

After 3 months of life, the likelihood of an infant initiating sleep with an epoch of REM sleep decreases precipitously. Sleep-onset REM periods are normal but become increasingly uncommon, through the first year of life. A notable feature of active/REM sleep is the reduction in total REM sleep volume as the infant sleep stages redistribute. NREM sleep remains generally static but the amount of REM sleep appears to be replaced by increasing wake times in the 24-hour cycle.[22,23]

Figure 1.15 summarizes many of the developmental EEG changes across the age spectrum.

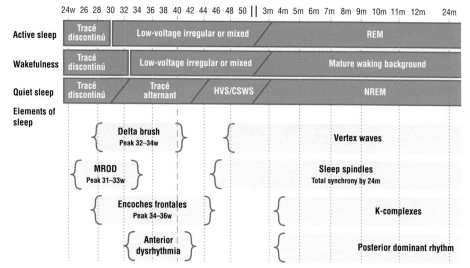

Fig. 1.15   This figure demonstrates expected changes in the sleep and wakefulness EEG as expected based on corrected gestational age from 24 to 50 weeks, then 3 months to 12 months, and at 24 months. This includes elements of sleep, including neonatal graphoelements, as well as the timing of the emergence of the posterior dominant rhythm in wakefulness. *CSWS,* Continuous slow wave sleep; *HVS,* high-voltage slow; *MROD,* monomorphic rhythmic occipital delta; *NREM,* non–rapid eye movement sleep; *REM,* rapid eye movement sleep.

Future Research and Other Clinical Perspectives

FETAL PERSPECTIVES

While we have discussed our current understanding of the ontogeny of the sleep EEG in the *ex utero* child, there are fascinating research paradigms past and present to consider the prenatal assessment of the biobehavioral state of sleep. The first study of human fetal EEG study by Borkowsi and Bernstine in 1955 utilized needle EEG in two surgically removed, nonviable fetuses at GAs of approximately 45 and 77 days, respectively.[24] These EEGs showed low-voltage (0.5 to 2 Hz) electrical activity with interceding (2 to 8 Hz) activity as well as a waveform which the authors suggested was a sleep spindle in one recording, and other rare fast frequencies. Based on the previous discussions in this chapter and the waveform morphology, this "sleep spindle" likely represented a delta brush instead; it is difficult to appraise a possible biobehavioral state such as sleep (a period of reversible quiescence) in a nonviable fetus being born in extremis and monitored until brain death.

This proof-of-concept does support early electrical activity but does not support a clear delineation of different biobehavioral states. This would be exceedingly challenging to replicate due to the exceptionally invasive nature of the aforementioned study and the limitations of typical EEG, even with advanced artifact resolution software, to accurately assess fetal EEG. Instead, there is a growing body of literature on fetal magnetoencephalography (MEG), a noninvasive neurophysiological monitoring parameter that may record EEG activity from the fetus.[25-29] MEG records magnetic signals generated by electrical currents in biological tissue and is not distorted by different layers of biological tissue (e.g., maternal abdominal muscles, uterine musculature). These data-rich recordings require a great deal of postprocessing to remove artifacts to parse out the small magnetic fields generated by the fetal brain. These *in utero* studies have demonstrated comparable EEG patterns to our *ex utero* scalp EEGs, including discontinuity, sharp transients, and delta brushes. Fetal MEG has also had seen use in monitoring at-risk pregnancies on a research basis and even detected pathological states such as burst suppression in an early infantile epileptic encephalopathy.[30]

There is the consideration of applying these modalities to understand differences in biobehavioral states of the active and inactive (i.e., awake and asleep) fetus. Haddad et al in 2011 attempted to address these correlates in 28 fetuses aged 30 to 37 weeks' gestation by comparing fetal MEG and actocardiograms, analytic plots of fetal gross body movements, and fetal heart rate patterns.[27] They found that the majority of their patients had behavioral states that have been correlated to neonatal quiet and active sleep. A major limitation presently in understanding fetal MEG data is the absence of true normative data and that most studies are limited to fetuses greater than 28 weeks' gestation. The first fetal movements may be appreciated by the mother between 16 and 25 weeks' gestation, reflexive and spontaneous movements may be detected as early as 7 to 10 weeks' gestation, and periods of transient activity and quiescence have been shown at approximately 20 weeks' gestation. These state changes may correspond to specific EEG patterns as detected via fetal MEG and further define the ontogeny fetal sleep EEG networks. It is difficult to predict if our understanding of normal predicted EEG development in the extremely premature neonate is a reasonable facsimile of normal *in utero* EEG development and if there are other patterns to uncover other than the (state notwithstanding) hypersynchronous discontinuity of the extremely preterm neonate via fetal MEG.

SLEEP SPINDLES *REDUX*

Sleep spindles represent one of the most easily identifiable pieces of sleep EEG architecture throughout human life. The specific functions of sleep spindle have been long hypothesized under the auspices of general sleep function hypotheses (e.g., memory, encoding, learning, neural plasticity). In more recent years, the influence of spindles as a correlate to memory consolidation has grown. Sleep spindle activity in infants has supported formation of generalized and language-specific memories during sleep.[31,32] Slow spindles have been correlated with visual perceptual learning,[33] whereas fast spindles have been correlated with more complex processes such as fluid intelligence, learning, and word-location associations.

We do not have clear differentiation of the origin or function of different spindles, from the "slow" spindles range most often seen in frontal EEG derivations in childhood and the "fast" spindles most often seen in the centroparietal EEG derivations.[19] Presumably there are complex networks of thalamocortical circuitry that result in these scalp-based frequency differences. The differentiation of these spindles into predictive biomarkers of pathological disease state has not been established.

Automated spindle detection using machine learning algorithms in 4-month-old infants with GAs greater than 37 weeks has been recently validated.[17] Utilizing increasingly available digital analyses of spindles may provide higher resolution of previously time-intensive and highly specialized work. These may better differentiate "slow" and "fast" spindles, create spindle-specific metrics and normative data across age spectrums, and help to further identify pathological states. Spindle analyses have been utilized in certain pathological states, such as correlating low spindle density to seizure burden in childhood epilepsy with centrotemporal spikes (formerly known as "benign rolandic epilepsy" and now termed "self-limited epilepsy with centrotemporal spikes")[34] and autism spectrum disorders.[18] Unconjugated hyperbilirubinemia in term infants has also been shown to be associated with decreased spindle density, duration, and frequency[35]; this study supported a possible thalamoreticular insult and hypothesized further use of spindle indices in neurodevelopmental monitoring. Sleep spindles have been sought to be used as a biomarker of outcome prediction in infantile spasms; however, these have demonstrated mixed results likely due to the heterogeneity of the causes of this incipient epileptic encephalopathy and the small sample sizes assessed.[36,37]

With disrupted sleep as an exceptionally common co-occurrence in autism spectrum disorder, many have argued that sleep disruption should be among the diagnostic criteria. Many research groups are actively using EEG to identify biomarkers which may predict (and more importantly propose potential interventions) an eventual diagnosis of autism.[38,39] Recent efforts have shown young children with autism spectrum disorder have decreased fast spindles, as well as decreased fast theta oscillations and increased beta oscillations, compared to healthy controls[40] (Page et al., 2020). Differences in sleep EEG features such as spindle indices may be a key biomarker in autism spectrum disorder.

IN UTERO TO EX UTERO SLEEP IN PREMATURITY AND THE NICU

Our review of the normal and expected ontogeny of the background EEG in very premature infants and even full-term neonates comes with a great caveat—many of the neonates undergoing continuous EEGs or PSGs are doing so due to some suspected pathology. There are legion pathological entities, including intraventricular hemorrhage, infections, congenital brain and/or upper airway malformations, and genetic disorders, which may prompt this monitoring. It is rare that the "well" 30-week CA neonate is getting a neurophysiologic recording otherwise. Premature delivery may have multifactorial maternal and fetal origins.

A curious concept is that certain maternal conditions and/or the medications expectant mothers take may have significant influences on normal sleep architecture in infants. A PSG study of 32 full-term "high-risk" infants born to mothers with depression compared to 32 full-term "low-risk" infants born to mothers without a personal history of depression found high-risk infants with altered sleep architecture at birth and at 6 months. Infants of depressed mothers had significantly lower quiet sleep percentage and fewer arousals but spent significantly more time awake than the low-risk group of infants.[41] Prior studies have found similar features of assessing maternal depression and finding less quiet/deep sleep in the depressed group. While this study had no differences in maternal antidepressant use between high-risk and low-risk groups, other studies have suggested neonates exposed to maternal antidepressant use have short-term sleep-related perinatal adverse effects including increased sleep disturbance and decreased quiet sleep.[42] Depression and maternal antidepressant use are quite common and may be considered models for maternal variables that may influence normal sleep developmental in neonates and infants. This poses the consideration of other maternal factors that are less prevalent and/or less well studied, such as the influence of maternal epilepsy and/or maternal antiseizure medication exposure on subsequent neonatal sleep development; we know that prenatal valproate exposure increases the risks of autism spectrum disorders and has a dose-dependent association with reduced cognition,[43,44] but we do not know the exact mechanisms of this interaction. Moving beyond fetal exposure, there is also the consideration of other potentially bioactive substances that are secreted in breastmilk, which may alter typical sleep architectural patterns and have continued reexposures.

Once our premature neonates have been born, many may have to spend some time in the NICU acclimating to the *ex utero* world. The most stable of these neonates have the majority of their care focused on "feeding and growing." However, even the most stable premature infants can have frequent apneas and bradycardias as well as poor temperature control; thus they are intensively monitored. The extrauterine developing brain environment, particularly one occupying a NICU, is not flawless facsimile to the intrauterine milieu. NICUs are often a loud, boisterous environment with a cycled light environment rather than the quiet, 24-hour "dark" condition provided by the uterus. Typical medical care and monitoring alarms provide jarring stimuli, which disrupts the natural progression of sleep-wake cycle development. The explicit effects these cares have on neurodevelopmental outcomes, or how mitigating these stimuli when appropriate would have on such outcomes, has yet to be elucidated.[45] We have observed that preterm infants are at higher risk for neurodevelopmental disabilities and some studies suggest these children are at higher risk of disordered sleep later in life.[46,47] But the influence of their prematurity or the associated environment on the normal development of the sleep network is not well defined in spite of efforts in varying pathologies, such as hypoxic-ischemic injury.[48] Some of this latter work highlights some key research tools to better understand neonatal sleep and its consequences in the NICU. Rather than relying upon the more extensive EEG montages, a limited array of electrodes permitted analysis of quantitative EEG. Amplitude-integrated EEG has long been utilized in NICUs for bedside assessment of seizures and other cerebral pathology, but utilizing this and other quantitative EEG tools (e.g., alpha-delta ratios, suppression indices) may provide new avenues toward understanding neonatal sleep development without relying on conventional pattern recognition.

CYCLIC ALTERNATING PATTERN AND ODDS RATIO PRODUCT

Cyclic alternating pattern (CAP) is an EEG marker of sleep instability and has been utilized as a research tool for investigation of pathologic brain processes and brain maturation since its first descriptions in 1985.[49] CAP is observed in shifts between sleep stages and from sleep to wakefulness and the CAP rate (percentage of CAP time to NREM time) is a marker of NREM sleep instability. There are specific "A" phase subtypes (A1, A2, and A3) based on the degree of synchronization/desynchronization observed in a transitory variation in frequencies and amplitudes of basal EEG activity lasting between 2 and 60 seconds, which are separated by an interval "B" phase. Infants as young as 46 and 55 weeks CA demonstrate oscillating slow EEG activities reminiscent of CAP.[50-52] CAP rates increase during the first 2 years of life in conjunction with sleep depth (i.e., the highest values are observed in slow-wave sleep) and infants have a higher index and percentage of the A1 (most synchronized) subtype.[52-56] This A1 subtype decreases between 5 and 16 months of life as a hypothesized maturation of the cortical arousal networks.[54] This increasing desynchronization has been hypothesized to correspond to a decreased risk of sudden infant death syndrome in the aging infant. Unfortunately, there are not many studies on CAP evaluating young children and these studies are small in study participants; much of its work has been in adults and in understanding various sleep disorders such as sleep apnea and insomnia. A meta-analysis has sought to accumulate normative CAP data across the age spectrum,[56] although significant work needs to be done to better extrapolate the developmental significance of CAP in the ontogeny of sleep and its relationship to normal and aberrant neurodevelopmental states.

The odds-ratio product (ORP) is a recently described continuous metric of sleep depth from 0 (deepest sleep) to 2.5 (full wakefulness) that assesses every 3 seconds of EEG data on the basis of likelihood of remaining asleep or transitioning to wakefulness in the following 3-second epoch.[57] This is an exciting paradigm shift in the conceptualization of sleep quality and depth in objective terms, and already work on establishing normative data and influence of pathological entities (e.g., obstructive sleep apnea, sedative exposure in ICUs) has been published.[58,59] Unfortunately the data for ORP in children is minimal[60] and absent in neonates and infants. Establishing normative data in pediatric populations may serve as a new source of sleep EEG biomarkers for a host of neurodevelopmental disorders.

Conclusions

The developmental trajectory of the sleep EEG from the premature neonate to term and into late infancy is highly dynamic and understanding a snapshot-in-time EEG or PSG requires an appreciation of that dynamism in the context of the developing brain. There is much work left to pursue to better appreciate the developmental consequences of aberrant sleep development in neonates and infants and how our well-intentioned interventions (e.g., the NICU) may negatively influence this. The fledgling field of pediatric sleep EEG research is ripe with opportunities to better understand predictive biomarkers of disease entities. Digital and quantitative analyses of EEG sleep data should continue to be developed, validated, and implemented toward clinical utility for our youngest patients.

References

1. Berger H. Über das elektroenkephalogramm des menschen. *Arch Psychiatr Nervenkr.* 1929;87(1): 527-570.
2. Libenson MH. The electroencephalogram of the newborn. In: Libenson MH, ed. *Practical Approach to Electroencephalography.* 1st ed. Saunders Elsevier; 2010:301-327.
3. Engle WA, American Academy of Pediatrics Committee on Fetus and Newborns. Age terminology during the perinatal period. *Pediatrics.* 2004;114(5):1362-1364.
4. Berry RB, Quan SF, Abreu AR, et al.; for the American Academy of Sleep Medicine. *The AASM Manual for the Scoring of Sleep and Associated Events: Rules, Terminology and Technical Specifications.* Version 2.6. American Academy of Sleep Medicine; 2020.
5. Hrachovy RA. Development of the normal electroencephalogram. In: Levin KH, Lüders HO, eds. *Comprehensive Clinical Neurophysiology.* WB Saunders; 2000:387-413.
6. Clancy RR, Bergqvist AGC, Dlugos DJ, et al. Normal pediatric EEG: neonates and children. In: Ebersole JS, Husain AM, Nordli DR, eds. *Current Practice of Clinical Electroencephalography.* 4th ed. Wolters Kluwer Health; 2014:125-212.
7. Tsuchida TN, Wusthoff CJ, Shellhaas RA, et al. American Clinical Neurophysiology Society standardized EEG terminology and categorization for the description of continuous EEG monitoring in Neonates: report of the American Clinical Neurophysiology Society Critical Care Monitoring Committee. *J Clin Neurophysiol.* 2013;30(2):161-173.
8. Den Ouden L, Rijken M, Brand R, et al. Is it correct to correct? Developmental milestones in 555 "normal" preterm infants compared with term infants. *J Pediatr.* 1991;118(3):399-404.
9. Girsen A, Do Sz, El-Sayed YY, et al. Association between small-for-gestational age and neurocognitive impairment at two years of corrected age among infants born at preterm gestational ages: a cohort study. *J Perinatol.* 2017;37(8):958-962.
10. Tekgul H, Bourgeois B, Gauvreau K, Bergin AM. Electroencephalography in neonatal seizures: comparison of a reduced and a full 10/20 montage. *Pediatr Neurol.* 2005;32(3):155-161.
11. Alix JJP, Ponnusamy A, Pilling E, Hart AR. An introduction to neonatal EEG. *Paediatr Child Health.* 2016;27(3):135-142.
12. Grigg-Damberger M, Gozal D, Marcus CL, et al. The visual scoring of sleep and arousal in infants and children. *J Clin Sleep Med.* 2007;3(2):201-240.
13. Grigg-Damberger M. The visual scoring of sleep in infants 0 to 2 months of age. *J Clin Sleep Med.* 2016;12(3):429-445.
14. Douglass LM, Wu JY, Rosman NP, Stafstrom CE. Burst suppression electroencephalogram pattern in the newborn: predicting the outcome. *J Child Neurol.* 2002;17(6):403-408.
15. Abdul Awal M, Lai MM, Azemi G, et al. EEG background features that predict outcome in term neonates with hypoxic ischaemic encephalopathy: a structured review. *Clin Neurophysiol.* 2016;127(1): 285-296.
16. Lenard HG. The development of sleep spindles in the EEG during the first two years of life. *Neuropadiatrie.* 1970;3:264-276.
17. Wei L, Ventura S, Mathieson S, et al. Spindle-AI: sleep spindle number and duration estimation in infant EEG. *IEEE Trans Biomed Eng.* 2022;69(1):465-474.
18. Farmer CA, Chilakamarri P, Thurm AE, et al. Spindle activity in young children with autism, developmental delay, or typical development. *Neurology.* 2018;91(2):e112-e122.
19. Gruber R, Wise MS. Sleep spindle characteristics in children with neurodevelopmental disorders and their relation to cognition. *Neural Plast* 2016;2016:4724792.
20. Kurth S, Ringli M, Geiger A, et al. Mapping of cortical activity in the first two decades of life: a high-density sleep electroencephalogram study. *J Neurosci.* 2010;30:13211-13219.
21. Novelli L, D'Atri A, Marzano C, et al. Mapping changes in cortical activity during sleep in the first 4 years of life. *J Sleep Res.* 2016;25:381-389.
22. Galland BC, Taylor BJ, Elder DE, Herbison P. Normal sleep patterns in infants and children: a systematic review of observational studies. *Sleep Med Rev.* 2012;16(3):213-222.
23. Agostini A, Centofanti S. Normal sleep in children and adolescence. *Child Adolesc Psychiatr Clin N Am.* 2021;30(1):1-14.
24. Borkowski WJ, Bernstine RL. Electroencephalography of the fetus. *Neurology.* 1955;5(5):362-365.

25. Eswaran H, Haddad NI, Shihabuddin BS, et al. Non-invasive detection and identification of brain activity patterns in the developing fetus. *Clin Neurophysiol.* 2007;118(9):1940-1946.
26. Lowery CL, Govindan RB, Preissl H, et al. Fetal neurological assessment using noninvasive magnetoencephalography. *Clin Perinatol.* 2009;36:701-709.
27. Haddad N, Govindan RB, Vairavan S, et al. Correlation between fetal brain activity patterns and behavioral states: an exploratory fetal magnetoencephalography study. *Exp Neurol.* 2011;228:200-205.
28. Vairavan S, Govindan RB, Haddad N, et al. Quantification of fetal magnetoencephalographic activity in low-risk fetuses using burst duration and interburst interval. *Clin Neurophysiol.* 2014;125:1353-1359.
29. Vasung L, Turk EA, Ferradal SL, et al. Exploring early human brain development with structural and physiological neuroimaging. *NeuroImage.* 2019;187:226-254.
30. Wacker-Gussmann A, Alber M, Abele H, et al. Fetal suppression burst pattern in Ohtahara syndrome visualized by fetal magnetoencephalography. *Int J Gynaecol Obstet.* 2013;120(1):96-98.
31. Friedrich M, Wilhelm I, Born J, Friederici AD. Generalization of word meanings during infant sleep. *Nat Commun.* 2015;6:6004.
32. Friedrich M, Mölle M, Friederici AD, Born J. The reciprocal relation between sleep and memory in infancy: memory-dependent adjustment of sleep spindles and spindle-dependent improvement of memories. *Dev Sci.* 2019;22(2):e12743.
33. Bang JW, Khalilzadeh O, Hämäläinen M, et al. Location specific sleep spindle activity in the early visual areas and perceptual learning. *Vision Res.* 2014;99:162-171.
34. Kramer MA, Stoyell SM, Chinappen D, et al. Focal sleep spindle deficits reveal focal thalamocortical dysfunction and predict cognitive deficits in sleep activated developmental epilepsy. *J Neurosci.* 2021; 41(8):1816-1829.
35. Gürses D, Kiliç I, Sahiner T. The effects of hyperbilirubinemia on sleep-spindle characteristics in infants. *Sleep.* 2005;28(5):644-648.
36. Altunel A, Altunel EO, Sever A. The utility of the hypsarrhythmia paroxysm index and sleep spindles in EEG for predicting cognitive outcomes in a case series of infantile spasms. *J Neurol Neurophysiol.* 2015;6(5):319.
37. Boulloche J, Dautreme P, Le Luyer B, et al. A prognostic study of cryptogenic infantile spasms. *Ann Pediatr (Paris).* 1991;38(2):71-74.
38. Gabard-Durnam LJ, Wilkinson C, Kapur K, et al. Longitudinal EEG power in the first postnatal year differentiates autism outcomes. *Nat Commun.* 2019;10(1):4188.
39. Levin AR, Carvin KJ, O'Leary HM. EEG power at 3 months in infants at high familial risk for autism. *J Neurodev Disord.* 2017;9(1):34.
40. Page J, Lustenberger C, Fröhlich F. Nonrapid eye movement sleep and risk for autism spectrum disorder in early development: a topographical electroencephalogram pilot study. *Brain behav.* 2020;10(3):e01557.
41. Bat-Pitault F, Sesso G, Deruelle C, et al. Altered sleep architecture during the first months of life in infants born to depressed mothers. *Sleep Med.* 2017;30:195-203.
42. Suri R, Lin AS, Cohen LS, Altshuler LL. Acute and long-term behavioral outcome of infants and children exposed in utero to either maternal depression or antidepressants: a review of the literature. *J Clin Psychiatry.* 2014;75(10):e1142-e1152.
43. Christensen J, Grønborg TK, Sørensen MJ, et al. Prenatal valproate exposure and risk of autism spectrum disorders and childhood autism. *JAMA.* 2013;309(16):1696-1703.
44. Meador KJ, Baker GA, Browning N, et al. Fetal antiepileptic drug exposure and cognitive outcomes at age 6 years (NEAD study): a prospective observational study. *Lancet Neurol.* 2013;12(3):244-252.
45. Van den Hoogen, Teunis CJ, Shellhaas RA, et al. How to improve sleep in a neonatal intensive care unit: a systematic review. *Early Hum Dev.* 2017;113:78-86.
46. Yiallourou SR, Wallace EM, Whatley C, et al. Sleep: a window into autonomic control in children born preterm and growth restricted. *Sleep.* 2017;40:zsx1.
47. Bennet L, Fyfe KL, Yiallourou SR, et al. Discrimination of sleep states using continuous cerebral bedside monitoring (aEEG) compared to polysomnography in infants. *Acta Paediatr.* 2016;105:e582-e587.
48. Shellhaas RA, Burns JW, Hassan F, et al. Neonatal sleep-wake analyses predict 18-month neurodevelopmental outcomes. *Sleep.* 2017;40:zsx144.
49. Terzano MG, Macia D, Salati MR, et al. The cyclic alternating pattern as a physiologic component of normal NREM sleep. *Sleep.* 1985;8:137-145.
50. Parrino L, Ferri R, Bruni O, et al. Cyclic alternating pattern (CAP): the marker of sleep instability. *Sleep Med Rev.* 2012;16:27-45.

51. Bruni O, Ferri R, Miano S, et al. Sleep cyclic alternating pattern in normal school-age children. *Clin Neurophysiol*. 2002;113:1806-1814.
52. Bruni O, Ferri R, Miano S, et al. Sleep cyclic alternating pattern in normal preschool-aged children. *Sleep*. 2005;28:220-230.
53. Miano S, Piavilla M, Blanco D, et al. Development of NREM sleep instability-continuity (cyclic alternating pattern) in healthy term infants aged 1 to 4 months. *Sleep*. 2009;32:83-90.
54. Miano S, Peraita-Adrados R, Montesano M, et al. Sleep cyclic alternating pattern analysis in healthy children during the first year of life: a daytime polysomnographic study. *Brain Dev*. 2011;33:421-427.
55. Alves GR, Rosa A, Brito M, et al. Cyclic alternating pattern in normal children aged 12 to 24 months. *Arq Neuropsiquiatr*. 2010;68:689-693.
56. Migueis DP, Lopes MC, Ignacio PSD, et al. A systematic review and meta-analysis of the cyclic alternating pattern across the lifespan. *Sleep Med*. 2021;85:25-37.
57. Younes M, Ostrowski M, Soiferman M, et al. Odds ratio product of sleep EEG as a continuous measure of sleep state. *Sleep*. 2015;38(4):641-654.
58. Penner CG, Gerardy B, Ryan R, Williams M. The odds ratio product (an objective sleep depth measure): normal values, repeatability, and change with CPAP in patients with OSA. *J Clin Sleep Med*. 2019; 15(8):1155-1163.
59. Georgopoulos D, Kondili E, Alexopooulou, Younes M. Effects of sedatives on sleep architecture measured with odds ratio product in critically ill patients. *Crit Care Explor*. 2021;3(8):e0503.
60. Ricci A, He F, Fang J, et al. Maturational trajectories of non-rapid eye movement slow wave activity and odds ratio product in a population-based sample of youth. *Sleep Med*. 2021;83:271-279.

CHAPTER 2

Circadian Development and Homeostatic Sleep Pressure

Kate C. Chan ▦ Chun Ting Au

Introduction

Sleep is a behavioral state characterized by decreased motor activity and reduced interaction with the external environment with easy reversibility. It is one of the most vital primary activities of the brain during infancy and plays an important role in neurocognitive and psychosocial development in early life. Current theoretical models suggest that there are two independent but interacting regulatory processes that control the timing, intensity, and duration of sleep: circadian sleep process and homeostatic sleep process. It is also known as the two-process model of sleep regulation, which accounts for the sleep-wake patterns in humans and their alertness during the day. Although these two sleep processes are the major intrinsic biologic drivers of an individual's sleep-wake pattern, sleep behaviors in children are also significantly influenced by the environment, cultural values, parental and social beliefs.[1] Sleep also has its internal rhythmic organization, as known as ultradian rhythms, which includes sleep cycles of rapid eye movement (REM) sleep and non-rapid eye movement (NREM) sleep. All these physiologic processes change over the life course, especially in the first few years of life. Understanding how sleep processes evolve and the factors influencing the development is important to define the normality of sleep across early childhood and to investigate the associations between sleep and neurodevelopment. An understanding of sleep physiology and regulation is also critical for effective parent counseling and sleep interventions for children with problematic sleep or sleep disorders. This chapter will review the sleep characteristics, circadian development, and homeostatic sleep process in infancy.

Sleep and Ultradian Rhythms in Infancy

Human sleep is composed of ultradian cycles between REM sleep and NREM sleep. In older children and adults, these two main sleep stages can be easily captured by monitoring the brain waves, eye movements, and chin muscle tone in a standard polysomnography (PSG). However, REM and NREM sleep in early infancy, also known as active sleep (AS) and quiet sleep (QS), respectively, may be difficult to be differentiated from each other based on these physiological signals because our brains in early life are not mature enough to produce the key features of REM and NREM sleep. The characteristics of REM and NREM during infancy are described in Table 2.1. Apart from EEG, EOG, and chin EMG, additional characteristics, including breathing regularity and behavioral observations for body, limb, or facial movements, provide essential information for the differentiation between REM and NREM sleep. Therefore, an audio-video recording synchronized with standard PSG is recommended for the sleep studies in infancy. Nonetheless, there is still a substantial proportion of sleep time that cannot be definitely categorized into REM or NREM sleep, owing to the concurrent occurrence of both REM and NREM features in the same epoch. These uncertain epochs, which mostly occur during wake-sleep

TABLE 2.1 ■ Characteristics of Sleep Stages in Early Infancy

	Characteristics			
Stage	Behavioral	Respiration	EEG	EOG and Muscle Tone
Awake	Calm or active with eyes open, scanning eye movements Brief eye closure can occur with crying	Irregular, rapid, and shallow	Low voltage irregular: continuous low voltage mixed-frequency activity with delta and predominantly theta activity Both high voltage slow and low voltage poly-rhythmic components; these are intermingled with little periodicity	Eye blinks, REMs, scanning eye move-ments; transient eye closures may be seen in wakefulness especially when the infant is crying
Active sleep (REM sleep)	Eyes closed, REM seen under closed eyelids, squirming, suck-ing, grimacing, small movements of the face or limbs	Irregular, some central pauses (may or may not meet criteria for apnea)	Low voltage, irregular or mixed frequency	Eyes closed with REMs; absence of muscle tone, frequent muscle twitches and body jerks that break through the muscle inhibition of infant REM sleep
Quiet sleep (NREM sleep)	Eyes closed, few movements, sucking can occur	Regular	Low frequency, high voltage; trace alternant (high-voltage slow activity interrupted by near electrical silence) in 37–44 weeks post conceptional age	Eyes closed, not moving; low muscle tone

EEG, Electroencephalography; EOG, electrooculography; NREM, non-rapid eye movement; REM, rapid eye movement.

and REM-NREM transitions, are labeled as transitional sleep (also known as indeterminate sleep, IS). The emergence of different sleep states is one of the most significant aspects of early brain maturation.[2] Premature infants and neonates also show distinct oscillatory features, such as trace alternant, delta brush, and temporal theta, which are age and region dependent.[3]

The origin of sleep and ultradian development is found during the fetal period. As early as by 32 weeks of gestation, AS and QS could be differentiated while a large amount of time is spent in IS. Between 32 and 40 weeks postconceptional age, QS significantly increases, and IS decreases without significant change in AS. Preterm birth per se does not appear to change the time course of the sleep development, which suggests this is an endogenous brain mechanism and a measure of brain maturation.[2]

In the first few months postterm, infants' sleep is divided evenly between AS and QS. By the second half of the first year postterm, AS and QS gradually transition into more mature form of REM sleep and NREM sleep, respectively. When young infants fall asleep, the initial sleep episode is typically REM sleep. At 3 months postterm, sleep-onset REM periods become replaced by the adult pattern of sleep-onset NREM periods. The proportion of REM sleep also decreases during early childhood. Active/REM sleep is 50% of sleep at term, 40% at 3 to 5 months postterm, and

close to the adult level of 25% to 30% of nocturnal sleep by about 1 year of age. The cyclic alterna-
tions of REM and NREM sleep throughout the night are known as ultradian rhythm. The ultradian cycle is about 45 to 60 minutes in infancy and gradually increases to 90 to 110 minutes by
school age. During the first weeks of life, power spectrum analysis of electroencephalography
(EEG) shows higher delta activity during QS when compared to AS. However, different stages of
NREM sleep, such as stage N1, N2, and slow wave sleep (SWS), cannot be classified. Sleep
spindles rapidly develop during the first 3 months postterm, likely reflecting developmental
changes in thalamocortical activity. A recent study identified an independent EEG band of 10 to
16 Hz (corresponding to sleep spindle frequencies) using principal component analysis at 41 weeks
postconceptional age, suggesting that sleep spindle development may start at the first week postterm.[4] Slow waves become visible between 2 and 5 months postterm, and the development of
which is the principal component for lengthening the duration of QS or NREM sleep in infancy.[5]
By 6 months postterm, the discrete electronical patterns of REM and NREM sleep progressively
resemble those seen in adults.[1] Sleep spindles (stage N2) and SWS during NREM sleep become
classifiable. However, the development of REM and NREM sleep may begin before these EEG
features become visually identifiable. A study using multiscale permutation entropy to quantify
EEG signal complexity demonstrated that EEG during both REM and NREM sleep become
more complex from 2 to 5 weeks of age,[6] suggesting that the brain wave begins to develop in the
first weeks of life.

The sleep and wakefulness of newborns are distributed equally across day and night. Subsequently, sleep becomes gradually consolidated toward the nighttime with an increase in the
nocturnal sleep duration and a decrease in the daytime sleep. The development of the 24-hour
rhythm in sleep-wake behavior during infancy is driven by the emergence of both circadian and
homeostatic sleep pressure, as well as by daily activities such as feeding patterns. Over the first
few months, the ability to retain calories increases, with a decrease in the caloric need and growth
relative to size. Infants gradually become able to consume adequate calories during the day and
require fewer nighttime meals.[7] Simultaneously, the biological rhythms that contribute to sleep
regulation mature, with decreased sleep fragmentation and increased sleep consolidation, making
infants capable of sleeping through the night. Most infants eventually begin sleeping through the
night by the age of 6 to 9 months.[1] A consolidated sleep through the nighttime is considered a
major developmental milestone and is a crucial area of infant care.

Circadian Development

Circadian rhythm is a near 24-hour periodicity found in every physiological process, including sleep,
in the human brain and body. It is endogenously synchronized by the circadian system, and adjusted
through the influence of exogenous factors.[7] The underlying endogenous circadian mechanisms
have a distinct neuroanatomic locus in the suprachiasmatic nuclei (SCN) of the hypothalamus,
known as the biologic clock, which sets the timing of rhythms by regulating neuronal activity, body
temperature, and hormonal signals.[8] This clock is synchronized by daily exogenous environmental
cues known as zeitgebers, and the most powerful zeitgeber is light.[7] Light activates photoreceptors
in the retina inhibiting pineal gland secretion of the sleep-promoting hormone, melatonin. Moreover, various molecular and genetic components of the clock have been identified.[8-10]

In animal studies, rhythms of metabolic activity and gene expression are evident in the SCN of
rodents and nonhuman primates by mid-to-late gestation.[8] In humans, melatonin and dopamine
receptors appear as early as gestational age 18 weeks in the fetal SCN, suggesting melatonin and
dopamine may serve as the primary communicators of circadian development in fetus.[8] Melatonin
from the mother readily passes through the placenta and the fetal blood-brain barrier and appears
to be the predominant relay of circadian information to the fetus.[8] The origin of circadian rhythm
development has been observed since the fetal period and believed to be entrained by the mother

to the light-dark cycle.[2] A day-night rhythm of fetal heart rate synchronized with maternal rest-activity, heart rate, cortisol, melatonin, and body temperature is found in humans.[11,12] The lack of circadian rhythm in an anencephalic fetus despite the day-night rhythm in the maternal heart rate supports that fetal brain is necessary for the development of this endogenous rhythm.[2] Fetal and early neonatal circadian rhythms are important as they prepare the infant for the later adaptation to the environmental light-dark cycle. Previous animal studies reported that exposing pregnant nonhuman primates to constant light suppresses the emergence of melatonin and body temperature rhythms in their offspring following birth.[8] Gestational circadian disruption also promotes social avoidance and hyperactivity behaviors in mice.[13] These findings highlight the importance of maternal circadian stability during pregnancy for the early development of fetal circadian systems.

Early childhood is a critical time period when consolidation of sleep-wake patterns over the 24-hour period occurs.[14] Newborns (0–3 months) do not have an established circadian rhythm. Episodes of sleep and waking seem randomly distributed across day and night. Moreover, day and night reversal is common in the first few weeks after birth. In fact, infants are born with low levels of maternally transferred melatonin, which dissipates by 1 week. Endogenous melatonin does not rise to detectable levels until approximately 6 weeks after birth, and circadian rhythm emerges by 2 to 3 months of age. Melatonin levels are still very low at 12 to 16 weeks, but by 6 months they become a stable part of the sleep-wake cycle. Nighttime sleep consolidation develops between the age of 4 and 12 months, while daytime sleep decreases progressively. The number of naps commonly decreases from 2 naps to once by 18 months, with discontinuation of daytime sleep typically by the age of 5 years.

Besides sleep-wake patterns, biological rhythms integral to the circadian cycle also include changes in body temperature and circadian-driven hormones such as melatonin and cortisol. A nocturnal trough of body temperature, which is a good marker of human circadian rhythms, is already present at 6 to 12 weeks of age in term infants.[2] Endogenous production of melatonin and cortisol also begins to cycle in a 24-hour rhythm at the first 3 months of age, although the exact timing of the development of hormonal circadian rhythm remains controversial. Kennaway et al. found no evidence of circadian rhythm in melatonin before 9 to 12 weeks of age in term infants. A delay of 2 to 3 weeks in development of melatonin circadian rhythm in preterm versus term infants was also reported.[15] On the other hand, a study in term infants demonstrated the development of cortisol circadian rhythm by 8 to 12 weeks of age.[16] Another longitudinal study in preterm infants (gestational age 31–34 weeks) showed circadian rhythm in salivary cortisol level in more than half of the infants at 2 to 8 weeks of life.[17] This group as a whole developed circadian rhythm of cortisol between 8 and 12 postnatal weeks similar to term infants. A more recent longitudinal study of 130 healthy full-term infants with monthly saliva sampling demonstrated that circadian rhythm of salivary cortisol secretion is already established by one month of age.[18] Similar findings were obtained in preterm infants in a subsequent study which showed that salivary cortisol circadian rhythm is established by one month corrected age.[19] Despite the inconsistency shown in previous studies, it is widely agreed that the biological rhythms and their synchronization with the times of day develop rapidly over the first 6 months of life, highlighting the importance of effective behavioral routines that reinforce this development early in infancy.[7]

The early development of circadian rhythms is based on specific maturation processes of the brain, set by both genetic and environmental factors.[8] There are individual differences in the development of circadian rhythms. The length of circadian cycle can be affected by circadian gene variants.[20] For the first few months after birth, nocturnal sleep onset is typically coupled with sunset and then to family bedtime thereafter, suggesting that the circadian system is initially entrained by light but is subsequently also entrained by other environmental and social factors. The factors that potentially affect the development of circadian rhythms include feeding (scheduled versus on-demand, mother's milk versus formula milk), environmental lighting (indoor versus outdoor, regular versus irregular light-dark cycle), and chronological or postconceptional age of the infant. Therefore, the results of circadian research in human infancy are often signifi-cantly confounded by maternal and/or environmental factors as well as by the recording methods.

Whether environmental factors can influence the time course of circadian rhythm maturation is controversial. A study by McMillen et al. found that in a group of infants discharged home with a setting of regular day-night cycle, a single caregiver and on-demand feeding, circadian rhythm of sleep adaptation occurred after 6 to 10 weeks regardless of whether the infants were preterm or term.[21] There was an inverse relationship between gestational age and the postnatal age at when the entrainment occurred in preterm infants, suggesting this postnatal delay in entrainment of the more preterm infants to be secondary to the longer period of nonentraining stimulation in the neonatal nursery environment. Regular environmental entrainment factors appear to be more important than preterm/term delivery in later adaptation of the infants to a light-dark cycle. However, in other studies, no differences were observed for the time of entrainment to day-night rhythm in infants exposed to differently lighted environments (a cycled light nursery versus con-tinuous dim nursery; or preterm infants exposed to continuous light in the NICU versus varying light intensity at home).[22,23] The exposure of preterm infants to continuous lighting for several weeks before discharge home does not appear to retard the development of sleep-wake circadian rhythms if an appropriate lighting regime is experienced at home.[23] Despite the controversy, however, there is no rationale that would justify a chaotic noncircadian environmental approach in the neonatal nursery. In fact, some studies demonstrate that nursing premature infants under regular light-dark schedules in the neonatal intensive care unit leads to greater weight gain when compared to constant bright light or dim light.[24-26] A systematic review concluded that cycled light seems to shorten the length of hospital stay, although the evidence is hampered by the small sample size and the inability to blind the intervention.[24] The lack of circadian rhythmicity, not only in light but also in the pattern of noise, parental care, may subject the infant's developing circadian rhythm to conflicting temporal cues. Regular light-dark schedules support the matura-tion of rest-activity, sleep-wake, and melatonin rhythms earlier in premature infants.[27] Further-more, if the SCN is responsive as early as 28 weeks of gestation, cycled light at this time until discharge home may influence circadian organization. Continuing regular day-night rhythm at home as well as maximizing the day-night differences by minimizing nighttime caregiver inter-vention, including feeding, may benefit the development of preterm and term infants. The American Academy of Pediatrics also recommends that parents should start promoting good sleep hygiene, with a sleep-promoting environment and a bedtime routine in infancy, and throughout childhood, to promote health and to prevent and manage sleep problems.[7] Larger multicenter randomized trials will be needed to determine the extent to which different light-dark schedules might improve long-term health outcomes in both preterm and term infants.

Homeostatic Sleep Process

Homeostatic sleep process, known as process S, represents a sleep-wake-dependent homeostatic component of sleep. It describes the body's internal neurophysiologic drive toward either sleep or wakefulness. The homeostasis is governed by the principles of equilibrium. Process S builds up as a function of wakefulness and decreases after sleep onset. There is a neurophysiologic drive to sleep after periods of wakefulness, and similarly a drive to wake after periods of sleep.[7] Re-search has indicated that the homeostatic sleep drive may be produced by sleep-promoting substances, somnogens, that accumulate during prolonged wakefulness and are depleted during sleep.[7,28,29] Adenosine is widely known as one of these somnogens. It is a byproduct of biological activity in the brain from dephosphorylation of adenosine triphosphate, and therefore accumu-lates with activity, and then dissipates with rest and sleep. Adenosine promotes sleep by inhibit-ing arousal, it activates the hypothalamic ventrolateral preoptic nucleus neurons that inhibit arousal-promoting centers.

In adults, the time course of the homeostatic process is often derived from EEG slow wave activity (SWA) (EEG delta power in the frequency range 0.75–4.5 Hz) during NREM sleep. EEG delta power during NREM sleep is in a quantitative relationship with prior sleep-wake history. It increases during early NREM sleep proportionally with increasing wake duration.[30] SWA decreases during subsequent sleep cycles in the night in adults and children.[31] However, relevant data in infant sleep regulation and homeostasis are relatively scarce. Sleep demonstrates substantial age-related changes. During early development, both animal and human studies showed that the ultradian sleep cycle is characterized by an alternating pattern of SWS in every other sleep cycle.[5] In human infants, it was also found that NREM sleep with high levels of low-frequency delta activity (0.75–1.75 Hz) is present in alternate NREM sleep episodes across the night, together with an age-dependent increase in the low-delta activity likely secondary to the vast increase in cortical connectivity due to increasing synaptogenesis.[5,32] This alternating pattern was most prominent at 6 months of age, and no decline in the low-frequency delta activity across the night was observed.[32] In contrast, theta activity (6.5–9 Hz) progressively declines over consecutive NREM episodes, suggesting that theta activity may better reflect the dissipation of sleep pressure during infancy than SWA.[32] A study found a negative correlation between the rate of process S diminishing and prior wakefulness in infants during the first year of life. However, delta latency was not correlated to prior wakefulness.[33] Therefore, SWA alone may not be an appropriate marker for sleep homeostatic pressure in infants. The exact age at which SWA becomes the sleep homeostatic marker is not known. On the other hand, more recent studies demonstrate that slow waves, when originating from a particular location, travel across the cortex to involve more populations of cortical neurons. Changes in sleep pressure affect the alternating firing pattern of cortical neurons and the level of synchronization among populations of cortical neurons represents a cellular counterpart of the homeostatic sleep regulation.[34] The slope of slow waves, as measured in the EEG, may be a marker of this neuronal synchronization and thus a marker of sleep pressure.[34] Fattinger et al. demonstrated a decrease in the amplitude and the slope of slow waves from the first to the last hour of NREM sleep in infants, suggesting that the level of neuronal synchronization decreases across the night in infants.[5] These findings support that the homeostatic sleep regulation develops early in infancy.

The dynamics of sleep homeostatic mechanisms slow down in the course of development.[35] In infants, several studies have demonstrated that the accumulation rate of homeostatic sleep pressure with waking during the day, and its dissipation during sleep are faster than in older children and adults.[1,36] The quicker accumulation of sleep pressure in infants and younger children necessitates longer and more frequent daily daytime naps and also accounts for shorter nap sleep-onset latencies. While homeostatic sleep pressure accumulates more slowly across development, older children become able to sustain wakefulness for longer periods of time, fewer naps and shorter nap durations, and eventually a consolidated sleep-wake pattern. A more recent study also demonstrated a developmental increase in wakefulness across the vulnerable preterm period, which occupied 15% of the time by full-term age.[37]

Interaction Between Circadian Processes and Sleep Homeostasis

Circadian and sleep homeostatic processes are independent but complexly interacting regulatory mechanisms, which control vigilance during wakefulness, sleep timing, and maintenance. During wakefulness, the cumulative increase in the homeostatic sleep pressure is opposed by the increasing circadian alertness to maintain constant levels of vigilance. On the other hand, during sleep, the increasing circadian sleep tendency counteracts the declining homeostatic sleep pressure to maintain sleep. The developing interaction of the two processes likely contributes significantly to determine the sleep-wake behavior in early childhood. However, data regarding how the two processes interact in infancy are scarce. As the dynamics of sleep homeostatic mechanisms are believed to be different during infancy when compared to older children and adults, the development of a circadian-dependent alerting signal in the absence of the opposing sleep homeostatic process during the first few months of life may explain the tendency for some infants to express crying behavior preferentially at certain times of day, such as in the evening hours.[1] Moreover, a misalignment of the two processes may be the culprit to the problems at sleep onset, nocturnal awakenings, difficulties awakening in the morning, or daytime sleepiness, which are common sleep problems during childhood. More future research will be needed in this regard to provide additional insights.

Sleep and Early Development

Sleep is a critical window for brain development and maturation in early human life. Evidence supports that sleep homeostasis is involved in aspects of learning and neural plasticity. REM sleep is believed to be important in brain development and growing and strengthening of new neural connections. It has been suggested that infants have proportionally more REM sleep that stimulates structural development, neural differentiation, and the development of neural pathways during the neonatal period.[7] During the first year of life, the amount of REM sleep decreases, while NREM sleep becomes the predominant state. The topographic distribution of SWA during NREM sleep and the local SWA maxima parallel the time course of synaptic density, cortical gray matter and behavioral maturation during childhood and adolescence.[38-42] These findings suggest that SWA is a good marker not only for sleep homeostasis but also for cortical plasticity and maturation during brain development.[1] During infancy, memory retention after the exposure to an artificial language was found to be associated with greater fronto-central SWA.[43] On the contrary, another study showed that SWA during nap did not correlate with event-related potentials during the memory test that involved the encoding of novel word meanings.[44] Therefore, the role of SWA in declarative memory during infancy needs to be clarified. Besides SWA, sleep spindle is another NREM feature that is known to reflect neural plasticity, myelination, and brain maturation.[45] More specifically, sleep spindle activity during infancy correlated with the offline generalization of new word meanings, supporting the role of sleep spindles for aggregating recent memories and for anchoring new knowledge into semantic long-term memory.[44,46] A recent study assessing the associations between the SWA and sigma powers and psychomotor development measured by Bayley-III in 36 infants at the age of 8 months showed that the occipital SWA and centro-occipital sigma power correlated with cognitive scales, and the frontal and occipital SWA and centro-occipital sigma power correlated with language and fine motor scales.[47] In fact, SWA and sleep spindles are implicated in various neurodevelopmental disorders, including autism spectrum disorder (ASD) and attention-deficit hyperactivity disorder (ADHD).[45]

Circadian disruptions may promote vulnerability to or the progression of certain disorders, particularly in a developmental context.[8] Dysfunction in circadian rhythms and sleep disturbance are often associated with childhood neurodevelopmental disorders. Unaffected parents of children with ASD have lower evening melatonin levels and lower activity of the acetylserotonin methyltransferase (ASMT) enzyme, which converts N-acetylserotonin to melatonin.[48] These findings suggest a genetic basis for impaired melatonin synthesis in ASD. Moreover, melatonin is a potent antioxidant. Therefore, reductions in melatonin during early development may lead to an accumulation of oxidative stress, causing harm to the developing brain and increase the risk of neurodevelopmental disorders such as ASD.[49] Treatments and interventions that target the circadian rhythms may improve clinical symptoms and daily functioning for the individual, for example, regular sleep and activity schedules seem to ameliorate daytime sleepiness and daytime behavioral problems in children and adolescents with ASD or ADHD.[8]

Summary

Infant sleep development is a highly complex and dynamic process in parallel to rapid neurocognitive and physical growth. It is regulated by circadian and homeostatic processes, which change across the lifespan with the most prominent change observed during childhood. Little is known about the interaction between the two processes during infancy. While there is a high interindividual and intraindividual variability in sleep development, how variations in sleep relate to developmental outcomes and the mediation by environmental and social factors in healthy infants remain to be elucidated. Further research is needed to enhance our understanding of the maturational change and the functional role of sleep during early development.

References

1. Jenni OG, Carskadon MA. Sleep behavior and sleep regulation from infancy through adolescence: normative aspects. *Sleep Med Clin*. 2012;7(3):529-538.
2. Mirmiran M, Maas YGH, Ariagno RL. Development of fetal and neonatal sleep and circadian rhythms. *Sleep Med Rev*. 2003;7(4):321-334.
3. Wallois F, Routier L, Heberlé C, Mahmoudzadeh M, Bourel-Ponchel E, Moghimi S. Back to basics: the neuronal substrates and mechanisms that underlie the electroencephalogram in premature neonates. *Neurophysiol Clin*. 2021;51(1):5-33.
4. Corsi-Cabrera M, Cubero-Rego L, Ricardo-Garcell J, Harmony T. Week-by-week changes in sleep EEG in healthy full-term newborns. *Sleep*. 2020;43(4):zsz261.
5. Fattinger S, Jenni OG, Schmitt B, Achermann P, Huber R. Overnight changes in the slope of sleep slow waves during infancy. *Sleep*. 2014;37(2):245-253.
6. Wielek T, Del Giudice R, Lang A, Wislowska M, Ott P, Schabus M. On the development of sleep states in the first weeks of life. *PLoS One*. 2019;14(10):e0224521.
7. Bathory E, Tomopoulos S. Sleep regulation, physiology and development, sleep duration and patterns, and sleep hygiene in infants, toddlers, and preschool-age children. *Curr Probl Pediatr Adolesc Health Care*. 2017;47(2):29-42.
8. Logan RW, McClung CA. Rhythms of life: circadian disruption and brain disorders across the lifespan. *Nat Rev Neurosci*. 2019;20(1):49-65.
9. Carskadon MA, Acebo C, Jenni OG. Regulation of adolescent sleep: implications for behavior. *Ann N Y Acad Sci*. 2004;1021:276-291.
10. Albrecht U, Eichele G. The mammalian circadian clock. *Curr Opin Genet Dev*. 2003;13(3):271-277.
11. Mirmiran M, Lunshof S. Perinatal development of human circadian rhythms. *Prog Brain Res*. 1996;111:217-226.
12. Lunshof S, Boer K, Wolf H, van Hoffen G, Bayram N, Mirmiran M. Fetal and maternal diurnal rhythms during the third trimester of normal pregnancy: outcomes of computerized analysis of continuous twenty-four-hour fetal heart rate recordings. *Am J Obstet Gynecol*. 1998;178(2):247-254.
13. Smarr BL, Grant AD, Perez L, Zucker I, Kriegsfeld LJ. Maternal and early-life circadian disruption have long-lasting negative consequences on offspring development and adult behavior in mice. *Sci Rep*. 2017;7(1):3326.
14. Jiang F. Sleep and early brain development. *Ann Nutr Metab*. 2019;75(1):44-54.
15. Kennaway DJ, Stamp GE, Goble FC. Development of melatonin production in infants and the impact of prematurity. *J Clin Endocrinol Metab*. 1992;75(2):367-369.
16. Mantagos S, Moustogiannis A, Vagenakis AG. Diurnal variation of plasma cortisol levels in infancy. *J Pediatr Endocrinol Metab*. 1998;11(4):549-553.
17. Antonini SR, Jorge SM, Moreira AC. The emergence of salivary cortisol circadian rhythm and its relationship to sleep activity in preterm infants. *Clin Endocrinol (Oxf)*. 2000;52(4):423-426.
18. Ivars K, Nelson N, Theodorsson A, Theodorsson E, Ström JO, Mörelius E. Development of salivary cortisol circadian rhythm and reference intervals in full-term infants. *PLoS One*. 2015;10(6):e0129502.
19. Ivars K, Nelson N, Theodorsson A, Theodorsson E, Ström JO, Mörelius E. Development of salivary cortisol circadian rhythm in preterm infants. *PLoS One*. 2017;12(8):e0182685.

20. Hsu PK, Ptáček LJ, Fu YH. Genetics of human sleep behavioral phenotypes. *Methods Enzymol.* 2015;552:309-324.
21. McMillen IC, Kok JS, Adamson TM, Deayton JM, Nowak R. Development of circadian sleep-wake rhythms in preterm and full-term infants. *Pediatr Res.* 1991;29(4 Pt 1):381-384.
22. Mirmiran M, Ariagno RL. Influence of light in the NICU on the development of circadian rhythms in preterm infants. *Semin Perinatol.* 2000;24(4):247-257.
23. Shimada M, Takahashi K, Segawa M, Higurashi M, Samejim M, Horiuchi K. Emerging and entraining patterns of the sleep-wake rhythm in preterm and term infants. *Brain Dev.* 1999;21(7):468-473.
24. Morag I, Ohlsson A. Cycled light in the intensive care unit for preterm and low birth weight infants. *Cochrane Database Syst Rev.* 2016;2016(8):CD006982.
25. Vásquez-Ruiz S, Maya-Barrios JA, Torres-Narváez P, et al. A light/dark cycle in the NICU accelerates body weight gain and shortens time to discharge in preterm infants. *Early Hum Dev.* 2014;90(9):535-540.
26. Hazelhoff EM, Dudink J, Meijer JH, Kervezee L. Beginning to see the light: lessons learned from the development of the circadian system for optimizing light conditions in the neonatal intensive care unit. *Front Neurosci.* 2021;15:634034. Available at: https://www.frontiersin.org/article/10.3389/fnins.2021.634034.
27. Rivkees SA, Mayes L, Jacobs H, Gross I. Rest-activity patterns of premature infants are regulated by cycled lighting. *Pediatrics.* 2004;113(4):833-839.
28. Kong J, Shepel PN, Holden CP, Mackiewicz M, Pack AI, Geiger JD. Brain glycogen decreases with increased periods of wakefulness: implications for homeostatic drive to sleep. *J Neurosci.* 2002;22(13):5581-5587.
29. Porkka-Heiskanen T, Alanko L, Kalinchuk A, Stenberg D. Adenosine and sleep. *Sleep Med Rev.* 2002;6(4):321-332.
30. Hubbard J, Gent TC, Hoekstra MMB, et al. Rapid fast-delta decay following prolonged wakefulness marks a phase of wake-inertia in NREM sleep. *Nat Commun.* 2020;11:3130.
31. Bes F, Schulz H, Navelet Y, Salzarulo P. The distribution of slow-wave sleep across the night: a comparison for infants, children, and adults. *Sleep.* 1991;14(1):5-12.
32. Jenni OG, Borbély AA, Achermann P. Development of the nocturnal sleep electroencephalogram in human infants. *Am J Physiol Regul Integr Comp Physiol.* 2004;286(3):R528-R538.
33. Fagioli I, Salzarulo P. Prior spontaneous nocturnal waking duration and EEG during quiet sleep in infants: an automatic analysis approach. *Behav Brain Res.* 1998;91(1-2):23-28.
34. Vyazovskiy VV, Olcese U, Lazimy YM, et al. Cortical firing and sleep homeostasis. *Neuron.* 2009;63(6):865-878.
35. Jenni OG, LeBourgeois MK. Understanding sleep–wake behavior and sleep disorders in children: the value of a model. *Curr Opin Psychiatry.* 2006;19(3):282-287.
36. Salzarulo P, Fagioli I. Post-natal development of sleep organization in man: speculations on the emergence of the "S process." *Neurophysiol Clin.* 1992;22(2):107-115.
37. Georgoulas A, Jones L, Laudiano-Dray MP, Meek J, Fabrizi L, Whitehead K. Sleep–wake regulation in preterm and term infants. *Sleep.* 2021;44(1):zsaa148.
38. Kurth S, Ringli M, Geiger A, LeBourgeois M, Jenni OG, Huber R. Mapping of cortical activity in the first two decades of life: a high-density sleep electroencephalogram study. *J Neurosci.* 2010;30(40):13211-13219.
39. Huttenlocher PR, Dabholkar AS. Regional differences in synaptogenesis in human cerebral cortex. *J Comp Neurol.* 1997;387(2):167-178.
40. Gogtay N, Giedd JN, Lusk L, et al. Dynamic mapping of human cortical development during childhood through early adulthood. *Proc Natl Acad Sci.* 2004;101(21):8174-8179.
41. Sowell ER, Thompson PM, Leonard CM, Welcome SE, Kan E, Toga AW. Longitudinal mapping of cortical thickness and brain growth in normal children. *J Neurosci.* 2004;24(38):8223-8231.
42. Luna B, Sweeney JA. The emergence of collaborative brain function: FMRI studies of the development of response inhibition. *Ann N Y Acad Sci.* 2004;1021:296-309.
43. Simon KNS, Werchan D, Goldstein MR, et al. Sleep confers a benefit for retention of statistical language learning in 6.5month old infants. *Brain Lang.* 2017;167:3-12.
44. Friedrich M, Wilhelm I, Born J, Friederici AD. Generalization of word meanings during infant sleep. *Nat Commun.* 2015;6(1):6004.

45. Page JM, Wakschlag LS, Norton ES. Nonrapid eye movement sleep characteristics and relations with motor, memory, and cognitive ability from infancy to preadolescence. *Dev Psychobiol.* 2021;63(8):e22202.
46. Friedrich M, Wilhelm I, Mölle M, Born J, Friederici AD. The sleeping infant brain anticipates development. *Curr Biol.* 2017;27(15):2374-2380.e3.
47. Satomaa AL, Mäkelä T, Saarenpää-Heikkilä O, Kylliäinen A, Huupponen E, Himanen SL. Slow-wave activity and sigma activities are associated with psychomotor development at 8 months of age. *Sleep.* 2020;43(9):zsaa061.
48. Melke J, Goubran Botros H, Chaste P, et al. Abnormal melatonin synthesis in autism spectrum disorders. *Mol Psychiatry.* 2008;13(1):90-98.
49. Jin Y, Choi J, Won J, Hong Y. The relationship between autism spectrum disorder and melatonin during fetal development. *Molecules.* 2018;23(1):198.

CHAPTER 3

Infant Respiratory Physiology During Sleep

Yeilim Cho ▪ Alisha George ▪ Ignacio E. Tapia

Introduction

Sleep is a vital process, characterized by decreased consciousness with inhibited motor activity and rapid reversibility. Respiratory physiology during sleep undergoes a multitude of maturational changes during childhood, especially in infancy.

Overview of Infant Breathing During Sleep

Since infants spend most of their time sleeping, understanding normal patterns and maturation of breathing during sleep is crucial. It is equally important to recognize the difference in breathing physiology between sleep and wakefulness as well as between different sleep stages, namely rapid eye movement (REM) and non-REM (NREM) sleep. For example, a decrease in functional residual capacity (FRC) in sleep is particularly marked in REM. In REM sleep (versus NREM), respiratory rate (RR) is higher and more variable. Ventilatory responses to hypoxia and hypercapnia are attenuated in sleep, particularly in REM (versus NREM) sleep.[1,2]

Maturation of sleep architecture takes place over several years of early childhood. In newborn infants, sleep stages can be categorized into REM versus NREM sleep, which are equivalent to "active" and "quiet" sleep, respectively, which represent a more organized sleep architecture. During quiet sleep, breathing is regular and manifests episodic sighs that are followed by oscillatory breathing. The response to sigh or recovery of tidal volume to presigh values is stable but slow in the first few days of life in newborns. During the period between 4 to 8 days and 3 to 4 months of life, the oscillatory period decreases, and respiration becomes potentially more stable. By 3 to 4 months, the response becomes more stable with a rapid response time.[3]

In active/REM sleep, breathing is irregular in terms of RR and tidal volume, with a variable oscillatory pattern. In newborn infants, pauses in breathing of up to 10 seconds are common, particularly in active sleep and the frequency of this decreases with age.[4] During active sleep (REM), muscle tone is diminished. Low intercostal muscle tone then leads to paradoxical movement of rib cage that is partially compensated by increased diaphragmatic work of breathing but at the expense of potential diaphragmatic fatigue in REM sleep.[5] As a result, so-called "expiratory braking" can be lost. In the immediate newborn period, the first breaths tend to be deeper and longer than subsequent breaths and are characterized by a short deep inspiration followed by a prolonged expiratory phase.[6] This expiratory braking helps to develop and maintain FRC in the newborn period when the chest wall is very compliant.[7] These series of breathing changes make REM sleep the most vulnerable stage for respiratory disturbances. Moreover, diminished muscle tone in upper airway muscles makes infants susceptible to airway obstruction in REM sleep, especially in infants with anatomical susceptibility such as macroglossia and micrognathia.[8]

NREM/quiet sleep is characterized by a generally regular breathing pattern, punctuated by intermittent sigh breaths. During NREM sleep, there is a decrease in RR and depth compared with the awake state, resulting in decreased minute ventilation.[9] REM sleep, on the other hand, is characterized by more irregular breathing, in both RR and tidal volume. During REM sleep, there is inhibition of skeletal muscle tone affecting the intercostal muscles and leading to thoracoabdominal asynchrony and increased diaphragmatic work of breathing. This paradoxical incursion of the rib cage with inspiration is often seen with younger postnatal age and can be expected up to 3 years of age.[10]

Normal values for hemoglobin oxygen saturation (SpO_2) reach at least 80% within 10 minutes of birth in term and healthy preterm infants without oxygen supplementation.[11] Arterial partial pressure of oxygen (PaO_2) values of 50 to 80 mmHg are sufficient to meet the metabolic demand in the newborn partly owing to the high proportion of fetal hemoglobin (HbF). Normative data for preterm infant are scarce. In one study that included a group of preterm infants during the first days of life, oxyhemoglobin desaturation episodes (SpO_2 <80%) were found on 10 of 55 recordings.[12] Baseline values during regular breathing ranged from 90% to 100%. Most oxyhemoglobin desaturation events are related to apneic episodes. The number of episodes diminishes with time.[13] Lower baseline O_2 levels at first week of postnatal age than at 1 month may be due to age-related differences in intrapulmonary and intracardiac shunting. Decrease in minute ventilation, combined with reduced intercostal muscle tone and supine positioning, all contribute to reduced oxygenation.

In full-term infants, the mean SpO_2 in REM sleep is approximately 4% less than that in NREM sleep at 1 week of age. This is due to low O_2 tensions, high incidence of apnea, high metabolic consumption, and a decrease in the O_2 stores in REM sleep. End-tidal CO_2 ($ETCO_2$) monitoring is limited at this age due to technical issues related to elevated RR that preclude a good $ETCO_2$ signal plateau. Schafer et al. found no changes in transcutaneous CO_2 measurements ($tcCO_2$) with postnatal age in newborns but the mean and maximum CO_2 decreases with time during the first 18 months of life.[14] The lower values of $tcCO_2$ in REM than NREM may be due to paradoxical sleep coupled with increased O_2 consumption.

Chest Wall and Lung Mechanics

Growth accompanies changes in chest wall geometry. Hence, the chest wall undergoes several maturational changes in the first few years of life, summarized below.

There is a striking difference in the cross-sectional shape of the infant rib cage compared to older children and adults. The chest wall shape of an infant almost resembles a circle, and with age, becomes more ovoid. The adult chest wall shape is achieved by roughly 3 to 5 years of age.[15]

The positioning of the ribs affects chest expansion in infancy. The relatively horizontal position of the ribs results in inefficient expansion of the chest wall. Then, when the hemidiaphragms contract in the setting of horizontal ribs, there is worsening distortion of the compliant infant chest wall.[15] In older children and adults, on the other hand, ribs are downward sloping which allows for greater chest expansion by lifting the anterior ribs.[16]

In both the prenatal and postnatal periods, the diaphragm undergoes developmental changes in terms of muscle fiber composition and neuronal properties, impacting its contractility and endurance.[17] In early infancy, the left hemidiaphragm dome is positioned around vertebral level 8. However, this hemidiaphragm descends to around level T11 as a child approaches 3 years of age. Throughout life, the right hemidiaphragm is typically positioned approximately half a vertebral level higher.

Changes in Compliance

Compliance, defined as the change in volume (L) per unit change in pressure (cm H_2O), can be measured for the lungs, chest wall, and total respiratory system. The lungs and chest wall have distinct, nonlinear relationships between volume and pressure. Compliance can be further broken down into static compliance and dynamic compliance. Static compliance can be ascertained at a fixed volume, while dynamic compliance is measured with normal breathing.

The lungs become inflated with inspiration and then recoil inward due to their elastic properties. Conversely, the chest wall exerts outward recoil. The FRC denotes the point at which the inward recoil of the lungs is equal to the outward recoil of the chest wall, and it is dependent on the passive elastic properties of the respiratory system. Lung compliance does not significantly change with age, even when adjusted for body size. However, the highly compliant chest wall of the neonate leads to a lower passive resting lung volume compared to older children and adults.[18]

In infancy and in later stages of life, FRC is reduced during sleep relative to the awake state; this is more pronounced during REM sleep. However, the compliance of the chest wall of newborns and infants is easily compromised when the diaphragm is contracted or when the intercostal muscles are inhibited, as occurs during REM sleep. In REM sleep, as previously mentioned, phasic inspiratory diaphragm contractions coupled with the decreased intercostal muscle tone cause paradoxical breathing; the rib cage moves inward rather than outward. In full-term newborns, rib cage distortion occurs nearly 100% of REM sleep periods.

Changes in Control of Breathing

In newborns, peripheral chemoreceptors play a central role in initiating the ventilatory, cardiovascular, and arousal responses to hypoxia or asphyxia. Dramatic resetting of the peripheral chemoreceptors occurs in early postnatal life especially during the first 2 weeks of life.

The hypoxic ventilatory response (HVR) refers to change in minute ventilation in response to hypoxia. Newborns exhibit biphasic HVR; transient increase in ventilation, followed by a decrease to or below baseline levels.[19] Interestingly, however, in infants born at 32 to 37 weeks, hyperventilation response to hypoxia does not occur in a cool environment. This biphasic response is thought to be due to central depression (versus peripheral chemoreceptors), decrease in metabolic rate, and changes in lung mechanics.[20] Premature infants may show a biphasic HVR response up to 25 days after birth.

The hypercapnic ventilatory response (HCVR) is the ventilatory response to CO_2, also expressed as changes in minute ventilation (L/minute) by mmHg of CO_2 (PCO_2). Conceptually, it measures CO_2 sensitivity. HCVR is influenced by age, sex, weight, body surface area, vital capacity, and genetic polymorphism.[21-23] The HCVR corrected for weight decreases with age.[23] HCVR is reduced in premature infants mostly due to a limited RR response to increased CO_2 despite a more substantial tidal volume response to CO_2. The HCRV increases as the infants mature.[24-26] For the HCVR measurement, controlled setting such as rebreathing or steady state is needed.[21]

HCRV is reduced in premature infants of less than 33 weeks gestational age. HCRV increases as 40 weeks postconceptional age is approached. In one study, HCRVs (unadjusted for body size) were 0.044 L/min/mmHg for <33 weeks, 0.174 for 33 to 36 weeks, and 0.292 for 37 to 40 weeks infants.[26] In full term infants, the HCRV mostly increases over the first 2 days but continues to mature over 8 weeks of life.[27] In the study by Søvik et al., 26 healthy term infants were assessed for ventilatory response to hypercapnia, hypoxia, and hypercapnic hypoxia in a randomized sequence. Although response magnitude to hypercapnia did not change, response rate to hypercapnia increased over 8-week period, suggesting ventilatory response continues to mature between postnatal between birth and 8 weeks in term infants.[27]

Obtaining HVR and HCVR during sleep is more complicated during sleep than during wakefulness even more so in infants as they do not have the developmental ability to express distress and cooperate with the measurements. Therefore, most available sleep data come from neonatal animal model.[28]

Ventilatory drives are important in the maintenance of ventilation during sleep but both HVR and the HCRV decrease during sleep. Reduction in HVR is more pronounced in REM versus NREM sleep in adults.[29] This may explain the REM-associated hypoxemia in both healthy infants and in those with cardiopulmonary disease. Minimal data exist on the effect of sleep stage on the HVR in infants due to the difficult set-up that such a test entails in noncooperative subjects. One study showed that HVR is more variable during REM than NREM sleep when assessed at 2 to 5 weeks, 2 to 3 and 5 to 6 months.[30]

HCRV markedly decreases in sleep in infants.[31] The degree of HCRV decrease appears to be similar between REM and NREM sleep.[32] In one study where the effect of CO_2 on the ventilatory pattern of 18 normal infants was assessed during sleep through the age of 4 months, the percent increase from base line in instantaneous minute ventilation during REM sleep was similar to that during NREM sleep.[32]

There has been a suggestion that sleep position can affect ventilatory response. In prematurely born infants, some studies have shown that respiratory control can be more vulnerable in supine sleep. In one study including premature infants (mean post conceptional age 35 weeks), the supine position was associated with a higher RR and lower SpO_2 than the prone position. HCVR was lower in the supine than in the prone position. Rib cage contribution to ventilation in the supine was less than in the prone position.[33] Ventilatory and arousal responses to mild asphyxia (hypercapnia/hypoxia) did not differ between supine and prone position in healthy infants at newborn but the response was diminished in prone position at 3 months of age, particularly in active sleep.[34] In contrast, some studies reported opposite findings that propose position is associated with impaired ventilatory response to CO_2 challenge in preterm infant asserting that such compromise in prone position may make preterm infant vulnerable to the SIDS.[35] In a study that included preterm infants with symptomatic apnea and bradycardia (gestational age of 26.9 weeks), no difference in the incidence of clinically significant apnea, bradycardia, or desaturation between supine and prone positions was seen. Thus, there is an ongoing debate about which sleep position is more disadvantageous to breathing and whether sleep position-related breathing instability contributes to the SIDS.

CENTRAL AND OBSTRUCTIVE APNEAS

Central pauses, or central apneas, in the form of periodic breathing are commonly observed in newborns. With increasing postnatal age, the frequency of central apnea decreases due to a more mature respiratory drive, increased FRC, and a less compliant chest wall.[36,37] While longer central apneas can occur in term infants in the first month or so of life, they are more frequently seen in preterm babies.[38] Periodic breathing, defined by 3 central pauses lasting at least 3 seconds in a period of respiration of 20 seconds or less, is commonly observed in the first few months of life but tends to decline in frequency after about 4 to 5 months of age.[37] Periodic breathing is also more pronounced in warm settings.[39] The frequency, mean, and maximum durations of apnea were correlated with the body heat loss in preterm neonate.[39] However, in a case control setting, one study found that infants who later died of SIDS had experienced significantly more frequent episodes of obstructive and mixed sleep apnea than control group preceding SIDS.[40] However, whether apnea of infancy is simply a marker (versus causal) of prematurity rather than the causal factor of SIDS is unclear.[41]

Infants have both anatomical and physiological properties subjecting them to tendency of airway obstruction and gas exchange abnormalities.[42] The newborn trachea and larynx are relatively superiorly positioned making epiglottis and soft palate proximal to each other. The infant mandible is nearly horizontal at birth resulting in a propensity toward posterior displacement. Adenotonsillar hypertrophy may become an important contributor to OSA in infants after 6 months of age. Besides these anatomical features, high chest wall compliance, ventilation-perfusion mismatching, and ventilatory control instability all contribute to the risk of OSA in infants. Congenital abnormalities of the airway, beyond the scope of this chapter, such as laryngomalacia, will have further effects on airway patency.

Conclusion

Both sleep and breathing are physiological processes that undergo progressive changes during infancy. Major changes for both sleep and breathing occur during the first months after birth. Breathing and ventilatory responses become more stable in the first months of life, and REM sleep represents the most vulnerable stage for respiratory instability. Respiratory events, including apneas, are more common in infants and decrease in healthy children.

References

1. Carse EA, Wilkinson AR, Whyte PL, Henderson-Smart DJ, Johnson P. Oxygen and carbon dioxide tensions, breathing and heart rate in normal infants during the first six months of life. *J Dev Physiol.* 1981;3(2):85 100.
2. Gaultier C. Cardiorespiratory adaptation during sleep in infants and children. *Pediatr Pulmonol.* 1995;19(2):105-117. doi:10.1002/ppul.1950190206.
3. Fleming PJ, Goncalves AL, Levine MR, Woollard S. The development of stability of respiration in human infants: changes in ventilatory responses to spontaneous sighs. *J Physiol.* 1984;347:1-16. doi:10.1113/jphysiol.1984.sp015049.
4. Ramanathan R, Corwin MJ, Hunt CE, et al. Cardiorespiratory events recorded on home monitors: comparison of healthy infants with those at increased risk for SIDS. *JAMA.* 2001;285(17):2199-2207. doi:10.1001/jama.285.17.2199.
5. Muller N, Gulston G, Cade D, et al. Diaphragmatic muscle fatigue in the newborn. *J Appl Physiol Respir Environ Exerc Physiol.* 1979;46(4):688-695. doi:10.1152/jappl.1979.46.4.688.
6. te Pas AB, Wong C, Kamlin CO, Dawson JA, Morley CJ, Davis PG. Breathing patterns in preterm and term infants immediately after birth. *Pediatr Res.* 2009;65(3):352-356. doi:10.1203/PDR.0b013e318193f117.
7. Mortola JP, Fisher JT, Smith B, Fox G, Weeks S. Dynamics of breathing in infants. *J Appl Physiol.* 1982;52(5):1209-1215. doi:10.1152/jappl.1982.52.5.1209.
8. Standards and indications for cardiopulmonary sleep studies in children. American Thoracic Society. *Am J Respir Crit Care Med.* 1996;153(2):866-878. doi:10.1164/ajrccm.153.2.8564147.
9. Ross KR, Rosen CL. Sleep and respiratory physiology in children. *Clin Chest Med.* 2014;35(3):457-467. doi:10.1016/j.ccm.2014.06.003.
10. Heraghty JL, Hilliard TN, Henderson AJ, Fleming PJ. The physiology of sleep in infants. *Arch Dis Child.* 2008;93(11):982-985. doi:10.1136/adc.2006.113290.
11. Dawson JA, Kamlin CO, Vento M, et al. Defining the reference range for oxygen saturation for infants after birth. *Pediatrics.* 2010;125(6):e1340-e1347. doi:10.1542/peds.2009-1510.
12. Richard D, Poets CF, Neale S, Stebbens VA, Alexander JR, Southall DP. Arterial oxygen saturation in preterm neonates without respiratory failure. *J Pediatr.* 1993;123(6):963-968. doi:10.1016/s0022-3476 (05)80395-6.
13. Poets CF, Stebbens VA, Alexander JR, Arrowsmith WA, Salfield SA, Southall DP. Arterial oxygen saturation in preterm infants at discharge from the hospital and six weeks later. *J Pediatr.* 1992;120(3): 447-454. doi:10.1016/s0022-3476(05)80919-9.
14. Schäfer T, Schäfer D, Schläfke ME. Breathing, transcutaneous blood gases, and CO2 response in SIDS siblings and control infants during sleep. *J Appl Physiol (Bethesda, MD: 1985).* 1993;74(1):88-102. doi:10.1152/jappl.1993.74.1.88.
15. Openshaw P, Edwards S, Helms P. Changes in rib cage geometry during childhood. *Thorax.* 1984;39(8): 624-627. doi:10.1136/thx.39.8.624.
16. Kaneko H, Horie J. Breathing movements of the chest and abdominal wall in healthy subjects. *Respir Care.* 2012;57(9):1442-1451. doi:10.4187/respcare.01655.

17. Mantilla CB, Sieck GC. Key aspects of phrenic motoneuron and diaphragm muscle development during the perinatal period. *J Appl Physiol (1985)*. 2008;104(6):1818-1827. doi:10.1152/japplphysiol.01192.2007.
18. Agostoni E. Volume-pressure relationships of the thorax and lung in the newborn. *J Appl Physiol*. 1959; 14:909-913. doi:10.1152/jappl.1959.14.6.909.
19. Miller HC, Behrle FC. The effects of hypoxia on the respiration of newborn infants. *Pediatrics*. 1954;14(2):93-103.
20. Davis GM, Bureau MA. Pulmonary and chest wall mechanics in the control of respiration in the newborn. *Clin Perinatol*. 1987;14(3):551-579.
21. Goldberg S, Ollila HM, Lin L, et al. Analysis of hypoxic and hypercapnic ventilatory response in healthy volunteers. *PloS One*. 2017;12(1):e0168930. doi:10.1371/journal.pone.0168930.
22. Jones RL, Neary JM, Ryan TG. Normal values for the hypercapnic ventilation response: effects of age and the ability to ventilate. *Respiration*. 1993;60(4):197-202. doi:10.1159/000196199.
23. Marcus CL, Glomb WB, Basinski DJ, Davidson SL, Keens TG. Developmental pattern of hypercapnic and hypoxic ventilatory responses from childhood to adulthood. *J Appl Physiol*. 1994;76(1):314-320. doi:10.1152/jappl.1994.76.1.314.
24. Frantz ID III, Adler SM, Thach BT, Taeusch Jr HW. Maturational effects on respiratory responses to carbon dioxide in premature infants. *J Appl Physiol*. 1976;41(1):41-45. doi:10.1152/jappl.1976.41.1.41.
25. Rigatto H, Brady JP, de la Torre Verduzco R. Chemoreceptor reflexes in preterm infants: II. The effect of gestational and postnatal age on the ventilatory response to inhaled carbon dioxide. *Pediatrics*. 1975; 55(5):614-620.
26. Krauss AN, Klain DB, Waldman S, Auld PAM. Ventilatory response to carbon dioxide in newborn infants. *Pediatr Res*. 1975;9(1):46-50. doi:10.1203/00006450-197501000-00009.
27. Søvik S, Lossius K. Development of ventilatory response to transient hypercapnia and hypercapnic hypoxia in term infants. *Pediatr Res*. 2004;55(2):302-309. doi:10.1203/01.pdr.0000106316.40213.db.
28. Putnam RW, Conrad SC, Gdovin MJ, Erlichman JS, Leiter JC. Neonatal maturation of the hypercapnic ventilatory response and central neural CO2 chemosensitivity. *Respir Physiol Neurobiol*. 2005;149(1-3): 165-179. doi:10.1016/j.resp.2005.03.004.
29. Douglas NJ, White DP, Weil JV, et al. Hypoxic ventilatory response decreases during sleep in normal men. *Am Rev Respir Dis*. 1982;125(3):286-289. doi:10.1164/arrd.1982.125.3.286.
30. Richardson HL, Parslow PM, Walker AM, Harding R, Horne RSC. Variability of the initial phase of the ventilatory response to hypoxia in sleeping infants. *Pediatr Res*. 2006;59(5):700-704. doi:10.1203/01.pdr.0000214978.94064.66.
31. Phillipson EA, Kozar LF, Rebuck AS, Murphy E. Ventilatory and waking responses to CO2 in sleeping dogs. *Am Rev Respir Dis*. 1977;115(2):251-259. doi:10.1164/arrd.1977.115.2.251.
32. Haddad GG, Leistner HL, Epstein RA, Epstein MA, Grodin WK, Mellins RB. CO2-induced changes in ventilation and ventilatory pattern in normal sleeping infants. *J Appl Physiol Respir Environ Exerc Physiol*. 1980;48(4):684-688. doi:10.1152/jappl.1980.48.4.684.
33. Martin RJ, DiFiore JM, Korenke CB, Randal H, Miller MJ, Brooks LJ. Vulnerability of respiratory control in healthy preterm infants placed supine. *J Pediatr*. 1995;127(4):609-614. doi:10.1016/s0022-3476(95)70125-7.
34. Galland BC, Bolton DP, Taylor BJ, Sayers RM, Williams SM. Ventilatory sensitivity to mild asphyxia: prone versus supine sleep position. *Arch Dis Child*. 2000;83(5):423-428. doi:10.1136/adc.83.5.423.
35. Smith APR, Saiki T, Hannam S, Rafferty GF, Greenough A. The effects of sleeping position on ventilatory responses to carbon dioxide in premature infants. *Thorax*. 2010;65(9):824-828. doi:10.1136/thx.2009.127837.
36. Ramanathan R, Corwin MJ, Hunt CE, et al. Cardiorespiratory events recorded on home monitors: comparison of healthy infants with those at increased risk for SIDS. *JAMA*. 2001;285(17):2199-2207. doi:10.1001/jama.285.17.2199.
37. Kelly DH, Stellwagen LM, Kaitz E, Shannon DC. Apnea and periodic breathing in normal full-term infants during the first twelve months. *Pediatr Pulmonol*. 1985;1(4):215-219. doi:10.1002/ppul.1950010409.
38. Hodgman JE, Gonzalez F, Hoppenbrouwers T, Cabal LA. Apnea, transient episodes of bradycardia, and periodic breathing in preterm infants. *Am J Dis Child*. 1990;144(1):54-57. doi:10.1001/archpedi.1990.02150250064032.

39. Tourneux P, Cardot V, Museux N, et al. Influence of thermal drive on central sleep apnea in the preterm neonate. *Sleep*. 2008;31(4):549-556. doi:10.1093/sleep/31.4.549.
40. Kato I, Groswasser J, Franco P, et al. Developmental characteristics of apnea in infants who succumb to sudden infant death syndrome. *Am J Respir Crit Care Med*. 2001;164(8):1464-1469. doi:10.1164/ajrccm.164.8.2009001.
41. Brooks JG. Apnea of infancy and sudden infant death syndrome. *Am J Dis Child*. 1982;136(11):1012-1023. doi:10.1001/archpedi.1982.03970470056016.
42. Katz ES, Mitchell RB, D'Ambrosio CM. Obstructive sleep apnea in infants. *Am J Respir Crit Care Med*. 2012;185(8):805-816. doi:10.1164/rccm.201108-1455CI.

CHAPTER 4

Behavioral Changes in Sleep During the First 2 Years

Judith A. Owens ■ Jennifer Gingrasfield ■ Maile A. Moore

Developmental Changes in Sleep Behavior 0 to 24 Months

GENERAL CONSIDERATIONS

While there are general trends in normal sleep development across the first 2 years of life (and beyond) as expanded upon below, it is important to recognize that some degree of individual variability within these developmental trajectories is to be expected, including in sleep patterns and sleep needs. For example, the definition of "sufficient" sleep not only is based on the number of hours on a chart but also takes the functional context into consideration; for example, does the child awaken spontaneously at the expected time or need to be awakened by a caregiver? When given the opportunity to sleep more, does the child extend sleep beyond the typical duration? Are sleep quantity and quality linked temporally to negative changes in daytime mood and behavior?

Sleep and sleep problems especially in young children, represent a complex amalgam of basic sleep and circadian biology, genetic predispositions, environmental influences (including macro such as neighborhood safety and noise and household overcrowding and micro such as the sleeping space and bedding), family dynamics, parenting practices, child temperament, cultural beliefs, values and practices, family stress including caregiver mental illness, financial challenges and exposure to abuse/neglect and domestic violence, medical issues, and developmental concerns.[1,2]

There are a number of basic trends in sleep that occur during infancy and beyond that reflect the physiologic/chronobiologic, developmental, and social/environmental changes that are occurring across childhood. These trends may be summarized as the gradual assumption of more adult sleep patterns as children mature:

- Sleep is *the* primary activity of the brain during early development; for example, by age 2 years, the average child has spent 9500 hours (approximately 13 months) asleep versus 8000 hours awake, and between 2 and 5 years, the time asleep is equal to the time awake.
- There is a gradual decline in the average 24-hour sleep duration from infancy through adolescence, which involves a decrease in both diurnal and nocturnal sleep amounts.
- Sleep duration, especially in the first year of life, is reported to be quite variable in large epidemiological studies, although this may reflect variability in caregiver estimates of time in bed rather than actual sleep duration.[3]
- After 12 months, there seems to be a tendency for children to settle into and track on a "sleep duration percentile." For example, a child whose sleep duration is in the 10th percentile is more likely to continue to sleep for relatively lower less hours, similar to what would be seen in regard to growth (height and weight) percentiles.

- Cross-cultural studies have suggested that sleep duration in infants and toddlers may also be significantly different across regions around the globe; in general, parent-reported total sleep duration is much lower in predominantly Asian countries versus "Western" countries; this seems to be largely due to later bedtimes in the former areas. This may be in part related to cultural variations in caregiver reporting due to expectations regarding "normal" or "ideal" sleep amounts and sleep practices.
- The within-sleep ultradian cycle of sleep stages lengthens from about 50 minutes in the term infant to 90 to 110 minutes in the school-age child. This has clinical significance in that typically a brief arousal or awakening occurs during the night at the termination of each ultradian cycle. As the length of the cycles increases, there is a concomitant decrease in the number of these end-of-cycle arousals (night wakings).

Finally, an appreciation of fundamental principles such as importance of caregiver education about normal developmental changes in sleep as part of "anticipatory guidance," acknowledgment that many sleep behaviors are learned (and thus may be "taught" by caregivers), and recognition that sleep problems in young children also have a profound impact not only on caregivers, but on other family members is critical to successful prevention and intervention.

NORMAL SLEEP PATTERNS, SLEEP MILESTONES, AND BEHAVIOR: 0 TO 24 MONTHS

A summary of the normal developmental changes in sleep in the first 2 years of life is presented in Table 4.1. Additional details regarding specific developmental consideration are included below.[4]

TABLE 4.1 ■ Summary of the Normal Developmental Changes in Sleep in the First 2 Years of Life

Age	Total Sleep 24-Hour Range	Night/Naps	Frequency of Night waking	Developmentally Appropriate Features
Newborns 0–2 months	9–18 hours	Variable, strongly influenced by hunger, wakeful periods of typically 1–2 hours	Every 2–3 hours	Active versus quiet sleep. Frequent grimacing, sucking, crying in active sleep.
Infants 3–12 months	12–14 hours	3–4 months = 4 naps totaling 3–4 hours 4–6 months = 3 naps totaling 2.5–3.5 hours 6–15 months = 2 naps totaling 2.5–3.5 hours 12–18 months = 1 nap totaling 1.5–2.5 hours	Sleep consolidation between 3 and 5 months, most infants are physiologically able to wean from overnight feeding by 6 months of age	Circadian rhythms are more developed by 3 months and periods of wakefulness slowly increase throughout infancy. A regulated daily sleep schedule can be obtained by 3–5 months.
Toddlers 13–24 months	11–14 hours	9–11/1–2.5	Developmentally capable of "sleeping through the night"	Developmentally appropriate increased awareness, testing. Okay to offer a transitional object at 12 months of age.

Newborn 0 to 2 Months

Typical ranges in sleep duration are reported to be 9 to 18 hours per day. In early infancy sleep patterns are evenly distributed across the day and night without clear day-night differentiation. Sleep-wake cycles are greatly influenced by hunger and satiety. Due to slower digestion, formula-fed infants feed every 2 to 4 hours. Breast milk is digested more rapidly thus feeding may occur every 1 to 3 hours.[5] Newborns typically feed 8 to 12 times per day. At this age, sleep periods are often separated by 1- to 2-hour periods of wakefulness. Circadian rhythms are still developing in these early months.[6]

Common Sleep Considerations for Age

- Newborns grimace, cry, suck, twitch, and blink during active sleep. Teaching caregivers about this normal feature of infant sleep, instructing them to "pause" a few minutes to watch and see if this is a true waking or just a sleep state shift can lead to improved sleep consolidation and fewer "behavioral" sleep issues down the line.
- Educating caregivers about normal sleep variability, cycles, and routines is critical. Introducing the concept of allowing the infant to settle into sleep drowsy but awake is very helpful starting at around 3 months.
- Parental stress, maternal postpartum depression or anxiety, and chronic parental sleep deprivation must be assessed as potential contributing factors to infant sleep problems and the *perception* of problematic sleep by caregivers.
- Feeding problems/gastroesophageal reflux/colic may contribute to actual or perceived sleep problems and often set the stage for behavioral sleep issues in later infancy.
- Sudden unexpected infant death (SUID): Continual assessment and education should be provided throughout infancy (discussed later in chapter).

Infants 3 to 12 Months

Total sleep in later infancy continues to vary and ranges from 12 to 14 hours per day. By around 3 months of age, circadian rhythms are more developed and the duration of periods of wakefulness during the day slowly increases throughout infancy.[7] Periods of wakefulness are not evenly distributed; rather wakefulness periods tend to lengthen over the course of the day with the longest of period of wakefulness in the evening ("second wind"). A regulated sleep schedule can typically be implemented by 3 to 5 months of age. Naps decrease with age: at 3 to 4 months most infants nap 4 times, 4 to 6 months 3 times, 6 to 7 months 2 times, and by 12 to 18 months once per day. Healthy term infants do not require overnight feeding by 6 months of age from a nutritional standpoint.

There are two important sleep "milestones" that typically occur during this time period.[7] The first is that of *sleep consolidation*, which is defined as the transition from equal distribution of sleep across the 24-hour day to the preponderance of sleep occurring at night, with shorter discrete sleep periods ("naps") during the day. An additional feature is an increasingly long sustained period of nocturnal sleep, often defined as "sleeping through the night" (although this is a bit of a misnomer as it implies that the normal brief night wakings at the end of a sleep cycle are not a feature of "good sleep"). Sleep consolidation is largely a corollary of developmental changes in sleep homeostasis and circadian rhythms. The second milestone, that of *sleep regulation*, refers to the ability of the infant to fall asleep independently at bedtime and return to sleep without caregiver intervention during normal night wakings. It is essentially a learned skill that involves the establishment of appropriate sleep onset associations and is thus more dependent upon caregiver behavior.

Common Sleep Considerations for Age

- See section below regarding bed-sharing/cosleeping recommendations.
- The acquisition of developmental milestones may contribute to sleep disruptions. For example, when infants achieve object permanence, they may protest more at bedtime when

separation occurs, and they may become aware of sleep onset associations more than they did as younger infants as they begin to understand the nature of "cause and effect." In terms of gross motor skills acquisition, they may be driven, for example, to practice pulling to stand in the crib before falling asleep.

- Periods of "sleep regression" are common during this time. These could be likely due to a combination of factors including advancement in physiologic sleep, decrease in total sleep requirement, and social/emotional/physical development.
- "Self-soothing," or the ability to regulate physiologic and emotional states independently slowly develops in early infancy.[7] In terms of sleep, this is considered the ability to independently fall asleep or return to sleep at sleep-wake transitions with little to no crying/protest behavior. Self-soothing can be exclusively internal or externally one may see behaviors such as thumb sucking, rocking, or hair twirling.
- If caregivers base sleep times *only* on cues (or wake windows), this may result in high day-to-day variability. This lack of circadian stability leads to more sleep dysregulation. Sleep schedules should be set with both homeostatic and circadian function in mind.
- By 6 months of age, most infants do not require any overnight feeding; however, in practice, night feeding commonly continues for much longer. This is often driven by sleep onset associations with nursing or bottle used to promote sleep onset and learned hunger/ misdistribution of feedings during the overnight period. Excessive urination, bowel movements, and physiologic digestive processes may additionally contribute to more disrupted sleep. In addition, nighttime feedings may contribute to an increase in otitis media due to eustachian tube blockage and promote dental ("baby bottle") caries.
- A consistent bedtime routine is associated with better sleep. By about 3 months of age, it is helpful to follow a brief and consistent bedtime routine with dressing, feeding, snuggling or rocking, and goal of putting the infant into the crib/bassinet drowsy but awake.
- Transitional objects such as a pacifier without an attached stuffed animal or blanket are recommended per infant safe sleep recommendations as a wake-sleep transition aid. However, many children will not accept a pacifier.
- The American Academy of Pediatrics advises no screen time for children less than 18 to 24 months of age with exception of supervised video-chatting. Increasing prevalence, availability, and use rates of screen time continue across childhood including during infancy. Screen time is disruptive for social emotional development and sleep. Children should sleep in a screen-free environment. Research shows (among other negative correlates) that a higher amount of screen time is associated with reduced total sleep time.

Toddlers 12 to 24 Months

By this age, children should be on a consistent regular sleep schedule. There should be a set bedtime and bedtime routine that leads to putting the child in bed drowsy but still awake. If the goal is to have the child sleep independently, then the child should start the night in the desired sleep location and should fall asleep without caregiver intervention. From a developmental standpoint, the typical toddler has an ever-expanding expressive and receptive vocabulary, a drive toward independence and autonomy, and a peak of separation anxiety at around 18 months of age, all of which can contribute to sleep problems.

Common Sleep Considerations for Age

- In general, screen time use increases with age. While many toddlers have screen/media devices in the bedroom, this has been shown to be associated with overall increased screen time, and sleep issues such as reduced sleep amounts, increased time to fall asleep, and more disrupted sleep. For children aged 18 to 24 months, the AAP recommends coviewing for less than 1 hour per day of high-quality, slow-paced programming.[8] As always, screens should be off 1 hour before bed. Additionally, screen time should not be tied into the morning routine, as young children may cut sleep short in order to start the day with screen time.

■ Transition from crib to bed: Most toddlers under 2 years of age benefit from sleeping in a crib rather than transitioning to a bed too early. At times, safety concerns arise when a young toddler can climb out of the crib and therefore is at risk for fall-related injury. In the latter case, the sleep environment should be thoroughly child proofed. Installing a walk-through style gate on the bedroom door can provide additional safety.

■ Age-appropriate transitional objects such as a stuffed animal or small blanket can provide comfort and ease the process of separating from caregivers at bedtime and during the night, as well as at nap time.

SAFE SLEEP PRINCIPLES

SUID remains the third leading cause of infant mortality in the United States and accounts for more than 3500 deaths annually. It is the leading cause of infant death from 1 to 11 months of age.[9-11]

SUID is a term that includes three classifications of cause of death of infants under 1 year of age: Sudden infant death (SIDS), infant accidental suffocation and strangulation in bed, and all other unknown causes. Because SUID typically occurs during sleep, in many cases there is not enough known about the circumstances of the death to determine definite cause. SIDS is theorized as a "triple risk model." Infants with underlying vulnerability (e.g., genetic, neurological) experience an exposure to a trigger event/s (e.g., airflow obstruction or risk factor) during a time that is a vulnerable stage of development of the central nervous system or immune system. The majority of SIDS fatalities occur between ages 1 and 4 months and 90% occur by 6 months of age but infants are considered at risk until 12 months of age.[9-12]

Following the American Academy of Pediatrics (AAP) "Back to Sleep" campaign in the early 1990s, the number of SIDS-related infant fatalities significantly decreased, but this decline has plateaued since the early 2000s and data shows some increase in the incidence of other crib-related infant deaths (including suffocation, asphyxiation, and entrapment). Therefore, in 2016, the AAP expanded the recommendations to increase attention on a safe sleep environment with goal of reducing the risk of all sleep-related infant deaths including SIDS as well as accidental suffocation and strangulation.[10,12] The AAP updated their recommendations in 2022 to highlight noninclined sleep surfaces, short-term emergency sleep locations, use of cardboard boxes as a sleep location, bed sharing, substance use, home cardiorespiratory monitors, and tummy time.[12a]

These recommendations include the sleep environment (i.e., room sharing without bed sharing with caregivers until at least age 6 months), sleeping position and bedding (reinforcing supine positioning for all sleeping periods on a firm noninclined sleep surface and removal of loose bedding from the infant's sleep area), and sleep aids (avoidance of all soft objects such as stuffed animals and blankets, and recommendation for the use of a pacifier at sleep onset without a blanket or soft toy attached). Other recommendations to reduce SUIDs risk such as encouraging breastfeeding, up-to-date vaccinations, and limiting maternal exposure to tobacco smoke, alcohol, and illicit drugs as well as secondary smoke exposure are included.[9,11,12,12a]

Infants with gastroesophageal reflux should follow all recommendations for infant-safe sleep including sleeping supine with head of bed flat. Wedges and positioners are not effective in reducing reflux and are not recommended. Infants receiving nasogastric or orogastric feeds should also follow the AAP recommendations. Exceptions are only potentially applicable for infants with significant anatomical disorders such as type 3 or 4 laryngeal clefts in which risk of death from GERD outweighs risk of SIDS.[10,8,8a]

Despite these recommendations, studies suggest that less than half of infants are "always" placed supine and more than one-half of infants share the parental bed at 8 weeks of age.[10] In one study approximately 90% of infants surveyed had hazardous items such as loose bedding or stuffed toys in the sleep space.[13] Certain factors raise the risk for sleep-associated death, including male gender, Black and Native American/Alaska Native race/ethnicity, exposure to cigarette smoke pre- or postnatally, young maternal age (under 20 years), and infants with medical complications such as preterm birth, cardiorespiratory disorders, low birth weight, and neurological concerns.[10,12,14]

The majority of infant safe sleep education is provided at the delivery hospital. Unfortunately, infant safe sleep education and assessment is limited beyond the initial hospitalization at birth.[15] Research shows the majority of parents report receiving information from their infant's health care provider about supine sleep, but they are less likely to recall education about use of blankets, objects in the crib, or bedsharing.[16] Thus, initiatives to provide thorough safe sleep education at multiple touch points throughout infancy are likely to increase caregiver adherence.

Medical providers have a responsibility to continually assess and guide caregivers toward infant-safe sleep. At times, these conversations can be uncomfortable. Approaching the family with open-ended questions and a nonjudgmental tone is helpful in encouraging an honest discussion. It is also important to understand the family's reasons for following unsafe sleep practices: they may be unaware of the full scope of recommendations or there may be cultural differences regarding a family's approach to infant sleep, including definitions of "good parenting" and differences in intergenerational practices in the setting of multiple caregivers. Caregivers may adopt short-term potentially unsafe sleep practices such as cosleeping in order to address a sleep problem such as frequent night wakings, especially in the setting of caregiver sleep deprivation and exhaustion.

In the pediatric hospital setting, it is vital to model infant-safe sleep practices. While studies have found that caregivers replicate the practices they witness in the hospital, research has also demonstrated that safe sleep practices are frequently not used in the inpatient setting.[17,18] If medical necessity dictates exceptions, this should be specifically discussed with the caregiver as a temporary medical intervention that is only applicable in the hospital setting.

Finally, it is also important to note that many widely available consumer products are incongruent with infant-safe sleep practices. In bed sleepers, pillow-like loungers, incline seats/sleepers, wedges, pacifiers with stuffed animals, etc. attached are all readily available for purchase by well-meaning caregivers. Understandably, many caregivers assume that if these items are being sold in stores, they are safe. In addition, commercial home apnea/cardiorespiratory smart monitors marketed to reduce SIDS are not recommended, as they have not been demonstrated to be effective and may contribute both to parental anxiety or alternatively to laxity about safe sleep recommendations.[11,12]

The Family Context of Sleep

CAREGIVER STYLES AND VALUES

Different caregiver styles can impact a family's approach to infant sleep practices and the definition of "problem" sleep. In seminal work originally published in the 1960s but widely referenced today, Diana Baumrind defined four basic parenting styles[20]:

- **Authoritarian**—These caregivers tend to expect obedience. They set strict rules with consequences. Children are not included in decision making or problem solving and are often punished for noncompliance. These caregivers have high demandingness with low responsiveness.
- **Authoritative**—These caregivers verbalize clear rules and expectations but children are included in problem solving and decision making. Communication is bidirectional from caregiver to child. These caregivers validate the child's feelings and attempt to avoid personal criticism and shame. High expectations are backed by a supportive and nurturing style. A common term for this approach is "Positive Parenting."

- **Permissive**—These caregivers are lenient with very few rules, tend to be warm and responsive, and allow children to direct many decisions, but frequently fail to set boundaries, often acting more as "friend" than "parent." They often avoid setting limits in order to not upset the child. Caregivers in this category may use threats at times but rarely follow through with the stated consequence.

- **Uninvolved**—These caregivers are often more consumed by their own lives and minimally involved with their child/children. They neither set boundaries nor communicate expectations regarding standards. Children often have to manage their day-to-day needs independently. Caregivers may be uninvolved for many reasons, often these are unintentional. Lack of involvement may be secondary to family stress, including financial pressures, and to being overwhelmed by other issues such as mental health problems or substance abuse, inadequate housing, or lack of knowledge about child developmental needs.[20]

More recently described and oft-quoted parenting styles include the overprotective/over intrusive or "helicopter" parent, the strict authoritative with primary goal of raising high achieving children "tiger" parent, and the promoting of physical independence, reasonable risk-taking, with less than currently typical parental oversight, so-called "free range parenting."[25]

These parenting styles are not mutually exclusive and some families may fluctuate in the approach to caregiving as needs, circumstances, and the age of the child change over time. Caregiving style is also impacted by child-related factors such as the child's temperament or behavior and the relationship is therefore more accurately described as bidirectional. Thus, family systems theories are important in understanding how each individual member of the family impacts the style, behavior, and outcomes of the others. Parenting styles are also often influenced by incorporation of or reaction to the caregiver style in which the parent was raised; for example, parents from an authoritarian environment may attempt to implement a more responsive and nurturing environment for their own child as a compensatory mechanism, but as a result may fail to set developmentally appropriate limits.[20-24]

The various caregiver styles described above provide a useful construct when assessing infant/toddler sleep problems. For example, the permissive style caregiver is often unable to set clear and consistent boundaries and limits. These caregivers may describe being afraid of their toddler or infant's emotional response. They commonly cope by accommodating all the requests the child makes or "walking on egg shells" so as not to set off a tantrum or crying. They often use terms like the child "won't let me," "insists," or "demands." Some permissive caregivers turn to threats but often do not follow through on the stated consequence. "If you get out of bed one more time I am taking away your teddy bear." Permissiveness may also be caused by a knowledge deficit about typical child development, as well as the benefits of a nurturing relationship that includes clear boundaries.

The "helicopter" caregiver may worry excessively that their young child isn't getting the "right" amount of sleep and express concern that far into the future this will negatively impact academic success. This type of parent may purchase and obsessively view the data from the latest infant sleep monitoring products in an effort to reassure themselves that the child does not have any obvious sleep problems. The use of melatonin to "promote better sleep" in a child who does not display any sleep issues is another example of a well-meaning but misguided excessive focus on sleep.

As another example, research shows consistent developmentally appropriate bedtimes and bedtime routines correlate with fewer sleep problems, as well as improvements in a child's executive function, attention, working memory, and school readiness, among other measures.[19] However, some caregiving styles negatively impact the setting of bedtime routines or schedules. Permissive caregivers frequently allow the child to develop maladaptive sleep onset associations at bedtime, such as prolonged periods of rocking or taking the child on car rides in order to fall asleep; bedtime routines may be elaborate and lengthy and allow for too many choices. These caregivers often try to implement consistent sleep schedules and habits but are commonly inconsistent in following through. They often have a difficult time tolerating any protest behavior from the child during implementation of new sleep routines. The authoritarian caregiver, for example, may determine that 7 pm is bedtime regardless of whether or not the child's natural sleep onset coincides with the timing of lights out. This may lead to increased bedtime resistance or prolonged time to fall asleep and highly negative bedtime experiences for both child and caregiver. These caregivers may also be less willing to accommodate the child's sleep needs or even to accept input from their health care practitioner. The uninvolved caregiver, on the other hand, may not have a sleep schedule at all or have minimal involvement in a bedtime routine.

CAREGIVER MENTAL HEALTH ISSUES

Mental health affects how we think, feel, and act and it is important at every stage in life. Mental illnesses are among the most common health conditions in the United States. Sleep disturbances are common when someone is dealing with a mental health disorder and the relationship is inherently bidirectional. Thus, it is imperative that the interviewing process during a sleep evaluation include questions about mental health concerns of caregivers, as well as difficulties initiating and/or maintaining sleep, unrefreshing sleep, or daytime fatigue/sleepiness. Identifying and acknowledging these concerns not only helps to understand what concerns and limitations the caregiver may have in implementing a behavioral treatment plan for their child's sleep problem but can also highlight any need for social or other support during this process.

Most caregivers know that sleep is important to themselves and their children, and often report that when they get poor sleep it affects their mood, concentration, energy level, diet, and relationships with partners, family, or coworkers, as well as their ability to parent.[26] Evidence supports a critical role of caregiver behaviors in the caregiver-child interaction. Caregivers with children who are poor sleepers tend to be more anxious and depressed.[27] Furthermore, caregiver depression has been shown to be associated with an increased prevalence of children's sleep problems.[28] For example, a caregiver who is stressed and has limited coping skills for a variety of reasons including mental health issues may inadvertently maintain a sleep problem by failing to enforce appropriate limit setting to avoid precipitating child distress. If a child is resisting bedtime and unable to settle in bed because they want to continue to watch TV or play, the caregiver may then acquiesce to these demands in order to avoid a tantrum or extended crying, leading to a cycle of escalating demands.

Anxiety and depression can interfere with sleep by making it difficult to fall asleep or wake at night and remain awake in an anxious state until morning.[29] An anxious person may not sleep enough and then feel exhausted during the day, with subsequently increasing anxiety about not sleeping well at night, consequent nights. Caregivers with anxiety who also have to address the needs of a child who sleeps poorly may understandably feel unmotivated or unable to take on the challenges of implementing a behavioral plan. Alternatively, they may become overly focused on their infants' sleep as a compensatory mechanism; for example, one study found that mothers with anxiety disorders were overly involved in infant and toddler bedtime routines (i.e., cosleeping, sleep association), and these behaviors were associated with higher rates of child sleep problems.[29]

When making any plan to treat a childhood sleep disorder, it is important to consider caregiver anxiety and stress. In a clinical setting, oftentimes anxious caregivers present with more questions and concerns and may require both a more gradual approach to and support for changing their child's sleep behaviors, including more frequent follow-ups and reassurance. In the end, it is also important to recognize if the caregivers' anxiety is overwhelming and prevents any ability to make changes to their child's sleep behaviors as this would then involve helping the caregiver navigate what resources they need.

Maternal Postpartum Depression

Maternal postpartum (PPD) or postnatal depression (PND) is believed to be the most common postpartum complication. PND is a debilitating mental health disorder that manifests as disturbed sleep, mood swings, changes in appetite, unrealistic concerns about the health and safety of the baby, sadness and hopelessness, difficulty in concentrating, and extreme emotional responses to daily living events ranging from complete lack of interest to thoughts of death and suicide. In some cases there is also a weakened attachment to the baby or fears of harming the baby. Many studies have found the relationship of a previous history of depression and anxiety is among the factors that are associated with a higher risk of postpartum depression.[30]

PND has been associated with excessive infant crying, feeding, and sleeping problems. These mothers may also have a difficult time bonding with their infants and may be less sensitive to infant cues and have a harder time adjusting to motherhood. Studies have found that depression is not the only mental health problem seen regularly in postpartum mothers, but anxiety and stress are significant psychological comorbidities, particularly in postpartum women whose infants are admitted to the NICU.[30] Depressed mothers may have their own lack of daily structure and bedtime routine, which can contribute to infant sleeping problems. Furthermore, studies have also shown that up to one-third of mothers who are depressed during the early postpartum period still suffer from depressive symptoms at 2 years postpartum.[29]

Unfortunately, PDD can go undetected, this is especially true for developing countries where mental health is a stigma and not covered by most insurance programs or governmental agencies.[27] The recognition of PPD is vital during routine visits, so clinicians can provide necessary support and referrals.

Lastly, one must not forget about the other caregiver (partner, father). Depression in fathers of breastfed infants has also been associated with parenting distress, dysfunctional interactions with the child, decreased marital adjustment, and perceived low parenting efficacy.[28] Paternal involvement has been linked to improvement in children's and mothers' sleep consolidation.[28] It is important to take into account fathers or other partner's mental health concerns during the first year of a child's birth.

Substance Use

Insomnia is commonly associated with use and withdrawal from substances. We know that use of psychoactive substances can lead to development of insomnia and circadian rhythm disorders.[31] For example, alcohol use has initial sedating effects at sleep onset and may be used by caregivers as a "hypnotic" to induce sleep, but can subsequently disrupt sleep as blood alcohol levels drop during the night with resultant increased sleep fragmentation. Of course, in addition, daytime use of alcohol is associated with impaired decision making that involves childcare responsibilities. Studies have shown that parental substance use is associated with a myriad of family and social problems. There can be inconsistency in parenting and disruptions or lack of healthy family routines, structure, or rituals or parental conflict and stress.[31] In addition, there is clear evidence that prenatal exposure to substances such as alcohol, cocaine, and heroin is associated with an increased risk of neurobehavioral and cognitive problems such as hyperactivity and inattention, language delays, and learning disabilities, as well as sleep problems. This further sets the stage for parent-child conflicts and challenges in achieving healthy sleep routines and habits in these families and creates more barriers to implementing interventions for existing sleep concerns.

MARITAL/PARTNER CONFLICT AND COHESION: COPARENTING CHALLENGES

Caregivers with a newborn enter into a relationship in which they must now work together to manage childcare needs and become parents. Transitioning to parenthood can also cause a high level of stress; sleep disturbances such as nighttime awakenings and shorter sleep duration can affect marital relationships. Studies have found that maternal/primary caregiver's sleep is more often disturbed by children compared with paternal/partner caregiver's sleep.[32] During the first three years of life, studies have also shown that fathers are often less involved than mothers in bedtime rituals and less likely to get up with the infant/young child during night wakings.[33] Alternatively, other studies have found that when fathers are more involved in monitoring their children's sleep as well as in their overall care, infants and toddlers display more consolidated sleep patterns.[28] In addition, dividing caregiving tasks between caregivers, in turn, helps mothers/primary caregivers to achieve better sleep and may contribute to less night wakings.

When there is marital (partner) conflict it may lead to difficulty in coordination and cooperation when it comes to managing their child's sleep. Often times the focus on the child's sleep problem may be a way to deflect the underlying conflicts at home. This can lead to difficulty in consistent parenting values, responsibilities, and routines. As an example, one parent may actively undermine the other or become overly involved in the child's life, thus leaving the other parent feeling withdrawn or disconnected. Also, routine bed sharing of the child with one caregiver while the other caregiver is "made" to sleep in a separate room may mask underlying relationship issues. If conflict at home is not addressed first, then it may hinder and impact how each caregiver manages sleep routines and works together to resolve any sleep disruptions that their child is having. Research shows that fathers who report higher marital satisfaction and social support, and lower levels of parenting stress, seem to be more involved in caring for their children at bedtime.[39] Thus, mutual parental involvement and decreased stress may moderate children's sleep. In contrast, research shows that caregivers with poor sleepers tend to be more anxious and depressed and less happy in their relationship.[32]

Lastly, divorce or separation may significantly influence a child's sleep. In younger children, there may be an increase in separation anxiety or fear of abandonment by both parents. Sleep routines, schedules, and the type of sleeping arrangement can also vary depending on which household the child is sleeping in. There also may be conflict due to the broadly different parenting styles at each home, leading to a "good cop/bad cop" scenario. Going back and forth between households with different (and sometimes diametrically opposed) sleep rules can be demanding on the child. While sometimes challenging to achieve, studies show that the quality of the relationship between coparents can have a strong influence on the mental and emotional well-being of children, including their sleep.[28] In clinical practice, it not only is challenging to provide a treatment plan that both households can follow through with but can also become disruptive to any progress made in one household if the plan is not followed in the other. The provider can also be caught in the middle of any conflict between households, in which one caregiver's intention may be to put blame of a child's sleep disruption due to the other caregiver not following any treatment guidelines. It is important to recognize these conflicts and refer to appropriate support services for the family.

SIBLING INFLUENCE

Bringing home a new sibling can be a joyous and celebratory time but may also bring on some challenges when it comes to figuring out how to manage already existing sleep disruptions in the household (child or caregiver) or bedroom logistics.

Sleep problems may start from the time the separation from mother happens due to childbirth or hospitalization related to pregnancy complications. If the mother was primarily "in charge" of bedtime and the bedtime routine, then is suddenly no longer available at this time, especially unexpectedly, the child(ren) may develop trouble falling asleep or staying asleep with the change in routine and caregiver absence. This may also be manifested by an increase in separation anxiety upon mother's return for fear that she may leave again.[34]

As the time of arrival of a new baby, routines may be thrown off and any positive sleep changes that had been implemented prior to the birth may be put aside, whether it be from the exhaustion of caring for the newborn or caregiver guilt (feeling they need to give increased attention to the sibling if they are preoccupied with the newborn). Luckily, many toddlers, even after the birth of a sibling, continue on with life with little interest in the newborn. Children who are older are often more interested in a new sibling and may even try to "help" with care of the newborn. Planning ahead in terms of addressing existing sleep concerns and new challenges (e.g., the need for the older sibling to transition to a toddler bed, where the new sibling will sleep in the short-term and eventually, and if they will share a room with the sibling or have their own room) well in advance of the birth (e.g., several months) so that positive behaviors are well-established. Alternatively, these changes could be postponed until the family as a whole has settled in with the new sibling. This also makes any temporary regression in sleep habits easier to anticipate and manage. For example, a young child who is currently bed sharing or room sharing with caregivers may have the reaction that the "new baby took my crib/room" and it is important to acknowledge the legitimacy of these feelings and to anticipate and deal with them in a developmentally appropriate fashion. That being said, new parents of a second child often have concerns about sleep habits and begin anticipating. It is important that new parents continue to try to establish good sleep hygiene in the older child before the arrival of the new sibling. If they plan to transition to a toddler bed, do this with enough time before the arrival of the new sibling.[35] The sibling should have a if there is a plan to work on any behavioral insomnia treatment plan with the older sibling, encourage caregivers to do this in plenty of time prior to the new sibling arrival (1–2 months before).

In households with multiple children, caregivers may also put addressing sleep problems in one child on the back burner so it will not cause disruption to the other siblings' sleep. Initial attempts at instituting a behavioral intervention, if it results in awakening a sibling, may lead to abandoning the behavioral plan to avoid having the entire family awake during the night. What caregivers may not realize is that siblings often sleep through any noise their brother or sister might make, whether they sleep in a separate bedroom or share one; however, there are certainly circumstances in which the child's protesting is loud enough to disturb the sibling.[36] If caregiver attention to limit testing behaviors around sleep ends up inadvertently reinforcing negative behavior (i.e., if the child learns that screaming so loud will wake his sibling and he therefore gets a caregiver to sleep with him in order to avoid this). The situation may be helped by explaining the plan to the other sibling and motivating her/him to go back to sleep during the night, negotiating a later bedtime for an older sibling, or temporarily moving them to another room. Caregivers may also use a sibling to help the poor sleeping child to not feel frightened at night by having them sleep in the same room. A sibling should not be used to help overcome fears at night.[36] Often this does not resolve the underlying fears and can act as a temporary "Band-Aid" and issues will start up again. Encouraging parents to continue with stable routines, setting limits at bedtime and during the night, is important even when a sibling is involved.

When dealing with a family that has twins or multiples, this can also add an area of stress when it comes to sleep challenges. More often than not, twins may share a bedroom and if there is one twin that sleeps better than the other, then this adds a layer of difficulty when trying to implement any behavioral interventions as the fear of waking the other twin often defeats any attempts of trying to help resolve the sleep problem. Frequently, twins/multiples can also feed off each other during times when caregivers are trying to set limits around bedtime and during the night leading to more unnecessary behaviors and difficulty for caregivers to follow through with any limits they are trying to set. If necessary, removing one of the twins out of the room temporarily may be the only option in order for the caregiver to help the other twin sleep.

SLEEP IN ALTERNATIVE CARE SETTINGS

Alternative care settings for young children, including community settings such as foster care, kinship care, and shelters, may contribute to the risk for poor sleep health and sleep disparities.[37] A number of factors combine to create heightened sleep-related vulnerabilities in children in alternative care settings. For example, before entering the child welfare system, children commonly experience a number of known risk factors for sleep-wake dysregulation including poor maternal prenatal health, perinatal risks such as prematurity and drug exposure, poverty, unstable and chaotic home environments, caregiver mental health problems, domestic violence, and child maltreatment. The subsequent abrupt removal from a parent's care, no matter how unsafe circumstances may be, serves as an additional trauma. These early adverse experiences, particularly if unbuffered by a safe and sensitive caregiving relationship, can set off a cascade of biological stress responses known to give rise to disruptions in the quality and quantity of sleep. In fact, disturbances of sleep are among the most common symptoms of early trauma and do not necessarily subside over time.

Awareness of these vulnerabilities and provision of support services and education to alternative care providers are critical to preventing or mitigating sleep disruptions in these families. Safe and stable home environments and the development of secure attachment to primary caregivers provide the necessary infrastructure for good sleep health, but education regarding developmentally appropriate sleep habits and behavioral approaches to managing sleep problems are also key. This point is deserving of particular emphasis, as greater levels of caregiver-reported sleep disruption in children are associated with more time spent in foster care, a greater number of placements, and higher levels of caregiver distress, in addition to the many established negative outcomes associated with poor sleep health in general.

References

1. Mindell J, Owens J. *A Clinical Guide to Pediatric Sleep: Diagnosis and Management of Sleep Problems.* 3rd ed. Philadelphia, USA: Wolters Kluwer; 2015.
2. Colvin J, Collie-Akers V, Schunn C, Moon R. Sleep environment risks for older and younger infants. *Pediatrics.* 2014;134(2):e406-e412.
3. Magee C, Gordon R, Caputi P. Distinct developmental trends in sleep duration during early childhood. *Pediatrics.* 2014;133(6):e1561-e1567.
4. Galland B, Taylor B, Elder D, Herbison P. Normal sleep patterns in infants and children: a systematic review of observational studies. *Sleep Med Rev.* 2012;16(3):213-222.
5. Altmann T. *"Feeding Your Baby", Your Baby's First Year.* American Academy of Pediatrics; 2020.
6. Mindell JA, Owens JA. *A Clinical Guide to Pediatric Sleep: Diagnosis and Management of Sleep Problems.* Philadelphia: Lippincott Williams & Wilkins; 2003.
7. Paavonen J, Saarenpää-Heikkilä O, Morales-Munoz I, et al. Normal sleep development in infants: findings from two large birth cohorts. *Sleep Med.* 2020;69:145-154. Available at: https://doi.org/10.1016/j.sleep.2020.01.009.
8. Council on Communications and Media. Media and young minds. *Pediatrics.* 2016;138(5):e20162591. doi:10.1542/peds.2016-2591.
9. Centers for Disease Control and Prevention. *Sudden Unexpected Infant Death and Sudden Infant Death Syndrome.* December 4, 2021. Available at: https://www.cdc.gov/sids/about/index.htm.
10. Centers for Disease Control/NCHS. National Vital Statistics System, *Period Linked Birth/Infant Death Data.* Rates calculated via CDC WONDER using latest available data by subpopulation. 2019. Available at: https://www.cdc.gov/sids/data.htm.
11. National Institutes of Health, U.S. Department of Health and Human Services. *Safe to Sleep Public Education Campaign.* December 4, 2021. Available at: https://safetosleep.nichd.nih.gov/.

12. Moon RY, Task Force on Sudden Infant Death Syndrome. SIDS and other sleep-related infant deaths: evidence base for 2016 updated recommendations for a safe infant sleeping environment. *Pediatrics.* 2016;138(5):e20162940. Available at: https://doi.org/10.1542/peds.2016-2940.

12a. Moon RY, Carlin RF, Hand I, Task Force on Sudden Infant Death Syndrome and The Committee on Fetus and Newborn. Sleep-related infant deaths: updated 2022 recommendations for reducing infant deaths in the sleep environment. *Pediatrics.* 2022;150(1):e2022057990. doi:10.1542/peds.2022-057990.

13. Bombard JM, Kortsmit K, Warner L, et al. Vital signs: trends and disparities in infant safe sleep practices   United States, 2009–2015. *MMWR Morb Mortal Wkly Rep.* 2018;67(1):39-46. Available at: https://doi.org/10.15585/mmwr.mm6701e1.

14. Batra EK, Teti DM, Schaefer EW, Neumann BA, Meek EA, Paul IM. Nocturnal video assessment of infant sleep environments. *Pediatrics.* 2016;138(3):e20161533. Available at: https://doi.org/10.1542/peds.2016-1533.

15. Moon RY, Hauck FR, Colson ER. Safe infant sleep interventions: what is the evidence for successful behavior change? *Curr Pediatr Rev.* 2016;12(1):67-75. Available at: https://doi.org/10.2174/1573396311666151026110148.

16. Hirai AH, Kortsmit K, Kaplan L, et al. Prevalence and factors associated with safe infant sleep practices. *Pediatrics.* 2019;144(5):e20191286. Available at: https://doi.org/10.1542/peds.2019-1286.

17. Mason B, Ahlers-Schmidt CR, Schunn C. Improving safe sleep environments for well newborns in the hospital setting. *Clin Pediatr.* 2013;52(10):969-975. Available at: https://doi.org/10.1177/0009922813495954.

18. Frey E, Hamp N, Orlov N. Modeling safe infant sleep in the hospital. *J Pediatr Nurs.* 2020;50:20-24. Available at: https://doi.org/10.1016/j.pedn.2019.10.002.

19. Kitsaras G, Goodwin M, Allan J, Kelly MP, Pretty IA. Bedtime routines child wellbeing & development. *BMC Public Health.* 2018;18(1):386. doi:10.1186/s12889-018-5290-3.

20. Berkowitz CD. *"Discipline", Berkowitz's Pediatrics: A Primary Care Approach.* Published April, 2021.

21. Huh D, Tristan J, Wade E, Stice E. Does problem behavior elicit poor parenting? A prospective study of adolescent girls. *J Adolesc Res.* 2006;21(2):185-204. doi:10.1177/0743558405285462.

22. Power TG, Sleddens EF, Berge J, et al. Contemporary research on parenting: conceptual, methodological, and translational issues. *Child Obes.* 2013;9(suppl 1):S87-S94. doi:10.1089/chi.2013.0038.

23. Wittig SMO, Rodriguez CM. Emerging behavior problems: bidirectional relations between maternal and paternal parenting styles with infant temperament. *Dev Psychol.* 2019;55(6):1199-1210. doi:10.1037/dev0000707.

24. Pizzo A, Sandstrom A, Drobinin V, Propper L, Uher R, Pavlova B. Parental overprotection and sleep problems in young children. *Child Psychiatry Hum Dev.* 2022;53:1340-1348. doi:10.1007/s10578-021-01199-2. Available at: https://doi.org/10.1007/s10578-021-01199-2.

25. Lindberg S. *Parenting Buzzwords and What They Mean.* Verywellfamily; January 29, 2022. Available at: https://www.verywellfamily.com/parenting-buzzwords-and-what-they-mean-4774339#toc-free-range-parenting.

26. De Stasio S, Boldrini F, Ragni B, Gentile S. Predictive factors of Toddlers' sleep and parental stress. *Int J Environ Res Public Health.* 2020;17(7):2494. Available at: https://doi.org/10.3390/ijerph17072494.

27. Sadler L, Banasiak N, Canapari C, et al. Perspectives on sleep from multiethnic community parents, pediatric providers, and childcare providers. *J Dev Behav Pediatr.* 2020;41(7):540-549. Available at: https://doi.org/10.1097/DBP.0000000000000799.

28. Ragni B, De Stasio S. Parental involvement in children's sleep care and nocturnal awakenings in infants and toddlers. *Int J Environ Res Public Health.* 2020;17(16):5808. Available at: https://doi.org/10.3390/ijerph17165808.

29. Petzoldt J, Wittchen HU, Einsle F, Martini J. Maternal anxiety versus depressive disorders: specific relations to infants' crying, feeding and sleeping problems. *Child Care Health Dev.* 2016;42(2):231-245. Available at: https://doi.org/10.1111/cch.12292.

30. Das A, Gordon-Ocejo G, Kumar M, Kumar N, Needlman R. Association of the previous history of maternal depression with post-partum depression, anxiety, and stress in the neonatal intensive care unit. *J Matern Fetal Neonatal Med.* 2021;34(11):1741-1746. Available at: https://doi.org/10.1080/14767058.2019.1647162.

31. Smith VC, Wilson CR, Committee on Substance Use and Prevention. Families affected by parental substance use. *Pediatrics.* 2016;138(2):e20161575. Available at: https://doi.org/10.1542/peds.2016-1575.

32. Gallegos MI, Jacobvitz DB, Sasaki T, Hazen NL. Parents' perceptions of their spouses' parenting and infant temperament as predictors of parenting and coparenting. *J Fam Psychol*. 2019;33(5):542-553. Avaiable at: https://doi.org/10.1037/fam0000530.

33. Bernier A, Bélanger ME, Bordeleau S, Carrier J. Mothers, fathers, and toddlers: parental psychosocial functioning as a context for young children's sleep. *Dev Psychol*. 2013;49:1375-1384. Available at: https://doi.org/10.1037/a0030024.

34. Trause MA, Voos D, Rudd C. Separation for childbirth: the effect on the sibling. *Child Psych Hum Dev*. 1981;12:32-39. Available at: https://doi.org/10.1007/BF00706671.

35. Kimball V. Family transitions: the birth of a two-child family. *Pediatr Ann*. 2015;44(6):224-227. Available at: https://doi.og/10.3928/00904481-20150611-03.

36. Ferber R. *Solve Your Child's Sleep Problems*. New York: Simon and Schuster; 2006.

37. Hash JB, Alfano CA, Owens J, et al. Call to action: prioritizing sleep health among US children and youth residing in alternative care settings. *Sleep Health*. 2022;8(1):23-27. doi:10.1016/j.sleh.2021.10.002.

Medical Sleep Disorders of Infancy

CHAPTER 5

Sudden Infant Death Syndrome

Thomas G. Keens ◼ Sally L. Davidson Ward

Introduction

"And this woman's son died in the night ..."

1 Kings 3: 19 (~950 B.C.)

Authors' note to the reader: This chapter describes and discusses the sudden and unexpected death of otherwise healthy infants. Given that this is the most common cause of death for infants between 1 month and 1 year of age, readers may have been personally impacted by such a death and this chapter may be disturbing to read.

For over 3000 years, people have known that apparently healthy babies could die suddenly and unexpectedly during their sleep. The usual clinical scenario is that a parent or caregiver places a baby down to sleep for an overnight sleeping period or a daytime nap. Sometime later, the infant is found to have died. Generally, these infants were healthy, and there was no sign that something was wrong with the baby or that death would occur. The baby was thought to have been asleep when death occurred. In some cases, the baby has been in the next room, within hearing distance of the parents, who came back to the baby within 30 minutes to find that the baby had died during that short period of time. Yet there was no noise, sound of struggle, or any indication that something was happening. There is no indication that the baby suffered.

When a baby dies suddenly, it precipitates a cascade of first responders. 911 is called. Police, fire, and paramedics respond to the scene. In most cases, the baby is obviously dead. A coroner's investigator performs an examination of the death scene. All states in the United States require that an autopsy be performed. Autopsies are used to determine the cause of death. An identifiable cause of death can only be found in 10% to 15% of sudden and unexpected infant deaths. This leaves the majority with no identifiable cause of death, and this is the group of babies whose deaths are attributed to sudden infant death syndrome (SIDS).

SIDS is defined as: "The sudden unexpected death of an infant, under one-year of age, with onset of the fatal episode apparently occurring during sleep, that remains unexplained after a thorough investigation, including performance of a complete autopsy, and review of the circumstances of death and the clinical history."[1] The key features of SIDS are that the death is unexpected and unexplained. SIDS is the most common cause of death between the ages of 1 month and 1 year, yet its cause remains unknown. Prior to 1990, the SIDS rate was 1 out of every 600 live births. Over time, the SIDS rate has fallen to less than 0.5 SIDS deaths per 1000 live births, but it is still the most common cause of postneonatal death.

SIDS has a unique age distribution. SIDS peaks at 2 to 4 months of age, with 95% of SIDS occurring before 6 months of age. Other natural causes of infant death peak near birth and decrease exponentially after that. This unique age distribution has led to the theory that SIDS is not just a collection of babies who died from causes that could not be determined, but rather, infants likely to have died from a similar mechanism.[2] SIDS also impacts different racial and ethnic populations disproportionately, occurring more frequently in infants from indigenous and

African-American backgrounds as compared to infants from non-Hispanic white, Hispanic, and Asian-Pacific Islander populations.[3]

Diagnosis

The diagnosis of SIDS can only be made in an infant who has died. There is no known "less severe" form of SIDS in a surviving infant, and SIDS can not be evaluated in any infant prior to death. In order to accurately identify SIDS, there should be an examination of the death scene performed by a qualified investigator and an autopsy performed by a qualified forensic or pediatric pathologist.[1,4-6] Death scene investigation protocols and autopsy protocols have been developed, and the use of these standardized protocols improves the accuracy and consistency of diagnosis.[1,5] The diagnosis of SIDS should be used as the cause of death when an infant meets this definition: (1) under 1 year of age; (2) death was sudden and unexpected; (3) death occurred when the infant was thought to be asleep; (4) examination of the death scene reveals no alternative cause of death; (5) autopsy reveals no identifiable cause of death; and (6) the case history does not indicate a medical problem which could have caused the death.[1,5]

There is some variation among medical examiners in the diagnoses which are used to define the cause of death in infants who die suddenly and unexpectedly during sleep.[7] Medical examiners and coroners may use SIDS or diagnoses such as sudden unexpected or unexplained infant death (SUID), sudden unexplained death in infancy (SUDI), undetermined, etc. However, it must be recognized that when diagnosing an individual infant's death, these terms all mean the same thing; that the death was unexpected and unexplained. In this chapter, the term "SIDS" will be used.[4,8] In epidemiological studies, SUID often includes infant deaths due to SIDS as well as asphyxiation, suffocation, and strangulation in bed (ASSB).

By definition, an identifiable cause of death is not found at postmortem examination in victims of SIDS. The autopsy of a victim of SIDS reveals no serious illness that could contribute to the death and no signs of significant stress. However, common postmortem findings include intrathoracic petechiae; pulmonary congestion and edema; minor airway inflammation (not severe enough to cause death); minimal stress effects in the thymus and adrenal glands; and normal nutrition and development.[1,5] These findings support that infants were generally healthy prior to death.

Research Into Possible Causes of SIDS

The cause of SIDS is unknown.[9] How are we to understand SIDS? Over the past 50 years, researchers have not been able to pinpoint a plausible abnormality in a physiological system to explain these deaths. Thus, we need to consider how the infant physiology interacts with potential stressors in the environment. Most SIDS researchers believe that SIDS occurs when an infant is in a potentially life-threatening situation, such as sleeping prone on soft bedding.[10] Most infants will lift or turn their head to avoid suffocation. If the infant cannot respond to this situation with a protective response, then there can be a progression through failure of arousal, hypoxic coma, bradycardia, and death. Most infants appear to rescue themselves, but some apparently do not, and they can die.

SIDS is best understood by the Triple Risk Model.[11] There are three overlapping circles representing development, infant vulnerability, and environment (Fig. 5.1). The size of the overlap is the chance of an infant dying from SIDS. Each circle can change in size, depending on the relative contribution of the effect. For example, SIDS is most common between 2 and 4 months of age, so a 3-month-old infant would have a larger developmental circle than an 11-month-old. Similarly, the other circles can change in size. The contributions and interactions between the three parts of the Triple Risk Model to SIDS are explained below.

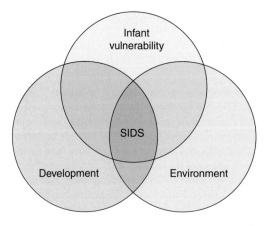

Fig. 5.1 The triple risk hypothesis of SIDS. SIDS is due to the interaction of many factors. The chance of an infant dying from SIDS is represented by the area of overlap of the *three circles*. Different infants may have different sized circles based on age, genetic variations, or other differences in physiology and environmental hazards. *(Modified from Filiano JJ, Kinney HC. A perspective on neuropathologic findings in victims of the sudden infant death syndrome: the triple-risk model. Biol. Neonate. 1994;65:194–197.)*

DEVELOPMENT

SIDS is most common in infants between 2 and 4 months of age,[2,9,12,13] at a time when other causes of infant mortality are waning. This distinct developmental pattern suggests that this is a unique time that promotes the risk of SIDS—a developmental window of physiologic vulnerability. The cardiorespiratory and neurologic systems are rapidly developing during the first six months of life. From an engineering point of view, systems in transition are intrinsically unstable. An unstable or immature respiratory control system, with or without high loop gain, can lead to apnea during sleep.[13] However, studies have shown that the developmental pattern of apneas in babies does not coincide with the peak age of SIDS.[14] Furthermore, infants who survive infancy can have long apneas and low oxygen (hypoxia) during sleep.[15] Therefore, the explanation for SIDS is not as simple as babies stopping breathing during sleep. SIDS deaths are increased in babies who reside at altitude over 8000 feet, suggesting that hypoxia may be a contributor to SIDS.[16] Is SIDS due to a catastrophic physiologic crisis? If normal infants do not precisely control breathing, heart rate, and oxygenation during sleep, then SIDS may not require catastrophic physiological crisis. Potentially, small perturbations in physiology or the surrounding environment are sufficient to result in death in an already vulnerable infant.

If an infant has a potentially dangerous exposure to hypoxia or hypercapnia during sleep, the most adaptive response is to move or wake up. Normal infants over 9 weeks of age were less likely to arouse in response to a hypoxic challenge than infants under nine weeks of age.[17] Fifty percent of normal infants studied longitudinally aroused in response to hypoxia at 1 month of age, compared to only ~10% at 3 months of age, and none at 6 months of age.[18] The loss of a potentially protective hypoxic arousal response coincides with the peak incidence of SIDS and there are changes in infant sleep-wake physiologic mechanisms which decrease this potentially protective physiologic response at the same age that the incidence of SIDS increases. This and other physiologic changes at this age may be a partial explanation for the increased risk of SIDS at around three months of age.

INFANT VULNERABILITY

Why do most infants arouse and turn or lift their heads in response to potentially dangerous conditions during sleep, but some do not? The neurotransmitter serotonin has been shown to be decreased in brainstems of infants who died from SIDS compared to those of babies dying from other causes.[19-22] Serotonin receptor binding sites were also decreased in SIDS.[19] Serotonin is an important neurotransmitter in the brainstem which controls life-support functions. This finding suggests that SIDS victims may have abnormal control of breathing, heart rate response to environmental challenges, and/or arousal. Further, serotonin was decreased both in SIDS infants who had no evidence of possible asphyxia or suffocation contributing to the death to the same extent as those in whom the death scene investigation suggested that asphyxia or suffocation might be present.[21,22] Thus, infants with normal brainstem serotonin may have been able to rescue themselves (unless the asphyxia was severe), whereas those who died may have been more vulnerable because of a brainstem neurotransmitter deficit. They may not have been able to mount a sufficiently robust response to rescue themselves.[10,21,22]

A continuum of brain abnormality from mild to severe may exist (Fig. 5.2). One could postulate that for an infant with normal brainstem physiology to die, the asphyxial insult must need to be severe. Conversely, for an infant to die without any asphyxial insult, the brain neurotransmitter system abnormality must have been severe. For most infants, who die in the presence of one or more SIDS risk factors or in an unsafe sleep environment, there is probably some brainstem dysfunction, though not enough to have caused death in the absence of environmental hazards.[21-23] The majority of babies dying suddenly today are found in a sleep environment with some risk factors, but not enough to cause death in every baby.[24-27] Here, biology interacts with the environment, requiring some increased vulnerability or inability to deal with environmental hazards in order for death to occur. At present, none of these abnormalities can be detected by newborn screening.

Other abnormalities in the hippocampus have also been found in some SIDS victims.[28] Research suggests that this abnormality is different than serotonin deficits. Both abnormalities were found in ~25% of SIDS victims studied, but most had only one or the other. This suggests that SIDS may have multiple biologic risk factors which can not presently be detected antemortem.[28]

Aside from abnormalities in the brain, certain cardiac disorders may also cause or contribute to death and increase an infant's vulnerability to SIDS. Cardiac arrhythmias may cause sudden unexpected death, yet not be detected at autopsy. For example, the prolonged QT interval syndrome (LQTS) is a condition, usually genetic in origin, which can cause a fatal ventricular arrhythmia.[29,30] Some babies who have died from SIDS may have died from LQTS, although the severity of LQTS can be variable and its result in SIDS will often require contribution from the environment or a secondary event, neonatal gene screening for cardiac ion channelopathies or screening ECGs to avoid these events could be challenging and costly.[30] Nevertheless, cardiac ion channel dysfunction, genetic and/or acquired, may be another mechanism to increase an infant's vulnerability toward death.

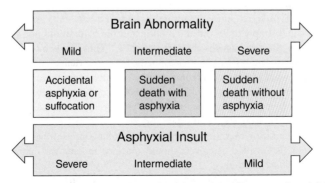

Fig. 5.2 The continuum of brain abnormality increasing infant vulnerability on *top* from *left* to *right* and increasing asphyxial contribution to death on the *bottom* from *right* to *left*. Many SIDS victims die in the presence of some environmental hazards, but these are often not enough to cause death in all babies. Those who die may have also had subtle brain abnormalities, increasing their vulnerability.

ENVIRONMENT

The infant sleep environment can pose unintended dangers to a sleeping baby. The majority of babies who die suddenly and unexpectedly have a number of risk factors identified at the time of death, and many of these are potentially modifiable.[24-27] Identifying and eliminating these modifiable risk factors has been associated with decreased SIDS deaths and a reduced risk of SIDS.[9] Risk factors are not causes: most babies with risk factors will not die, and some patients without risk factors will die. However, from an epidemiologic standpoint, those babies with environmental risk factors have an increased risk of dying. Safe infant sleep recommendations have decreased the SIDS rate but have not been sufficient to eliminate SIDS even when every recommendation is followed. There are biological contributors inherent in SIDS deaths which may not be eliminated by following safe infant sleep alone.[31]

Safe Infant Sleep Recommendations

Beginning in the 1980s, a number of environmental risk factors during sleep were discovered which could increase the risk of SIDS or other accidental causes of infant death during sleep. The majority of babies who die suddenly and unexpectedly during sleep do so in the presence of one or more risk factors.[24-27] In 2016, the American Academy of Pediatrics (AAP) redefined risk factors for unsafe infant sleep and made evidence-based recommendations for decreasing the risk of SIDS,[9,12] which are summarized below.

BACK TO SLEEP FOR EVERY SLEEP

To reduce the risk of SIDS, infants should be placed for sleep in a supine position for every sleep by every caregiver until the child reaches one year of age. Side sleeping is not safe and is not advised.[9,12]

Many studies have been performed over many years in many countries which show that prone sleeping is associated with an increased risk of dying from SIDS. Consequently, in 1992, the AAP first recommended that babies should not sleep prone. The prone sleeping rate fell from ~70% in 1992 to ~12% in 2010.[31] The SIDS rate has fallen in parallel fashion with the fall in prone sleeping.[32] Thus, most SIDS researchers equate the fall in SIDS deaths with the decrease in prone sleeping.[33] Side sleeping is unstable, and it is also associated with an increased SIDS risk compared to the supine position. In order to keep a baby sleeping on the side, one will need to prop the baby. Usually, the prop will be placed on the back, ensuring that the baby moves they will roll onto the stomach, which is the most dangerous position.

Prone sleeping was preferred in many cultures because if a baby spits up, the supposition was that the material could simply drain out the mouth, and the baby would not aspirate. However, in the prone position, the esophagus is above the trachea.[34] Thus, if a baby spits up, the material can travel by gravity into the trachea. In the supine position, the esophagus is below the trachea. So, spit up material would have to overcome gravity to enter the trachea. The supine sleeping position does not increase the risk of choking or aspiration, even in the presence of gastroesophageal reflux disease, where the supine sleep position is still recommended.

Once an infant can roll from supine to prone and from prone to supine, infants can be allowed to remain in the sleep position that they assume. Because rolling into soft bedding is an important risk factor for SIDS, parents and caregivers should continue to keep the infant's sleep environment clear of soft or loose bedding.

USE A FIRM SLEEP SURFACE

Infants should be placed on a firm sleep surface covered by a fitted sheet with no other bedding or soft objects.[9] Soft bedding and items in the crib increase the risk of SIDS 4 to 8 times.

BREASTFEEDING IS RECOMMENDED

Breastfeeding is associated with a reduced risk of SIDS.[9,35] Unless contraindicated or not possible, babies should breastfeed exclusively or be fed with expressed milk for 6 months. The protective effect of breastfeeding increases with exclusivity. However, any breastfeeding has been shown to be more protective against SIDS than no breastfeeding.

It is recommended that infants sleep in the parents' room, close to the parents' bed, but on a separate surface designed for infants, ideally for the first year of life, but at least for the first 6 months. The AAP recommends roomsharing, but not bedsharing.[9] Nevertheless, bedsharing is common. Nearly 40% of California parents of infants admitted to "bedsharing always or often."[36] Some have suggested that bedsharing has a survival advantage for babies. Considerable research has been performed in this area. Bedsharing does increase the frequency and duration of infant breastfeeding when compared to babies sleeping in another room.[37] However, when compared to babies who roomshare with their mother, but do not bedshare, there is no difference in the frequency or duration of breastfeeding.[38] Bedsharing does not improve an infant's breathing or decrease infant apnea.[39] There appear to be no physiologic benefits of bedsharing. On the other hand, there are many epidemiological studies which show an increased risk of SIDS with bedsharing compared to roomsharing without bedsharing.[26,27,40-44] Infant beds or cribs can be placed next to the parent's bed, to facilitate interaction, but provide the safety of an independent sleep space.

Bedsharing has an increased risk of SIDS, and it is not recommended.[9] Bedsharing is *especially unsafe* with:

- Infant less than 4 months of age.
- Parent cigarette smoking, even if they do not smoke in bed.
- Parent is excessively tired; such as with sleep deprivation; <4-hour sleep the previous night.
- Parent use of sedating drugs or alcohol.
- Bedsharing with a nonparent or multiple persons.
- Soft or unsafe bed.
- Duvets, pillows, or soft covers.
- Sleeping with the baby on a sofa, armchair, or couch. This is extremely dangerous, and it is associated with a 50 to 70 times increased risk of SUID.

Thus, the AAP specifically recommends[9] that roomsharing, with the infant in a crib in the parents' room next to the adult bed, is safest and is safer than bedsharing. Infants brought to bed for breastfeeding should return to a separate crib. Do not bedshare if parents smoke cigarettes. Do not bedshare if the parents' arousal is depressed (alcohol, drugs, sleep deprived <4-hour sleep the night before). Do not sleep with an infant on a sofa or chair.

Bedsharing in an adult bed is associated with a number of known risk factors, such as soft bedding, pillows, and blankets in the bed, etc. These alone can increase the SDS risk when bedsharing. Would bedsharing still be dangerous if all other risk factors were removed? Some health care agencies suggest that bedsharing might be safe when other risk factors are eliminated.[45] There are limited studies of bedsharing without other risk factors, but a few suggest that the risk of SIDS with bedsharing is still increased.[45]

What if parents insist on bedsharing? Based on current information, there is no safe way to bedshare. Public Health messages should not be altered because some people do not want to adhere.[45] Providers should remain firm in what is advised and what is safe. However, providers should be willing to work individually with families who insist on bedsharing to reduce the SIDS risk as much as possible.

Skin-to-skin care is encouraged right after birth and during subsequent days.[46] However, the mother should be awake and able to respond to her infant. The mother-infant dyad should be monitored during skin-to-skin care to assure that it is being done safely. Rooming-in for normal newborn nurseries is also encouraged, but bedsharing should be avoided when the mother is sleepy or not alert and unable to respond to her infant.[46] There is no evidence that placing infants on their side during the first few hours after delivery, rather than supine, promotes clearance of amniotic fluid and decreases the risk of aspiration.[47] Provide safe infant sleep education to parents of newborn infants prior to discharge and safe sleep modeling in the newborn nursery.

Keep soft objects and loose bedding away from the infant's sleep area to reduce the risk of SIDS, suffocation, entrapment, and strangulation.

Babies should sleep in an empty crib, without blankets or pillows, with nothing covering the head, and without bumper pads.[9]

CONSIDER OFFERING A PACIFIER AT NAP TIME AND BEDTIME

Although the mechanism is unclear, studies have reported a protective effect of pacifiers on the incidence of SIDS.[9] The protective effect of the pacifier is observed even if the pacifier falls out of the infant's mouth. Because of the risk of strangulation, pacifiers should not be hung around the infant's neck. Pacifiers that attach to infant clothing should not be used with sleeping infants.

AVOID SMOKE EXPOSURE DURING PREGNANCY AND AFTER BIRTH

Both maternal smoking during pregnancy and smoke in the infant's environment after birth are major risk factors for SIDS.[9] Maternal cigarette smoking during pregnancy is associated with a 3 to 15 times increased risk of SIDS. The more cigarettes the mother smokes per day during pregnancy, the higher the risk.[48] After the baby is born, exposure to second-hand cigarette smoke is also associated with an increased risk for SIDS. Because mothers usually spend more time with infants than fathers, maternal smoking after birth carries 6 to 22 times increased risk of SIDS, and paternal smoking after pregnancy carries a 3 to 4 times increased risk.[49] The more hours/day a baby is exposed to second-hand cigarette smoke, the higher the SIDS risk. Babies exposed to 8 hours/day of cigarette smoke have a 10 times increased risk of dying from SIDS.[48] Data regarding second-hand e-cigarette smoke (vaping) are lacking, but this exposure may prove to be even more dangerous than tobacco smoke, as the vapor particles are small and may deposit further into the lungs than particulate tobacco smoke.

AVOID ALCOHOL AND ILLICIT DRUG USE DURING PREGNANCY AND AFTER BIRTH

There is an increased risk of SIDS with prenatal and postnatal exposure to alcohol or illicit drug use. Mothers should abstain from alcohol and illicit drugs periconceptionally and during pregnancy.[50,51]

AVOID OVERHEATING AND HEAD COVERING IN INFANTS

Infants should be dressed appropriately for the environment, with no greater than one layer more than an adult would wear to be comfortable in that environment. Parents and caregivers should evaluate the infant for signs of overheating, such as sweating or the infant's chest feeling hot to the touch. Overbundling and covering of the face and head should be avoided.[9]

PREGNANT WOMEN SHOULD OBTAIN REGULAR PRENATAL CARE

There is substantial epidemiologic evidence linking a lower risk of SIDS for infants whose mothers obtain regular prenatal care. Pregnant women should follow guidelines for frequency of prenatal visits.

INFANTS SHOULD BE IMMUNIZED IN ACCORDANCE WITH RECOMMENDATIONS OF THE AAP AND CENTERS FOR DISEASE CONTROL AND PREVENTION

There is no evidence that there is a causal relationship between immunizations and SIDS. Immunized infants have about half the SIDS rate as those who are not immunized.[52]

Avoid the use of commercial devices that are inconsistent with safe sleep recommendations. Be particularly wary of devices that claim to reduce the risk of SIDS. Examples include wedges and positioners. These have not been proven to be safe or effective. Some have been associated with strangulation of infants.[9]

DO NOT USE HOME CARDIORESPIRATORY MONITORS AS A STRATEGY TO REDUCE THE RISK OF SIDS

The use of cardiorespiratory monitors has not been documented to decrease the incidence of SIDS in healthy infants.[14] These devices are sometimes prescribed for use at home for infants with medical problems related to breathing and oxygenation.

SUPERVISED, AWAKE "TUMMY TIME" IS RECOMMENDED TO FACILITATE DEVELOPMENT AND TO MINIMIZE DEVELOPMENT OF POSITIONAL PLAGIOCEPHALY

Some prone positioning, or "tummy time," while the infant is awake and being observed, is recommended to help prevent flattening of the head and to facilitate development of the upper shoulder strength.[9] Some infants develop positional plagiocephaly from supine sleep. However, this generally resolves spontaneously by 2 years of age.[53]

There is no evidence to recommend swaddling as a strategy to reduce the risk of SIDS.

Infants **swaddled prone** have a 50 times increased risk of SIDS compared to unswaddled babies sleeping supine.[54] Swaddling should be avoided in:

- Infants over 2 to 3 months of age. There is a danger that when infants begin to roll from supine to prone, the swaddled prone infant cannot regain the supine position.

SUCCESS OF THE SAFE TO SLEEP PROGRAM IN REDUCING SIDS DEATHS

Since 1992, these Safe Infant Sleep recommendations have been phenomenally successful at reducing the SIDS rate.[9,34] Only one-third as many babies are dying now as once did. Informing parents about SIDS, and how the risks can be reduced, has been a huge success story in modern health care. However, many parents ignore and/or are unwilling to comply with safe infant sleep recommendations.[55] Part of the problem is that health care professionals do not consistently advocate for safe infant sleep to parents of infants.[55,56] Thus, the AAP recommends that "Health care professionals, staff in newborn nurseries and NICUs, and childcare providers should endorse and model the SIDS risk reduction recommendations from birth."[9] Parents of infants are more likely to adhere to safe infant sleep recommendations if they receive this advice consistently from their primary care provider and other health professionals.[55]

SUBSEQUENT SIBLINGS OF SIDS VICTIMS

When the parents of a baby who died of SIDS have a subsequent child, they often are afraid that this new baby may also die. These subsequent siblings of a baby who died from SIDS are not at increased risk for SIDS.[57] They have the same risk of SIDS as the general population. There is no testing, such as sleep studies, electrocardiograms, or genetic studies, which can predict if a subsequent sibling of a SIDS victim is at increased risk for SIDS. Thus, such tests are not recommended. Nevertheless, parents who have experienced the death of a baby from SIDS frequently ask what they can do to reduce the risk of their subsequent baby from also dying from SIDS. Parents should do everything that any parent does to optimize the health of their baby. Once the baby is born, parents should follow "Safe to Sleep" recommendations. These recommendations have been shown to decrease the number of babies dying from SIDS.[9]

Parent Grief

When a baby dies from SIDS, the health care team must recognize that the parents and families of these babies are additional victims of this tragedy. Although the death of any child is painful, SIDS deaths are unique. SIDS deaths come quietly, suddenly, and unexpectedly. These babies were usually happy and healthy. They were tucked safely into their cribs for an overnight sleep or a daytime nap. Sometime during that sleeping period, they died. Health care professional must be prepared to be a source of strong support for these families. Reaching out to the family who has experienced a SIDS death is critical. Newly bereaved SIDS parents are devastated and may be paralyzed by grief. The importance of the support and education from a trusted provider cannot be over-emphasized.

Many states require that public health nurses visit families who have had a SIDS death. The purpose of these visits is to provide grief support and SIDS education.[58] They are not part of an investigation into the possible cause of the baby's death. When done correctly, they are extremely important in helping SIDS parents in their grief journey. SIDS parent support groups also provide peer support. Most parents will say that talking to another parent who has experienced the same tragedy that they are going through is the most powerful and helpful source of support. When possible, newly bereaved parents should be referred to a local or online SIDS parent support group.

The death of a child is a death that is feared but not expected. A parent whose baby has died is one of the most traumatic losses any person can experience. This trauma is intensified by the final cause of death diagnosed as SIDS, which means that the infant's death was sudden, unexpected, and unexplained. The lack of an explanation for the death of a presumably healthy baby leaves parents, family members, and caregivers with intense feelings of grief, guilt, and confusion. Most parents experience profound and intense guilt, and they blame themselves for their baby's death.[58]

Because the SIDS death is unexplained, parents often scrutinize the pregnancy and the baby's brief life for things they may have done to cause the death, or at least not prevent it.[58] Almost always, the things parents identify and worry about have no relation to their baby's death.

Providing parents with a theoretical understanding of what is known about SIDS helps to reduce their guilt. The triple risk hypothesis helps parents to realize that their baby's death was not due solely to environmental hazards.[11] Many SIDS victims have subtle abnormalities of the brain.[21,22] Some vulnerable babies may never die if they are never challenged by environmental hazards. When a SIDS death is associated with risk factors, that baby may have had increased vulnerability or a decreased ability to deal with environmental challenges compared to other babies.[21,22] These factors are beyond the parent's or caregiver's control, and this is important to emphasize to reduce a parent's guilt.

Helping parents reduce their feelings of guilt and self-blame is the most important counseling action health professionals can take.[58] Anger and guilt are common emotions for parents of SIDS victims. They may feel angry with their God, their spouse, their children, or with others, whether involved or totally separate from the death. Grief is a natural and normal reaction to loss. It is a response that is physical, emotional, spiritual, and psychological. Newly bereaved parents need to know that all of these feelings and thoughts are normal, and they should decrease with time, especially with support.

In mothers of babies who died from SIDS, prolonged grief disorder (PGD) is common, and it may persist for many months after the infant's death.[59] Daily intrusive emotional pain or yearning was found in 68% of mothers, and yearning was significantly associated with emotional pain. Parents report difficulties discussing their experiences of loss and seeking assistance to support the grief. These findings are important to guide those helping to address a mother's grief months and even years after a SIDS death. The symptoms of PGD should not be considered as a "disorder," but rather they may be a normal or common expression of grief in these mothers.[59] Prolonged grief in the fathers of babies who die from SIDS has not been extensively explored and specific studies on same-sex parents and adoptive parents are similarly lacking. Anecdotally, providers who experience a SIDS death in their practice may also experience prolonged grief, questioning the adequacy of their care and wondering if they "missed" something that contributed to their patient's death.

Linking newly bereaved parents with other parents of SIDS victims is one of the most helpful things that one can do.[58] It allows newly bereaved parents and caregivers to talk with someone who has experienced a similar infant death. Speaking with a parent whose baby died years ago gives the newly bereaved parent hope that their highly emotional crisis state is temporary and that their pain will ease over time. The newly bereaved parents can see how other parents have coped with their grief. It shows them that their lives will not always be this sorrowful or this hard. However, these parents are forever changed. One parent said: "We all are changed by the loss of a child or grandchild. Our grief becomes a part of who we are now. It becomes our 'new normal.'"

Father's Grief: While mothers are often the main focus for support and expressions of sympathy, a father's loss is no less. Fathers typically develop very protective feelings about their families, so that the sudden death of their precious baby can feel overwhelming and undermine their self-esteem. Because traditional masculinity is characterized by strength, it leaves little room for grief, sadness, breaking down, or confusion.

Some fathers find that going back to work or resuming other activities helps. Other fathers may have great difficulty returning to work where they are expected to function productively. Dealing with other fellow workers, who do not understand grief, may just add strain and pressure.

Many fathers are helped by attending parent support meetings and being connected to other fathers who have also experienced infant loss. Similar to mothers, relating to other fathers who have experienced a death of an infant from SIDS allows them to not feel alone in their grief, and it also allows them to see that there is hope for a less painful future.

Sibling's Grief: When a baby dies from SIDS, and there are other children in the home, they will also experience grief. Some children need a chance to talk about what happened and how they are feeling. Children's questions about death should be answered as honestly as possible in an age-appropriate way; their questions should not be ignored. Children will create answers for questions not acknowledged. Children tend to cope with death by "acting out" their feelings and fears rather than talking about them. They may not always understand "why" they hurt, but they can clearly identify their pain. All children react differently, but some of the most common expressions of grief in children are anger, feelings of abandonment, guilt, temper outbursts, regression, increased dependency, silence, withdrawal, depression, behavior changes, and disinterest in previously engaging activities.

Siblings of SIDS victims need to be reminded that nothing they did, said, or thought caused the baby to die, and nobody is to blame. They should know that SIDS happens only to babies. It can not happen to them or to grown-ups.

A child's understanding of their sibling's death changes as they mature. Thus, children may ask the same questions at different ages but will need different answers as they mature.

Childcare Providers: Many parents return to work around 3 months after their baby's birth. This age is also the peak incidence of SIDS. Thus, many infants die in childcare when the parents were away from their infants.[60] Childcare providers will also experience guilt and loss, especially if there has been a longstanding relationship with the child and/or parents. However, there are additional implications for the childcare provider. If they are a licensed childcare provider, there will almost certainly be an investigation by childcare licensing. Depending on the findings, their childcare license may be at risk. Only a few states have childcare regulations enforcing safe infant sleep practices. Therefore, in some cases, a child may have died in a high-risk sleep environment. Childcare providers should universally receive education about safe infant sleep, and regulations enforcing these would also be beneficial.

When an infant death occurred in childcare, the relationship with the parents is highly variable. Because parents were not present when their baby died, they may have additional guilt, which may escalate the intensity of emotional reactions toward the childcare provider, both positive and negative. Sometimes, parents will blame the childcare provider for the death, especially if the baby was found in an unsafe sleep environment. Sometimes, the childcare provider also experiencing grief can be supportive to the parents. There is no roadmap about how to help both parents and childcare providers, and health care professionals will need to individualize their approach to support each.

Summary

In summary, SIDS is the most common cause of death in infants between the ages of 1 month and 1 year, yet the cause remains unknown. The cause is best understood as an interaction between development, infant vulnerability, and environmental hazards. This triple risk model, and recent research, suggests that SIDS deaths occur when these three elements coincide. Some vulnerable babies may never die if they were never challenged by environmental hazards. When a SIDS death is associated with risk factors, that baby may have had increased vulnerability or a decreased ability to deal with environmental challenges compared to other babies. These factors are beyond the family's control, and this is important to emphasize in order to reduce parental guilt. A SIDS death can not be predicted prior to death. SIDS can not be prevented. However, public health interventions have successfully decreased the number of babies dying from SIDS. SIDS has not been eliminated, and we still are faced with addressing the needs of parents of SIDS victims, surviving family members, and childcare providers when involved. All health care providers must feel empowered and responsible for sharing and modeling safe sleep recommendations.

References

1. Krous HF, Beckwith JB, Byard RW, et al. Sudden infant death syndrome (SIDS) and unclassified sudden infant deaths (USID): a definitional and diagnostic approach. *Pediatrics*. 2004;114:234-238.
2. Guntheroth W, Spiers PS. The triple risk hypotheses in sudden infant death syndrome. *Pediatrics*. 2002;110:e64. doi:10.1542/peds.110.5.e64.
3. CDC. 2018. Available at: https://www.cdc.gov/sids/data.htm.
4. Goldstein RD, Blair PS, Sens MA, et al. Inconsistent classification of unexplained deaths in infants and children hinders surveillance, prevention, and research: recommendations from the 3rd International Congress on Sudden Infant and Child Death. *Forensic Sci Med Pathol*. 2019;15(4):622-628. Available at: https://doi.org/10.1007/s12024-019-00156-9.
5. Bundock EA, Corey TS, eds. *Unexplained Pediatric Deaths: Investigation, Certification, and Family Needs*. San Diego, California: Academic Forensic Pathology International; 2019.
6. Shapiro-Mendoza CK, Pelusci VJ, Hoffman B, et al. Half century since SIDS: a reappraisal of Terminology. *Pediatrics*. 2021;148:e2021053746.
7. Shapiro-Mendoza CK, Parks SE, Brunstrom J, et al. Variations in cause-of-death determination for sudden unexpected infant deaths. *Pediatrics*. 2017;140:e20170087.

8. Cutz E. The disappearance of sudden infant death syndrome: has the clock turned back? *JAMA Pediatr.* 2016;170:315-316.
9. Moon RY, Darnall RA, Feldman-Winter L, et al. SIDS and other sleep-related infant deaths: updated 2016 recommendations for a safe infant sleeping environment. *Pediatrics.* 2016;138:e20162938.
10. Kinney HC, Thach BT. The sudden infant death syndrome. *N Engl J Med.* 2009;361:795-805.
11. Filiano JJ, Kinney HC. A perspective on neuropathologic findings in victims of the sudden infant death syndrome: the triple-risk model. *Biol Neonate.* 1994;65:194-197.
12. Moon RY, AAP Task Force on Sudden Infant Death Syndrome. SIDS and other sleep-related infant deaths: evidence base for 2016 updated recommendations for a safe infant sleeping environment: technical report. *Pediatrics.* 2016;138:e20162940. doi:10.1542/peds.2016-2940.
13. Fleming PJ, Levine MR, Long AM, Cleave JP. Postneonatal development of respiratory oscillations. *Ann N Y Acad Sci.* 1998;533:305-313.
14. Ramanathan R, Corwin MJ, Hunt CE, et al. Cardiorespiratory events recorded on home monitors: comparison of healthy infants with those at increased risk for SIDS. *J Am Med Assoc.* 2001;285:2199-2207.
15. Hunt CE, Corwin MJ, Lister G, et al. 1 Longitudinal assessment of hemoglobin oxygen saturation in healthy infants during the first six months of age. *J Pediatr.* 1999;135:580-586.
16. Katz D, Shore S, Bandle B, Niermeyer S, Bol KA, Khanna A. Sudden infant death syndrome and residential altitude. *Pediatrics.* 2015;135:e1442-e1449.
17. Ward SL, Bautista DB, Keens TG. Hypoxic arousal responses in normal infants. *Pediatrics.* 1992;89:860-864.
18. Hamutcu R, Bautista Bolduc D, Saeed MM, Ward SL, Keens TG. Effect of development and sleeping position on hypoxic and hypercapnic arousal responses. *Am J Respir Crit Care Med.* 2001;163(5):A953.
19. Paterson DS, Trachtenberg FL, Thompson EG, et al. Multiple serotonergic brainstem abnormalities in sudden infant death syndrome. *J Am Med Assoc.* 2006;296:2124-2132.
20. Duncan JR, Paterson DS, Hoffman JF, et al. Brainstem serotonergic deficiency in sudden infant death syndrome. *J Am Med Assoc.* 2010;303:430-437.
21. Randall BB, Paterson DS, Haas EA, et al. Potential asphyxia and brainstem abnormalities in sudden and unexpected deaths in infants. *Pediatrics.* 2013;132:e1616-e1625.
22. Kinney HC, Richerson GB, Dymecki SM, Darnall RA, Nattie EE. The brainstem and serotonin in the sudden infant death syndrome. *Annu Rev Pathol.* 2009;4:517-550.
23. Goldstein RD, Kinney HC, Willinger M. Sudden unexpected death in fetal life through early childhood. *Pediatrics.* 2016;137:e20154661.
24. Ostfeld BM, Esposito L, Perl H, Hegyi T. Concurrent risks in sudden infant death syndrome. *Pediatrics.* 2010;125:447-453.
25. Trachtenberg F, Haas EA, Kinney HC, Stanley C, Krous HF. Risk factor changes for sudden infant death syndrome after initiation of back-to-sleep campaign. *Pediatrics.* 2012;129:630-638.
26. Erck Lambert AB, Parks SE, Cottengim C, Faulkner M, Hauck FR, Shapiro-Mendoza CK. Sleep-related infant suffocation deaths attributable to soft bedding, overlay, and wedging. *Pediatrics.* 2019;143:e20183408.
27. Parks SE, Lambert AB, Hauck FR, Cottengim CR, Faulkner M, Shapiro-Mendoza CK. Explaining sudden unexpected infant deaths, 2011-2017. *Pediatrics.* 2021;147:e2020035873.
28. Haynes RL, Kinney HC, Haas EA, et al. Medullary binding deficits and hippocampal abnormalities in sudden infant death syndrome: one or two entities. *Front Pediatr.* 2021;9:762017. doi:10.3389/fped.2021.762017.
29. Schwartz PJ, Stramba-Badiale M, Segantini A, et al. Prolongation of the QT interval and the sudden infant death syndrome. *N Engl J Med.* 1998;338:1709-1714.
30. Davis AM, Glengarry J, Skinner JR. Sudden infant death: QT or not QT? That is no longer the question. *Circ Arrhythm Electrophysiol.* 2016;9:e003859.
31. Goldstein RD, Trachtenberg FL, Sens MA, Harty BL, Kinney HC. Overall postneonatal mortality and rates of SIDS. *Pediatrics.* 2016;137:e20152298.
32. CDC. 2018. Available at: https://www.cdc.gov/sids/data.htm.
33. Willinger M, Hoffman HJ, Wu KT, et al. Factors associated with the transition to nonprone sleep positions of infants in the United States: The National Infant Sleep Position Study. *J Am Med Assoc.* 1998;280:329-335.
34. NICHD. *SIDS Risk Reduction: Curriculum for Nurses.* NIH Publication No. 06-6005. 2006.
35. Hauck FR, Johnson JMD, Tanabe KO, Moon RY, Venneman MM. Breastfeeding and reduced risk of sudden infant death syndrome: a meta-analysis. *Pediatrics.* 2011;128:103-110.
36. Maternal Child and Adolescent Health Program, Center for Family Health, California Department of Public Health. *Maternal and Infant Health Assessment Survey.* 2011. Available at: http://www.cdph.ca.gov/data/surveys/MIHA/MIHAComparisonMaps/CompareRegBedshare2011.pdf.

37. McKenna JJ, Mosko SS, Richard CA. Bedsharing promotes breastfeeding. *Pediatrics.* 1997;100:214-219.
38. Ball HL, Ward-Platt MP, Heslop E, Leech SJ, Brown KA. Randomized trial of infant sleep location on the postnatal ward. *Arch Dis Child.* 2006;91:1005-1010.
39. Richard CA, Mosko SS, McKenna JJ. Apnea and periodic breathing in bedsharing and solitary sleeping infants. *J Appl Physiol.* 1996;84:1374-1380.
40. Blair PS, Fleming PJ, Smith LJ, et al. Babies sleeping with parents: case-control study of factors influencing the risk of the sudden infant death syndrome. CESDI SUDI Research Group. *Br Med J.* 1999;319:1457-1462.
41. McGarvey C, McDonnell M, Chong A, O'Regan M, Matthews T. Factors relating to the infant's last sleep environment in sudden infant death syndrome in the Republic of Ireland. *Arch Dis Child.* 2003;88:1058-1064.
42. Tappin D, Ecob R, Brooke H. Bedsharing, roomsharing, and sudden infant death syndrome in Scotland: a case-control study. *J Pediatr.* 2005;147:32-37.
43. Blair PS, Sidenbotham P, Evason-Coombe C, Edmonds M, Heckstall-Smith EMA, Fleming P. Hazardous cosleeping environments and risk factors amenable to change: case-control study of SIDS in south West England. *Br Med J.* 2009;339:b3666. doi:10.1136/bmj.b3666.
44. Blair PS, Sidenbotham P, Pease A, Fleming PJ. Bed-sharing in the absence of hazardous circumstances: Is there a risk of sudden infant death syndrome? An analysis from two case control studies conducted in the UK. *PLoS One.* 2014;9(9):e107799.
45. Tappin D, Mitchell EA, Carpenter J, Hauck F, Allan L. Bed-sharing is a risk for sudden unexpected death in infancy. *Arch Dis Child.* 2023;108(2):79-80. doi:10.1136/archdischild-2021-322480.
46. Feldman-Winter L, Goldsmith JP, AAP Committee on Fetus and Newborn, and AAP Task Force on Sudden Infant Death Syndrome. Safe sleep and skin-to-skin care in the newborn period for healthy term infants. *Pediatrics.* 2016;138:e20161889.
47. Tablizo MA, Jacinto P, Parsley D, Chen ML, Ramanathan R, Keens TG. Supine sleeping position does not cause clinical aspiration in neonates in hospital newborn nurseries. *Arch Pediatr Adolesc Med.* 2007;161:507-510.
48. Blair PS, Fleming PJ, Bensley D, et al. Smoking and the sudden infant death syndrome: results from 1993-5 case-control study for confidential inquiry into stillbirths and deaths in infancy. Confidential Enquiry into Stillbirths and Deaths Regional Coordinators and Researchers. *Br Med J.* 1996;313:195-198.
49. Mitchell EA, Tuohy PG, Brunt JM, et al. Risk factors for sudden infant death syndrome following the prevention campaign in New Zealand: a prospective study. *Pediatrics.* 1997;100:835-840.
50. Ward SL, Bautista D, Chan L, et al. Sudden infant death syndrome in infants of substance-abusing mothers. *J Pediatr.* 1990;117:876-881.
51. Elliott AJ, Kinney HC, Haynes RL, et al. Concurrent prenatal drinking and smoking increases risk for SIDS: Safe Passage Study report. *EClinicalMedicine.* 2020;19:100247. Available at: https://doi.org/10.1016/j.eclinm.2019.100247.
52. Vennemann MM, Hoffgen M, Bajanowski T, Hense HW, Mitchell EA. Do immunisations reduce the risk for SIDS: a meta-analysis. *Vaccine.* 2007;25:4875-4879.
53. Hutchison BL, Hutchison LA, Thompson JM, Mitchell EA. Plagiocephaly and brachycephaly in the first two years of life: a prospective cohort study. *Pediatrics.* 2004;114:970-980.
54. Pease AS, Fleming PJ, Hauck FR, et al. Swaddling and the risk of sudden infant death syndrome: a meta-analysis. *Pediatrics.* 2016;137:e20153275.
55. Hirai AH, Kortsmit K, Kaplan L, et al. Prevalence and factors associated with safe infant sleep practices. *Pediatrics.* 2019;144:e20191286.
56. Eron NB, Dygert KM, Squillace C, et al. The physician's role in reducing SIDS. *Health Promot Pract.* 2009;10:1-9.
57. Bacon CJ, Hall DBM, Stephenson TJ, Campbell MJ. How common is repeat sudden infant death syndrome? *Arch Dis Child.* 2008;93:269-270.
58. Stastny PF, Keens TG, Alkon A. Supporting SIDS families: the public health nurse SIDS home visit. *Public Health Nurs.* 2016;33:242-248.
59. Goldstein RD, Lederman RI, Lichtenthal WG, et al. The grief of mothers after the sudden unexpected death of their infants. *Pediatrics.* 2018;141:e20173651.
60. Moon RY, Patel KM, McDermott SJ. Sudden infant death syndrome in child care settings. *Pediatrics.* 2000;106:295-300.

CHAPTER 6

Evaluation of Obstructive Sleep Apnea in Infants: Including Polysomnography

Joanna E. MacLean

Introduction

The assessment of obstructive sleep apnea (OSA) in infants shares many similarities with older children. Polysomnography and clinical assessment are the cornerstones in both. Infants, however, have considerable changes in sleep and breathing across the first year of life, so establishing thresholds for testing results is a challenge. Given this challenge, establishing a firm diagnosis of OSA in an infant can be difficult. Polysomnography (PSG) is the accepted standard for the diagnosis of OSA across childhood, though is not available in many jurisdictions. Understanding how developmental changes in breathing may alter PSG interpretation as well as an understanding of alternative tools for evaluation is important for the identification of OSA in infants as well as considering treatment decisions.

Developmental Changes in Sleep and Breathing That May Impact OSA Evaluation

Sleep and breathing maturation is a crucial aspect of development and undergoes important changes in early infancy which may impact identification of abnormal sleep or breathing in the first years of life. Both sleep and breathing are evident as physiological processes as early as 25- and 10-weeks' gestational age, respectively.[1] Neither sleep nor breathing control systems are fully developed at birth and both are not likely to fully mature until late in the first decade of life or into adolescence.[1-5] With sleep occupying 16 to 18 h/day after birth and decreasing across the first year of life, it clearly plays an important function in early development.[1] Longitudinal studies of breathing response show that healthy infants have greater variability in change in ventilation and arousal from sleep in response to hypoxia at lower postnatal age, with this variability decreasing in the first months of life.[6] These changes in sleep and breathing in early life mean that what can be considered appropriate sleep and breathing changes across infancy.

While sleep and breathing are independent processes, the relationship between sleep and breathing is important to understand when assessing either separately or the interaction between the two. Sleep is divided into different stages, with infants having a predominance of rapid eye movement (REM, also called active in infants) sleep at birth; REM occupies 50% of total sleep time at birth, decreasing such that slow wave sleep (SWS, stage N3 sleep, or deep sleep) is the predominate stage by 1 year of age.[7,8] During REM sleep, there is a reduction of the tonic activity of the diaphragm and intercostal muscles that, along with a complaint chest wall, results in paradoxical inward rib cage movement associated with lower oxygen saturation.[6] Respiratory frequency and stability is more variable during REM sleep which, alongside changes in chest wall activity, means that respiratory events, including central, obstructive, and oxygen desaturation events, are more common during REM sleep than other sleep stages.[1] Changes in chest wall mechanics likely also explain lower and more variable oxygen saturations in REM compared to other sleep stages. Like REM sleep, the frequency of respiratory events in healthy infants decreases across the first year of life.[9-11] Arousals from sleep, an important protective mechanism, are also more common in REM sleep and decrease over the first year of life. Sleep is cyclical across the night with shorter cycles in infants. As nocturnal sleep is established after 3 months of age, there is also a shift such that SWS predominates during daytime sleep as well as in the first part of the night and REM in the later part of the night. These features mean that age-related changes predispose even healthy infants to higher numbers of respiratory events in early life which complicates the identification of OSA.

Primary Tools for Assessing Obstructive Sleep Apnea in Infants

The early interest and investigations of OSA in infants stemmed from a potential association between adult OSA or familial OSA and sudden infant death syndrome (SIDS) and subsequent interest in a potential association between OSA in infants and risk of SIDS.[12-14] Tools used to assess breathing during sleep in at-risk infants included different types of movement monitors connected to alarms to detect cessation of breathing movement, 12- to 24-hour polygraphy recording a combination of electroencephalograms (EEG), electrocardiograms (ECG), and/or respiratory activity, and transcutaneous O_2 and CO_2 monitoring[15-20] with less information about clinical or airway assessments. Today, attended in-laboratory polysomnography (PSG) and clinical assessment are the cornerstone to assessing OSA in infants.

Polysomnography: PSG is the accepted standard for the diagnosis of OSA in children including infants though whether different standards are needed for the definition of OSA in infants is controversial. The American Academy of Sleep Medicine (AASM) published infant sleep scoring criteria in 2015[21] completing the challenge of standardized rules from 0 to 17 years of age. The International Classification of Sleep Disorders (ICSD) 3rd edition defines pediatric OSA based on the presence of at least one symptom of OSA (i.e., snoring, labored/paradoxical/obstructive breathing during sleep, sleepiness/hyperactivity/behavioral/learning problems) and PSG results demonstrating at least one of: (1) an obstructive-mixed apnea-hypopnea index (OMAHI) >1 event/second; or (2) a pattern of obstructive hypoventilation (i.e., P_aCO_2 >50 mmHg for >25% of total sleep time) with snoring, flattening of the inspiratory nasal pressure waveform and/or paradoxical thoracoabdominal motion.[22] While the definition acknowledges that adult diagnostic criteria may be used for ages 13 to 18 years of age, infants are not considered separately. Other authors have recommended infant OSA definitions that include apnea-hypopnea index (AHI) >1 event/hour,[23-25] AHI ≥2 events/hour,[26] obstructive apnea-hypopnea index (OAHI) ≥2 events/hour,[27] mixed obstructive apnea index (MOAI) >3 events/hour,[28] obstructive mixed apnea-hypopnea index (OMAHI) >3 events/hour,[29] apnea index (AI) >5 events/hour,[30] obstructive respiratory distress index (ORDI) >5 events/hour, and AHI >10 events/hour.[31] The range of variables used to define OSA and cut-offs show variability in what is considered OSA in infants with values that overlap with data from otherwise healthy infants.

Normative PSG data in infants comes both from older studies, where definitions of respiratory events differ from the currently recommended standards, as well as studies that have defined respiratory events based on AASM criteria. In a review of normative PSG data by Ng and Chan the most common definition of apnea across studies was based on time (events ≥3 seconds) rather than the two missed breaths used in the AASM rules.[32,33] The authors note that this is in contrast to events considered significant in neonatology being ≥20 seconds.[34,35] Three of the included studies provided age-related trends for the apnea index and showed apnea indices were highest in the neonatal period with decreasing trends for obstructive, central, and mixed apneas indices with increasing age in the first year of life.[10,11,36] Median values for obstructive apnea index (OAI) were 0 events/hour across all studies with two studies reporting 90th percentiles of 0.6 to 0.7 events/hour from 2 weeks of age and 0.2 to 0.4 events/hour by 2 to 3 months of age. Of note, hypopneas are not included in these events. A more recent summary of PSG parameters is provided by Daftary and colleagues in their study of PSG values in healthy infants.[37] The results include ranges for typical PSG parameters that highlight the high degree of variability for healthy infants <30 days of age.[37] This includes AHI (1.0–37.7 events/hour), OAI (0.2–12.5 events/hour), central apnea index (0–27.2 events/hour), mixed apnea index (0–8.3 events/hour), and hypopnea index (0.7–12.9 events/hour). The authors provide a summary table comparing their results to those from three other studies and demonstrate a trend for decreasing respiratory events from <30 days of age to 1 to 2 years of age. Not all studies used the AASM criteria for collecting and scoring PSG data.[33] The three studies that included sleep staging showed a mean AHI of 14.9 events/hour <30 days, 21.4 events/hour <45 days of age, and 2.8 events/hour at 1 to 2 years of age.[37-39] There was less variation by age of the median duration of respiratory events. This decrease in respiratory events with age mirrors that described in the Childhood Home Monitoring Evaluation, where extreme events decreased from birth to 43 weeks gestational age in both term and preterm infants,[40] and what is describe in a study of infants <2 years of age undergoing PSG.[41] While further studies with the same measurement methodology are needed to more accurately define the upper limits of normal for different respiratory events, the results highlight variability in the number of respiratory events in otherwise healthy infants in early life as well as decreasing events from birth through the first years of life.

Clinical assessment: Clinical history alone is insufficient to distinguish OSA from non-OAS in snoring children.[42-44] Combining this clinical information with PSG results is important to add to the assessment of OSA risk and guide decisions around treatment, monitoring, and follow-up. Symptoms of OSA in infants differ in some respects from those of older children. Parents or caregivers may not identify noises made by an infant as "snoring" so probing about noisy or audible breathing during sleep may be needed.[45] The absence of snoring or noisy breathing does not rule out OSA as complete airway obstruction is silent. Apnea, while a primary feature of OSA, may be more difficult to recognize in infants because of more subtle respiratory effort.[46] Difficulties with feeding or tiring with feeding may be a sign of airway obstruction, given the challenge of coordinating suck and swallow with a compromised airway.[46] With infants sleeping for a large proportion of the 24 hour day, it may be difficult to appreciate a disruption in sleep duration or daytime sleepiness; inquiring about periods where an infant is awake and alert may be helpful to assess whether sleep is restorative even when awake periods are relatively short. Sweating during sleep is not uncommon in otherwise healthy infants though may be important in an infant with other features of OSA.[46] Similarly, restlessness can be difficult to assess in infants who have not yet developed suppression of muscle activity in REM sleep though may point to struggles to open an obstructed airway in an infant with other symptoms of OSA. Asking specifically about tolerance to different sleep positions is important as parents or caregivers may not admit to trying a position other than supine sleep given the recommendations for "back to sleep" because of SIDS risk. They may, however, admit if asked that they have noted differences in snoring, noisy breathing, or other OSA-related symptoms when the infant sleeps prone on their chest or otherwise supervised during sleep. Recurrent respiratory tract infections, which are also common in infants, can be related to OSA because narrower airways become congested more easily, and disrupted sleep may alter immune function. In a retrospective chart review of infants with OSA, the most common presenting symptoms were pauses in breathing (27%), followed by a combination of characteristics (22%) and snoring (18%). In another cohort of infants with OSA, snoring (53%) and nocturnal desaturations (24%) were the most common indications for PSG.[25] While there is a broad range of potential symptoms of OSA, focusing on the concerns of an individual infant can highlight important features of OSA in that infant.

Physical examination adds additional important information about OSA risk in infants. Growth measurements, ideally serial ones, are useful to assess growth as additional energy expended to support breathing during sleep or decreased oral intake related to difficulty in feeding can impact growth.[46] In an early study of 14 infants with OSA, failure to thrive was the main complaint for 20%.[45] Mid-face hypoplasia or retro/micrognathia may indicate a smaller airway that is more likely to be compromised during sleep.[46] This can be best assessed by looking at the infant from the side where the size of the lower jaw (mandible) can be more easily assessed in relationship to the upper jaw (maxilla). Tonsillar hypertrophy may be seen in infants beyond 3 months of age though is a less common feature in infants versus children with OSA.[47] Developmental milestones are important as impaired sleep may impact development, and impaired development may be a flag to other causes of developmental delay, including musculoskeletal and neurological conditions, that may heighten OSA risk. Poor weight gain or developmental progress may also influence decisions about follow-up when a diagnosis of OSA is unclear; early reassessment may be indicated for an infant with these concerns compared to an infant with the same symptoms and PSG results who has appropriate growth and development. The clinical assessment provides important information about the impact of OSA and the potential benefits of treatment to important measures of overall health.

Risk factors are important to consider, though not all infants with any particular risk factor will develop OSA. Common risk factors for OSA in infants include craniofacial anomalies, prematurity, gastroesophageal reflux, and adenotonsillar hypertrophy.[48] Hypotonia and central nervous system immaturity can each contribute to OSA risk because of their potential effect of compromising airway function and response to respiratory challenges, such as sleep and acute respiratory tract infection. In a study of 139 infants 0 to 17 months of age with OSA, the most common comorbidity was gastroesophageal reflux disease (GERD, 68%), followed by craniofacial disease (37%), neuromuscular disease (34%), prematurity (30%), genetic syndrome (30%), laryngo/tracheomalacia (27%), and epilepsy (17%). In another study, the most common risk factors for OSA were hypotonia (53%), GERD (30%), and laryngomalacia (24%), with 34% of infants having a genetic abnormality.[25] Understanding the risk factors for OSA may help to identify OSA earlier in its course, especially in infants with complex medical illnesses.

Additional Tools as Substitutes or Additional Assessment in Infants With Suspect OSA

While PSG is the accepted standard for the diagnosis of OSA in infants and children, access to PSG is limited, unavailable, or subject to long wait times in many jurisdictions. As a result, PSG may not be an option and alternative tools may be used to add objective or additional information to the clinical assessment of infants with suspected OSA.

Overnight Oximetry: Continuous overnight oximetry is a common tool used for the assessment of OSA in children with some challenges and fewer studies about its use in infants. Similar to other measures related to breathing, oxygen pulse saturations (S_pO_2) in healthy infants are more variable at younger age with the range between minimum and maximum S_pO_2 narrowing and shifting toward higher values from 2 weeks to 24 months of age (Fig. 6.1).[49] Based on S_pO_2 desaturation of $\geq3\%$, desaturations are more frequent at 2 weeks of age than 24 months, decreasing from a mean of 27.2 events/hour to 3.3 events/hour. Desaturations are typically 3% to 4% from baseline and 5 to 6 seconds in duration. Compared to term infants at the same postnatal age, infants born preterm spend longer at S_pO_2 <96% and have more desaturation events which are longer and deeper.[50] Of note, the cumulative frequency plots displayed in Fig. 6.1 are not the typical way that S_pO_2 is summarized in PSGs or other clinical testing. Cumulative frequency plots have the benefit of including measurement of the variability of S_pO_2 and can be used to look at S_pO_2 distribution as well as desaturation incidence, depth, and duration.[50] Regardless of how

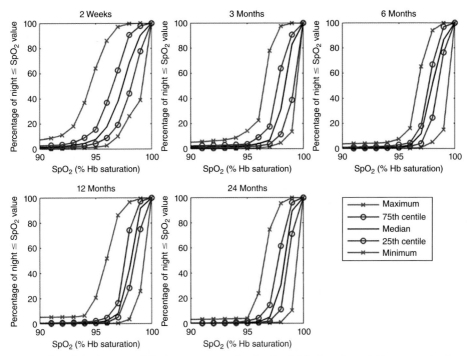

Fig. 6.1 Cumulative frequency (CF) reference-curves showing the distribution of overnight oxygen saturation from full nocturnal recordings from 2 weeks to 24 months of age. These plots describe the proportion of the recording spent at or below an integer oxygen saturation value. *(Reproduced with permission of the author from Nocturnal oxygen saturation profiles of healthy term infants. Terrill, PI, Dakin C, Hughes I, et al. Arch Dis Child 2015. with permission from BMJ Publishing Group Ltd.)*

S_pO_2 data are analyzed and displayed, understanding how the data will change across the first years of life is vital to what the data can tell you.

A commonly used S_pO_2 score, the McGill Oximetry score (MOS), was developed to identify OSA in children from overnight S_pO_2 recordings.[51] The dataset included children 6 months to 18 years of age and excluded children with comorbidities including central nervous system disease, airway and lung disease, neuromuscular disease, GERD, and other syndromes or genetic abnormalities. The MOS uses patterns of S_pO_2 decreases $\geq 4\%$ to classify overnight oximetry recordings as positive (3 or more desaturation clusters and at least 3 desaturations to <90%), negative (no desaturation to <90%), or inconclusive (did not meet criteria for positive or negative). Desaturation clusters are defined as 5 or more desaturations occurring in a 10- to 30-minute period. This scoring typically requires manual review of the S_pO_2 data across the night as desaturation clusters are not the same as the oxygen desaturation index (ODI) or desaturation index (DI; i.e., number of desaturation events/hour of recording time) which are commonly provided by S_pO_2 machine software. The scoring criteria were further modified to enable prioritization of adenotonsillectomy based on severity (Table 6.1) though it is unclear if infants were included in the validation portion of the study.[52] The MOS was compared to PSG results in a study of 53 infants under 1 year of age with laryngomalacia and clinical suspicion of OSA, 46 of whom had OSA, and included 14 infants with additional comorbidities.[53] Using a PSG definition of OSA of OAHI ≥ 2 events/hour, the MOS showed a sensitivity of 91% and specificity of 25% with

TABLE 6.1 ■ McGill Oximetry Score Criteria Including Criteria for Severity of Obstructive Sleep Apnea

			S_aO_2		
Score	Description	Clusters	# drop <90%	# drop <85%	# drop <80%
1	Normal/inconclusive	<3, baseline S_pO_2 >95%	<3	0	0
2	Mild OSA	≥3	≥3	≤3	0
3	Moderate OSA	≥3	≥3	>3	≤3
4	Severe OSA	≥3	≥3	>3	>3

OSA, Obstructive sleep apnea.
Reproduced with permission from Nixon GM, Kermack AS, Davis GM, et al. Planning adenotonsillectomy in children with obstructive sleep apnea: the role of overnight oximetry. *Pediatrics*. 2004;113(1):e19–e25. by the AAP

positive and negative predictive values of 91% and 0%, respectively. Using a revised MOS definition of two desaturation clusters and one desaturation to <90% worsened OSA prediction (sensitivity 89%, specificity 0%). The MOS provides a systematic way to evaluate overnight S_pO_2 recordings and its relatively high sensitivity and low specificity may be useful in ruling out OSA in infants with a negative test result though it should not be used to confirm OSA.

An alternative measure to the MOS for overnight oximetry data is the ODI. Two studies have compared the ODI and PSG results for the diagnosis of OSA in infants. This was included in the study of infants with laryngomalacia mentioned above and used two ODI (≥3% desaturation threshold) cut-offs.[53] The first was an ODI cut-off based on the best predictor of OAHI ≥2/hour which was 7.74 events/hour and yielded a sensitivity of 62% and specificty of 63% with positive and negative predictive values of 90% and 23%, respectively. The second cut-off was an ODI>2 events/hour which yielded a sensitivity of 96% and specificity of 0%. The second study included 38 infants <1 year of age who underwent both overnight oximetry and PSG within 3 months of each other, where OSA was defined by OAHI >1 event/hour.[54] Using an ODI (≥4% desaturation threshold) for events ≥0 seconds (ODI4$_0$) ≥3 events/hour showed a sensitivity of 87% and specificity of 43% with negative and positive predictive values of 43% and 83%, respectively. Increasing the OAHI cut-off to 2, 5, and 10 events/hour increased the sensitivity to 100% but decreased the specificity to 40%, 35%, and 24%, respectively. The results of using ODI as a predictor of OSA are like those of the MOS in that a negative result may be useful in ruling out OSA, while a positive result should not be used to confirm OSA.

Home Sleep Apnea Testing: The use of home sleep apnea testing (HSAT) in children is not recommended by the AASM.[55] The reasons for this recommendation include a lack of evidence comparing HSAT to PSG for the diagnosis of OSA in children under 18 years of age. That position paper cited few studies that addressed the feasibility or validity of HSAT use in children with only one study including children <2 years of age.[56] This study was a study of the feasibility of HSAT in children using a six-channel monitor (nasal flow, thoracic and abdominal movements, pulse oximetry, heart rate, and body position) and included children 0 to 15 years of age.[56] HSAT testing was completed at home or in hospital with a younger age in those undergoing hospital versus home studies (0.3 versus 3.8 years of age), suggesting infants may have been more likely to undergo HSAT in hospital. There was a 7% failure rate of studies with no difference in the failure rate of hospital versus home studies. However, the median age of the children with failed studies was 0.3 years (range 0–13.8 years), suggesting that infants had more failed studies than older children. Additional information that supports feasibility of HSAT in infants included a study of 562 healthy infants with a mean age of 1.1 ± 0.2 years who attempted home sleep cardiorespiratory monitoring (nasal pressure, oronasal thermistor, pulse oximetry, respiratory inductance plethysmography, actigraphy).[57] The results show that 91% of studies provided technically acceptable data with no loss of signal preventing data analysis of any parameter. Both studies had trained technicians set up the HSAT device on the night of testing which may have contributed to the high success rate. With demonstrated feasibility and reasonable validity of HSAT in older children,[58-61] HSAT testing may be a reasonable option to obtain additional data in infants with suspected OSA, although its accuracy compared to PSG in this age group has not yet been established.

Airway Assessment: Infants are more vulnerable to upper airway obstruction, at least in part, because of increased mobility of the mandible and tongue which can push the soft palate against the pharyngeal wall.[62] A variety of clinical upper airway assessments have been described, predominantly in infants with Robin sequence (RS). The most common method is bedside assessment, including observation of the infant in an upright and supine position as well as while feeding.[63] As airway closing pressures are markedly influenced by neck flexion, subtle changes in head angle may confirm risk of airway obstruction in a sleeping infant.[64] This is ideally done or guided by a clinician experienced with airway assessment in infants, such as an otolaryngologist.

Assessing airway obstruction by comparing supine and prone sleep positions can also be valuable. While a brief observation of an infant in supine and prone sleep positions may be useful, PSG or overnight oximetry provides objective data of the response to a change in sleep position. In a study of 21 infants with RS undergoing PSG, the OAI declined from 21 to 9 events/hour from supine to prone sleep, while ODI ($\geq$4% desaturation threshold) declined from 22 to 13 events/hour with no change in mean S_pO_2 or transcutaneous CO_2.[65] In a study of 67 infants with RS who underwent PSG, 16% did not require treatment of OSA and an additional 50% responded to prone sleep position.[66] OSA does not improve in all infants with a change in sleep position, so any change from the recommended safe sleep position of supine must be done with caution. Careful discussion with parents and caregivers of the risk as well as adherence to the other components of safe sleep recommendations, and, ideally, objective confirmation of improvements in airway obstruction in an alternative sleep position are needed prior to any recommendations of a sleep position other than supine sleep.

Anatomical assessment of airway size may provide additional information to support OSA. The challenge is that a small airway on its own may not be sufficient to cause OSA, as airway and ventilatory response mechanisms can compensate for an otherwise compromised airway. While radiographic studies have demonstrated smaller airways in infants with micrognathia compared to control infants, most infants with micrognathia (isolated 64%, with craniofacial differences 86%) had events that required stimulation during the first 6 months of life despite those with isolated micrognathia having airway measures that were more similar to controls than to those with craniofacial differences.[67] Given the high risk of airway obstruction in infants with micrognathia and the risk related to radiation exposure in early life, upper airway radiographs may be difficult to justify as part of an assessment for OSA. Upper airway endoscopy or MRI can localize sites of airway obstruction; this may be more relevant for infants who have failed to respond to initial treatment of OSA or in the context of surgical planning. A study of children who underwent fiberoptic endoscopy and had PSG findings consistent with OSA (AHI $\geq$1 event/hour) showed that all infants <1 year of age with normal muscle tone had dynamic abnormalities (either isolated or combined with fixed defects) as compared to 17% of children >2 years of age.[68] Only 15% of children with OSA had normal upper airway endoscopy and were presumed to have OSA on the basis of a dynamic disorder not demonstrated by endoscopy. Laryngomalacia was identified in 17 children (44%), 16 of whom had associated disorders, so the major mechanism of airway obstruction could not be isolated. In an MRI study of sites of airway narrowing in infants with and without OSA, the palate was found to be a major site of airway obstruction in those with OSA.[69] While the palate and retroglossal area are common sites of airway obstructions in adults, the study results showed that in a higher proportion of infants, the palate was the predominant site of airway obstruction compared to what has been reported in adults. Both endoscopy and MRI are likely to require sedation, which may alter airway tone and responses, and must be considered when deciding whether to use these tools for the assessment of OSA in infants.

Questionnaires: The use of questionnaires can be useful for serial assessments of symptoms of OSA, although infant-specific OSA questionnaires are lacking. The Brouillette score is a three-item scale that has been validated against PSG in children 1 to 10 years of age.[70] For the validation, OSA was defined by both PSG and clinical criteria including >30 apnea events in 7 hours of sleep (apnea index of approximately >4 events/hour), abnormal O_2 or CO_2, and clinically significant effects of sleep-related respiratory events. The scale correctly predicted OSA in 91% and 97% of two groups of children. The Pediatric Sleep Questionnaire (PSQ) may be the most commonly used scale for OSA in children.[71] The PSQ is a 22-item scale where positive responses to ≥33% (or 7) items are consistent with OSA. The scale was validated in children 2 to 18 years against a PSG diagnosis of OSA defined by an AHI ≥5 events/hour (moderate-severe OSA) with a sensitivity of 85% and specificity of 87%. The scale includes questions that may not be relevant or are considered normal in infants, especially young infants, such as "complain that they are sleepy during the day," "child usually takes a nap during the day," and "wakes up with headaches in the morning" making a total score invalid in infants. However, the PSQ may be useful as a means of tracking OSA symptoms. The brief infant sleep questionnaire (BRIEF, 10-items), including the revised version (BRIEF-R, 33-items), are not scales that assess OSA but rather assess sleep in infants.[72,73] While these tools cannot help with the identification of OSA, they can provide a means of identifying problems with sleep that could be related to OSA. Overall, the available questionnaires may provide a standardized way of tracking symptoms of OSA or sleep disruption caused by OSA which may aid in assessment and follow-up.

Testing Methods on the Horizon: The most promising evolving testing methods focus on using artificial intelligence or machine learning techniques to analyze components of physiological data that are part of existing tools. This includes analyzing S_pO_2,[74-79] ECG,[75] and airflow[80-82] as examples. While most of the reports so far have been of single data elements, the ability of novel analysis techniques to include multiple signals, which could account for the impact of changes in one signal on other measures, is exciting. With methods of data analysis that allow use of full scope of the data collected, the potential for safe, accurate testing methods that are minimally intrusive and can be easily carried out in the home is on the horizon.

Guidelines for the Diagnosis of OSA in Infants

Infants have been excluded or not considered separately in most guidelines developed for the diagnosis of OSA. The American Academy of Pediatrics Guideline for the diagnosis and management of uncomplicated OSA in children and the American Academy of Otolaryngology–Head and Neck Surgery Foundation clinical practice guideline on tonsillectomy excluded infants under 1 year of age.[83,84] The American Academy of Otolaryngology–Head and Neck Surgery Foundation clinical practice guideline on tonsillectomy recommend that children less than 2 years of age or those with specific comorbidities should be referred for PSG prior to tonsillectomy and clinicians should advocate for PSG prior to tonsillectomy for all children.[84] The guidelines of the American academy of Sleep Medicine[85] and the Australasian Sleep Association clinical practice guidelines for performing sleep studies in children[86] do not have separate recommendations for infants other than recommending that PSG is indicated in some infants who experience apparent life-threatening events. Infants were not considered in the guideline developed by a joint initiative of the Brazilian Medical Association and the Federal Council of Medicine.[87]

A European Respiratory Society Task Force developed a separate statement on obstructive sleep-disordered breathing for children 1 to 23 months of age.[88] This included PSG as an option for objective testing alongside video PSG, nap PSG, polygraphy, and overnight oximetry. The

Task Force defined OSA syndrome (OSAS) based on obstructive apnea-hypopnea index (OAHI) ≥1 event/hour with subcategorization of severity including mild (OAHI 1–5 events/hour), moderate (OAHI >5–10 episodes/hour), and severe (OAHI >10 events/hour) OSA. The statement includes an algorithm which progresses from "At risk for OSAS" through "Follow-up." Given that most of the recommendations are based on expert consensus, there is need for further work to provide data to support guidelines for the diagnosis of OSA in infants.

Summary

Infants represent a unique group with respect to the assessment of OSA. While the same tools that are used in older children are appropriate in infants, the interpretation of the results needs to consider the unique sleep and breathing of infants at the time of testing. With limited access to PSG, as the accepted standard for the diagnosis of OSA in all children, in many jurisdictions, there is a need for investment in the development of new methods, likely based on physiological data that is commonly collected, to improve access and accuracy of the assessment of OSA in infants.

References

1. MacLean JE, Fitzgerald DA, Waters KA. Developmental changes in sleep and breathing across infancy and childhood. *Paediatr Respir Rev.* 2015;16:276-284.
2. Fogel SM, Smith CT. The function of the sleep spindle: a physiological index of intelligence and a mechanism for sleep-dependent memory consolidation. *Neurosci Biobehav Rev.* 2011;35:1154-1165.
3. Schechtman VL, Harper RK, Harper RM. Distribution of slow-wave EEG activity across the night in developing infants. *Sleep.* 1994;17:316-322.
4. Gibbs EL, Lorimer FM, Gibbs FA. Clinical correlates of exceedingly fast activity in the electroencephalogram. *Dis Nerv Syst.* 1950;11:323-326.
5. Scholle S, Zwacka G, Scholle HC. Sleep spindle evolution from infancy to adolescence. *Clin Neurophysiol.* 2007;118:1525-1531.
6. Horne RS. Cardio-respiratory control during sleep in infancy. *Paediatr Respir Rev.* 2014;15:163-169.
7. Louis J, Cannard C, Bastuji H, Challamel MJ. Sleep ontogenesis revisited: a longitudinal 24-hour home polygraphic study on 15 normal infants during the first two years of life. *Sleep.* 1997;20:323-333.
8. Anders TF, Keener M. Developmental course of nighttime sleep-wake patterns in full-term and premature infants during the first year of life. I. *Sleep.* 1985;8:173-192.
9. Hunt CE, Brouillette RT, Hanson D, David RJ, Stein IM, Weissbluth M. Home pneumograms in normal infants. *J Pediatr.* 1985;106:551-555.
10. Kahn A, Groswasser J, Sottiaux M, et al. Clinical symptoms associated with brief obstructive sleep apnea in normal infants. *Sleep.* 1993;16:409-413.
11. Kato I, Franco P, Groswasser J, Kelmanson I, Togari H, Kahn A. Frequency of obstructive and mixed sleep apneas in 1,023 infants. *Sleep.* 2000;23:487-492.
12. Schwartz BA. Letter: sleep-induced apnea and sudden infant death. *N Engl J Med.* 1974;290:750.
13. Naeye RL. Pulmonary arterial abnormalities in the sudden-infant-death syndrome. *N Engl J Med.* 1973;289:1167-1170.
14. Strohl KP, Saunders NA, Feldman NT, Hallett M. Obstructive sleep apnea in family members. *N Engl J Med.* 1978;299:969-973.
15. Blake AM, Langham J, Collins LM, Reynolds EO. Clinical assessment of apnoea-alarm mattress for newborn infants. *Lancet.* 1970;2:183-185.
16. Caro CG, Bloice JA. Contactless apnoea detector based on radar. *Lancet.* 1971;2:959-961.
17. Smith JE, Scopes JW. A new apnoea alarm for babies. *Lancet.* 1972;2:545-546.
18. Deuel RK. Polygraphic monitoring of apneic spells. *Arch Neurol.* 1973;28:71-76.
19. Stein IM, Shannon DC. The pediatric pneumogram: a new method for detecting and quantitating apnea in infants. *Pediatrics.* 1975;55:599-603.
20. Rowe LD, Hansen TN, Nielson D, Tooley WH. Continuous measurements of skin surface oxygen and carbon dioxide tensions in obstructive sleep apnea. *Laryngoscope.* 1980;90:1797-1803.

21. Grigg-Damberger MM. The visual scoring of sleep in infants 0 to 2 months of age. *J Clin Sleep Med.* 2016;12:429-445.

22. Obstructive sleep apnea, pediatric. In: Sateia M, ed. *International Classification of Sleep Disorders Third Edition.* 3rd ed. Darien, IL: American Academy of Sleep Medicine; 2014:63-68.

23. Katz ES, Mitchell RB, D'Ambrosio CM. Obstructive sleep apnea in infants. *Am J Respir Crit Care Med.* 2012;185:805-816.

24. Rayasam S, Johnson R, Lenahan D, Abijay C, Mitchell RB. Obstructive sleep apnea in children under 3 years of age. *Laryngoscope.* 2021;131:E2603-E2608.

25. Ramgopal S, Kothare SV, Rana M, Singh K, Khatwa U. Obstructive sleep apnea in infancy: a 7-year experience at a pediatric sleep center. *Pediatr Pulmonol.* 2014;49:554-560.

26. Goffinski A, Stanley MA, Shepherd N, et al. Obstructive sleep apnea in young infants with Down syndrome evaluated in a Down syndrome specialty clinic. *Am J Med Genet A.* 2015;167A:324-330.

27. Khayat A, Bin-Hassan S, Al-Saleh S. Polysomnographic findings in infants with Pierre Robin sequence. *Ann Thorac Med.* 2017;12:25-29.

28. Buchenau W, Urschitz MS, Sautermeister J, et al. A randomized clinical trial of a new orthodontic appliance to improve upper airway obstruction in infants with Pierre Robin sequence. *J Pediatr.* 2007;151:145-149.

29. MacLean JE, Fitzsimons D, Fitzgerald DA, Waters KA. The spectrum of sleep-disordered breathing symptoms and respiratory events in infants with cleft lip and/or palate. *Arch Dis Child.* 2012;97:1058-1063.

30. Monasterio FO, Molina F, Berlanga F, et al. Swallowing disorders in Pierre Robin sequence: its correction by distraction. *J Craniofac Surg.* 2004;15:934-941.

31. Morice A, Soupre V, Mitanchez D, et al. Severity of retrognathia and glossoptosis does not predict respiratory and feeding disorders in pierre robin sequence. *Front Pediatr.* 2018;6:351.

32. Ng DK, Chan CH. A review of normal values of infant sleep polysomnography. *Pediatr Neonatol.* 2013;54:82-87.

33. *The AASM Manual for the Scoring of Sleep and Associated Events.* American Academy of Sleep Medicine; 2020. Available at: https://aasm.org/clinical-resources/scoring-manual/. Accessed January 3, 2022.

34. al-Saedi SA, Lemke RP, Haider ZA, Cates DB, Kwiatkowski K, Rigatto H. Prolonged apnea in the preterm infant is not a random event. *Am J Perinatol.* 1997;14:195-200.

35. Spear ML, Stefano JL, Spitzer AR. Prolonged apnea and oxyhemoglobin desaturation in asymptomatic premature infants. *Pediatr Pulmonol.* 1992;13:151-154.

36. Schlüter B, Buschatz D, Trowitzsch E. Polysomnographic reference curves for the first and second year of life. *Somnologie.* 2001;5:3-16.

37. Daftary AS, Jalou HE, Shively L, Slaven JE, Davis SD. Polysomnography reference values in healthy newborns. *J Clin Sleep Med.* 2019;15:437-443.

38. Duenas-Meza E, Bazurto-Zapata MA, Gozal D, Gonzalez-Garcia M, Duran-Cantolla J, Torres-Duque CA. Overnight polysomnographic characteristics and oxygen saturation of healthy infants, 1 to 18 months of age, born and residing at high altitude (2,640 meters). *Chest.* 2015;148:120-127.

39. Scholle S, Wiater A, Scholle HC. Normative values of polysomnographic parameters in childhood and adolescence: cardiorespiratory parameters. *Sleep Med.* 2011;12:988-996.

40. Ramanathan R, Corwin MJ, Hunt CE, et al. Cardiorespiratory events recorded on home monitors: comparison of healthy infants with those at increased risk for SIDS. *JAMA.* 2001;285:2199-2207.

41. DeHaan KL, Seton C, Fitzgerald DA, Waters KA, MacLean JE. Polysomnography for the diagnosis of sleep disordered breathing in children under 2 years of age. *Pediatr Pulmonol.* 2015;50:1346-1353.

42. Carroll JL, McColley SA, Marcus CL, Curtis S, Loughlin GM. Inability of clinical history to distinguish primary snoring from obstructive sleep apnea syndrome in children. *Chest.* 1995;108:610-618.

43. Xu Z, Cheuk DKL, Lee SL. Clinical evaluation in predicting childhood obstructive sleep apnea. *Chest.* 2006;130:1765-1771.

44. Sproson EL, Hogan AM, Hill CM. Accuracy of clinical assessment of paediatric obstructive sleep apnoea in two English centres. *J Laryngol Otol.* 2009;123:1002-1009.

45. Leiberman A, Tal A, Brama I, Sofer S. Obstructive sleep apnea in young infants. *Int J Pediatr Otorhinolaryngol.* 1988;16:39-44.

46. Ward SL, Marcus CL. Obstructive sleep apnea in infants and young children. *J Clin Neurophysiol.* 1996;13:198-207.

47. Greenfeld M, Tauman R, DeRowe A, Sivan Y. Obstructive sleep apnea syndrome due to adenotonsillar hypertrophy in infants. *Int J Pediatr Otorhinolaryngol.* 2003;67:1055-1060.
48. Arens R, Marcus CL. Pathophysiology of upper airway obstruction: a developmental perspective. *Sleep.* 2004;27:997-1019.
49. Terrill PI, Dakin C, Hughes I, Yuill M, Parsley C. Nocturnal oxygen saturation profiles of healthy term infants. *Arch Dis Child.* 2015;100:18-23.
50. Terrill PI, Dakin C, Edwards BA, Wilson SJ, MacLean JE. A graphical method for comparing nocturnal oxygen saturation profiles in individuals and populations: Application to healthy infants and preterm neonates. *Pediatr Pulmonol.* 2018;53:645-655.
51. Brouillette RT, Morielli A, Leimanis A, Waters KA, Luciano R, Ducharme FM. Nocturnal pulse oximetry as an abbreviated testing modality for pediatric obstructive sleep apnea. *Pediatrics.* 2000;105:405-412.
52. Nixon GM, Kermack AS, Davis GM, Manoukian JJ, Brown KA, Brouillette RT. Planning adenotonsillectomy in children with obstructive sleep apnea: the role of overnight oximetry. *Pediatrics.* 2004;113:e19-e25.
53. Makhout S, Boudewyns A, Van Hoorenbeeck K, Verhulst S, Van Eyck A. Nocturnal pulse oximetry as a possible screening method for obstructive sleep apnea in infants with laryngomalacia. *Sleep Med.* 2022;90:91-95.
54. Ehsan Z, He S, Huang G, Hossain MM, Simakajornboon N. Can overnight portable pulse oximetry be used to stratify obstructive sleep apnea risk in infants? A correlation analysis. *Pediatr Pulmonol.* 2020;55:2082-2088.
55. Kirk V, Baughn J, D'Andrea L, et al. American Academy of Sleep Medicine Position Paper for the use of a home sleep apnea test for the diagnosis of OSA in children. *J Clin Sleep Med.* 2017;13:1199-1203.
56. Brockmann PE, Perez JL, Moya A. Feasibility of unattended home polysomnography in children with sleep-disordered breathing. *Int J Pediatr Otorhinolaryngol.* 2013;77:1960-1964.
57. Vézina K, Mariasine J, Young R, et al. Cardiorespiratory monitoring data during sleep in healthy canadian infants. *Ann Am Thorac Soc.* 2020;17:1238-1246.
58. Revana A, Vecchio J, Guffey D, Minard CG, Glaze DG. Clinical application of home sleep apnea testing in children: a prospective pilot study. *J Clin Sleep Med.* 2022;18:533-540.
59. Withers A, Maul J, Rosenheim E, O'Donnell A, Wilson A, Stick S. Comparison of home ambulatory type 2 polysomnography with a portable monitoring device and in-laboratory type 1 polysomnography for the diagnosis of obstructive sleep apnea in children. *J Clin Sleep Med.* 2022;18:393-402.
60. Bhattacharjee R, Benjafield A, Blase A, et al. The accuracy of a portable sleep monitor to diagnose obstructive sleep apnea in adolescent patients. *J Clin Sleep Med.* 2021;17:1379-1387.
61. Ikizoglu NB, Kiyan E, Polat B, Ay P, Karadag B, Ersu R. Are home sleep studies useful in diagnosing obstructive sleep apnea in children with Down syndrome? *Pediatr Pulmonol.* 2019;54:1541-1546.
62. Stark AR, Thach BT. Mechanisms of airway obstruction leading to apnea in newborn infants. *J Pediatr.* 1976;89:982-985.
63. Reddy VS. Evaluation of upper airway obstruction in infants with Pierre Robin sequence and the role of polysomnography—Review of current evidence. *Paediatr Respir Rev.* 2016;17:80-87.
64. Wilson SL, Thach BT, Brouillette RT, Abu-Osba YK. Upper airway patency in the human infant: influence of airway pressure and posture. *J Appl Physiol Respir Environ Exerc Physiol.* 1980;48:500-504.
65. Coutier L, Guyon A, Reix P, Franco P. Impact of prone positioning in infants with Pierre Robin sequence: a polysomnography study. *Sleep Med.* 2019;54:257-261.
66. Kukkola HK, Vuola P, Seppa-Moilanen M, Salminen P, Kirjavainen T. Pierre Robin sequence causes position-dependent obstructive sleep apnoea in infants. *Arch Dis Child.* 2021;106:954-960.
67. Gunn TR, Tonkin SL, Hadden W, Davis SL, Gunn AJ. Neonatal micrognathia is associated with small upper airways on radiographic measurement. *Acta Paediatr.* 2000;89:82-87.
68. Goldberg S, Shatz A, Picard E, et al. Endoscopic findings in children with obstructive sleep apnea: effects of age and hypotonia. *Pediatr Pulmonol.* 2005;40:205-210.
69. Don GW, Kirjavainen T, Broome C, Seton C, Waters KA. Site and mechanics of spontaneous, sleep-associated obstructive apnea in infants. *J Appl Physiol.* 2000;89:2453-2462.
70. Brouilette R, Hanson D, David R, et al. A diagnostic approach to suspected obstructive sleep apnea in children. *J Pediatr.* 1984;105:10-14.
71. Chervin RD, Hedger K, Dillon JE, Pituch KJ. Pediatric sleep questionnaire (PSQ): validity and reliability of scales for sleep-disordered breathing, snoring, sleepiness, and behavioral problems. *Sleep Med.* 2000;1:21-32.

72. Sadeh A. A brief screening questionnaire for infant sleep problems: validation and findings for an Internet sample. *Pediatrics*. 2004;113:e570-e577.

73. Mindell JA, Gould RA, Tikotzy L, Leichman ES, Walters RM. Norm-referenced scoring system for the Brief Infant Sleep Questionnaire—Revised (BISQ-R). *Sleep Med*. 2019;63:106-114.

74. Alvarez D, Kheirandish-Gozal L, Gutierrez-Tobal GC, et al. Automated analysis of nocturnal oximetry as screening tool for childhood obstructive sleep apnea-hypopnea syndrome. *Annu Int Conf IEEE Eng Med Biol Soc*. 2015;2015:2800-2803.

75. Cohen G, de Chazal P. Automated detection of sleep apnea in infants: a multi-modal approach. *Comput Biol Med*. 2015;63:118-123.

76. Vaquerizo-Villar F, Alvarez D, Kheirandish-Gozal L, et al. Detrended fluctuation analysis of the oximetry signal to assist in paediatric sleep apnoea-hypopnoea syndrome diagnosis. *Physiol Meas*. 2018;39:114006.

77. Vaquerizo-Villar F, Alvarez D, Kheirandish-Gozal L, et al. Wavelet analysis of oximetry recordings to assist in the automated detection of moderate-to-severe pediatric sleep apnea-hypopnea syndrome. *PloS One*. 2018;13:e0208502.

78. Vaquerizo-Villar F, Alvarez D, Kheirandish-Gozal L, et al. Utility of bispectrum in the screening of pediatric sleep apnea-hypopnea syndrome using oximetry recordings. *Comput Methods Programs Biomed*. 2018;156:141-149.

79. Vaquerizo-Villar F, Alvarez D, Kheirandish-Gozal L, et al. A convolutional neural network architecture to enhance oximetry ability to diagnose pediatric obstructive sleep apnea. *IEEE J Biomed Health Inform*. 2021;25:2906-2916.

80. Barroso-Garcia V, Gutierrez-Tobal GC, Kheirandish-Gozal L, et al. Usefulness of recurrence plots from airflow recordings to aid in paediatric sleep apnoea diagnosis. *Comput Methods Programs Biomed*. 2020;183:105083.

81. Barroso-Garcia V, Gutierrez-Tobal GC, Gozal D, et al. Wavelet analysis of overnight airflow to detect obstructive sleep apnea in children. *Sensors*. 2021;21(4):1491.

82. Barroso-Garcia V, Gutierrez-Tobal GC, Kheirandish-Gozal L, et al. Bispectral analysis of overnight airflow to improve the pediatric sleep apnea diagnosis. *Comput Biol Med*. 2021;129:104167.

83. Marcus CL, Brooks LJ, Draper KA, et al. Diagnosis and management of childhood obstructive sleep apnea syndrome. *Pediatrics*. 2012;130:576-584.

84. Mitchell RB, Archer SM, Ishman SL, et al. Clinical practice guideline: tonsillectomy in children (update). *Otolaryngol Head Neck Surg*. 2019;160:S1-S42.

85. Aurora RN, Zak RS, Karippot A, et al. Practice parameters for the respiratory indications for polysomnography in children. *Sleep*. 2011;34:379-388.

86. Pamula Y, Nixon GM, Edwards E, et al. Australasian Sleep Association clinical practice guidelines for performing sleep studies in children. *Sleep Med*. 2017;36 suppl 1:S23-S42.

87. Zancanella E, Haddad FM, Oliveira LA, et al. Obstructive sleep apnea and primary snoring: diagnosis. *Rev Bras Otorrinolaringol*. 2014;80:S1-S16.

88. Kaditis AG, Alonso Alvarez ML, Boudewyns A, et al. ERS statement on obstructive sleep disordered breathing in 1- to 23-month-old children. *Eur Respir J*. 2017;50(6):1700985.

Management of Obstructive Sleep Apnea in Infants

Lance Feld ■ Zarmina Ehsan ■ Christopher M. Cielo

General Considerations

Historically, there have been more challenges in the evaluation and management of obstructive sleep apnea (OSA) in infants compared to older children, but more recently OSA has been increasingly recognized and studied in these youngest patients. OSA has been linked to age-specific comorbidities in this age group, including neurocognitive and developmental delays, failure to thrive, and even sudden infant death.[1] Infants are particularly vulnerable to OSA due to anatomical features and REM-predominant sleep distribution and are at further increased risk when there are underlying neurologic or neuromuscular conditions, or issues with respiratory mechanics and ventilatory control.[2] The management of OSA in infants is challenging due to limited age-specific outcome targets, a limited number of devices that would otherwise be appropriate for older children, and the higher proportion of comorbidities in this age group which requires more individualized treatment plans.[1] The limited evidence for treatment guidelines in infants has resulted in variability in management between centers. Even when a treatment plan is put in place, its effectiveness can be affected by various extraneous factors, such as rapid changes in required support due to growth and development.

The decision to initiate treatment for OSA in infants and which modality to utilize may be dependent on a variety of factors, including the child's age, presenting symptoms, etiology of upper airway obstruction, polysomnogram results, and the presence of additional comorbidities, either related to or in addition to OSA.[3] In this chapter, OSA management options will be reviewed, including nonsurgical and surgical, for infants less than 2 years of age (Table 7.1). Additionally, special considerations related to monitoring for treatment efficacy will be considered. Lastly, future directions for infant OSA management will be proposed.

The etiology of sleep-disordered breathing in infants is multifactorial and pathophysiology is unique from older children and adults.[2] Factors such as compromised upper airway anatomy, disadvantaged pulmonary mechanics, ventilatory control immaturity, lower arousal threshold, laryngeal chemoreflex, and a REM-predominant sleep state distribution make infants particularly vulnerable to OSA. Though not currently well described in the literature, OSA risk factors in infants can be conceptualized as discreet but sometimes overlapping endotypes (Fig. 7.1). Broadly speaking, these endotypic categories can be divided into (1) bone abnormalities, (2) soft tissue abnormalities, and (3) other abnormalities that can be targets of management strategies described below.

Medical Management of Infant OSA

Given the potential repercussions of untreated OSA in infants, clinicians must be aware of management options, especially for more severe OSA. Further challenging management, the natural

TABLE 7.1 ■ Summary of Common nonsurgical and Surgical Management Options for Obstructive Sleep Apnea in Infants

Treatment Modality	Mechanism of Action	Benefits	Challenges	Target Populations
Nonsurgical				
Positive airway pressure	Pressurized air acts as a pneumatic stent to maintain airway patency.	May be effective for even moderate-severe OSA. Use and efficacy can be monitored. Noninvasive. Strong evidence to support its efficacy in older patients.	Potential for increased risk of skin breakdown. Difficult to find well-fitting interfaces for infants. Desensitization may be challenging without adequate support. Increased use may predispose to midface hypoplasia.	Moderate-severe OSA when appropriate interface available.
High-flow nasal cannula	Heats and humidifies air, decreases dead space within the upper airway, and reduces upper airway collapse through a continuous stream of positive pressure.	Nasal prongs require less desensitization than PAP interface.	Potential risk for pneumothorax or pneumomediastinum due to air leak. May not be adequate for more severe OSA. Monitoring and titration limited.	Moderate OSA when PAP not available.
Supplemental oxygen	Reduce desaturation associated with obstructive events.	Widely available, nasal cannula more comfortable than PAP interface.	Insufficient for more severe OSA, possibility of blunting respiratory drive.	Mild-moderate OSA and/or hypoxemia without hypoventilation.
Oral/nasal appliances	Bypass oropharyngeal and nasopharyngeal obstruction, respectively.	Noninvasive. Less cumbersome compared to other nonsurgical methods.	Some not widely available. Mucosal irritation, ulcer formation, risk for infection.	Population depends on specific appliance; typically, infants with craniofacial conditions.
Prone positioning	Allows for anterior displacement of tongue base by gravity, relieving the obstruction.	Simple, requires no equipment or intervention.	Ineffective for more significant OSA. May increase risk for SIDS.	Adjunct in glossoptosis with mild OSA.
Surgical				
Adenotonsillectomy	Removal of obstructing adenoid and tonsillar tissue.	Highly effective first-line treatment for OSA related to adenotonsillar hypertrophy.	Infants may be at greater risk for significant postoperative complications. Most infants will not have adenotonsillar hypertrophy and will not be candidates.	Those with adenotonsillar hypertrophy as the primary cause of OSA.

Procedure	Description	Benefit	Complications/Considerations	Candidates
Tongue-lip adhesion (TLA)	Surgical fixation between the lip and tongue, a form of glossopexy. Meant to prevent posterior displacement of the tongue resulting in obstruction.	May negate the need for tracheostomy in patients with RS and severe OSA.	Higher rates of complications and residual OSA as compared to MDO. Less likely to prevent the need for tracheostomy, compared to MDO, in patients with RS and severe OSA.	Those with micro- or retrognathia and moderate-severe OSA from glossoptosis.
Mandibular distraction osteogenesis (MDO)	Involves bilateral osteotomies of the mandibular rami and distractor placement bilaterally, allowing for sequential lengthening of the hypoplastic mandible.	Highly effective in many patients, even with very severe OSA. May be associated with improved ability to feed.	Potential complications may include malunion or misalignment of the involved bones, and infection.	Those with micro- or retrognathia and moderate-severe OSA from glossoptosis.
Tongue reduction	Debulking of an enlarged tongue to reduce oropharyngeal obstruction.	May negate the need for invasive respiratory support.	No consensus on appropriate timing. Potential complications include wound dehiscence and surgical revision. May impact dental outcomes and dentoalveolar development.	Those with moderate-severe OSA related to macroglossia (i.e., Beckwith-Wiedemann syndrome).
Supraglottoplasty	Includes making an incision in the aryepiglottic folds releasing the epiglottis and removing redundant tissues which result in collapse of the larynx on inspiration.	May obviate the need for tracheostomy, previously the primary treatment for those with OSA and laryngomalacia.	Potential complications include cough and dysphagia. Potential need for surgical revision. Efficacy of procedure versus natural history of condition unclear.	Those with laryngomalacia.
Tracheostomy	Use of an adjunctive and artificial airway to bypass upper airway obstruction.	Definitive treatment to bypass upper airway obstruction. Improved symptoms in adult populations.	Invasive procedure with potential complications (i.e., tracheostomy tube occlusion, accidental decannulation).	Those with limited treatment options or OSA refractory to surgical intervention.

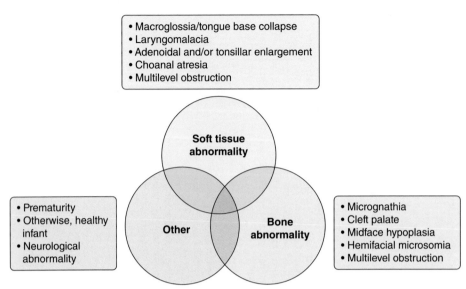

Fig. 7.1 Conceptual model of infant OSA endotypes.

history of OSA in some conditions associated with OSA in infants and young children is poorly understood, and the need for and type of intervention may change over time. For example, patients with nonsyndromic micrognathia may have severe OSA during the neonatal period, but mandibular growth is expected to occur. In these instances, temporizing therapies with a nasopharyngeal airway, positive airway pressure, or other nonsurgical therapies may be sufficient.[2] In contrast, infants with syndromic micrognathia such as Treacher Collins syndrome may not experience sufficient mandibular growth and may be more appropriately referred for surgical intervention, discussed below.

Ultimately, the decision about the most appropriate therapy should incorporate a variety of factors, including the severity of the OSA from objective testing, as well as accompanying comorbidities, the projected prognosis for the patient's underlying medical condition, and available treatment options. For mild OSA without significant clinical concerns, the decision to manage with watchful waiting may be appropriate. There are a variety of nonsurgical treatment options for infants with OSA, reviewed below.

POSITIVE AIRWAY PRESSURE

While adenotonsillectomy is considered first-line treatment for pediatric OSA,[4] positive airway pressure (PAP) is an acceptable option for those without adenotonsillar hypertrophy or where adenotonsillectomy is contraindicated.[5,6] PAP has previously been shown to improve symptoms in children with OSA and has led to improvements on polysomnogram including both decreased apnea-hypopnea indices and increased arterial oxygen saturation, as well as improved quality of life, and positive impacts on cardiovascular risk.[7-9] Adherence to PAP can be challenging and thus a multimodal approach can help ease this burden, particularly in infants.

PAP is prescribed as either continuous positive airway pressure (CPAP) or bilevel positive airway pressure. Auto-titrating PAP is available, but not currently appropriate for infants. PAP works by delivering pressurized air, acting as a pneumatic stent to maintain airway patency, preventing obstruction.[4] Most PAP devices for the treatment of OSA are designed for adults and

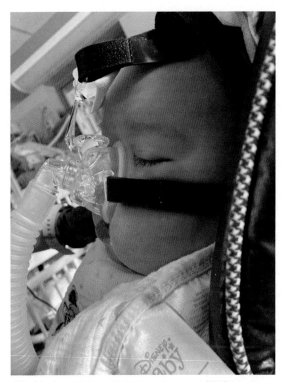

Fig. 7.2 Lateral view of infant wearing nasal CPAP interface.

larger children. In many cases, infants will not meet the minimum weight requirement for PAP machines and will require a portable home ventilator. When fitting a particular infant for an interface with which to supply the prescribed PAP, there are fewer options available and additional challenges for patients with craniofacial differences. Traditionally, nasal masks (Fig. 7.2) are the preferred option for infants due to availability, fit, and safety. While there are some naso-oral or full-face interfaces, there could be risk of harm by aspiration with these in the home environment, particularly if the child is not being directly observed. Another option is nonoccluding nasal prongs, although these come with their own challenges, including a lack of occlusion with air leak, resulting in lower pressures, and making this device less likely to be effective for more severe OSA.[10] After initiating PAP, polysomnography should be used to titrate to an effective pressure, as with older children and adults.

While there are a limited number of studies to objectively assess the utility of PAP in infants with OSA, there is some data to support its effectiveness. In an early report of 74 infants less than 12 months, followed closely for a mean duration of nearly 3 years, all but two were successfully able to use PAP.[11] Another study from 1999 evaluated a cohort of infants who underwent overnight polysomnography to assess the severity of their OSA and followed them longitudinally.[12] The authors found that CPAP was useful in preventing obstruction and improving sleep disturbance associated with OSA. Most of the cohort (18/24, 75%) used CPAP at home, in some cases for greater than 4 years. In a more recent retrospective study from our group, the efficacy of CPAP in 41 infants less than 6 months old was compared to a cohort of school-age children (5–10 years of age) with OSA underwent both baseline and titration polysomnography after having started PAP.[1] Despite having more severe baseline OSA, a similar proportion of infants were effectively titrated with PAP compared to their older counterparts, and machine downloads showed that infants used PAP more. Surprisingly, the barriers to use were similar between the two groups.

While PAP can be an effective treatment modality for infants with OSA, adherence can be a challenge, as with older patients. Identifying potential barriers to PAP use is important for the medical team to address, and caregiver efficacy is an important concept. Though studied in older children and adolescents, it has been shown that caregiver-reported self-efficacy plays an important role in predicting PAP adherence.[13] Additional challenges in infants include frequently changing infant sleeping patterns and rapid growth, which may necessitate changes in the interface as well as required pressures. For infants, our practice is to frequently reevaluate PAP use and barriers with families in the clinic and reevaluate the need for PAP and required pressures with titration studies in the sleep laboratory, particularly during the first year of life, when there can be frequent changes. Potential side effects of PAP in infants may include nasal congestion, sensitive skin, and an increased risk for skin breakdown.[14] With prolonged use, there is also a potential risk for midface hypoplasia, particularly in infants with craniofacial clefts. The long-term success of CPAP for infants lies within the abilities and capabilities of the medical team to not just prepare the child for home but the family as well.

HIGH-FLOW NASAL CANNULA

High-flow nasal cannula (HFNC) is a noninvasive treatment option that has been studied in both adults and children with respiratory insufficiency.[15] HFNC both heats and humidifies air, and its mechanism lies in both decreasing dead space within the upper airway and preventing upper airway collapse through substantial airflow that can provide positive pressure.[16] HFNC is delivered through a nasal cannula interface, sometimes occluding a greater portion of the nares than a traditional low-flow cannula.

HFNC could be an alternative to PAP in young children and infants, particularly when there is not a PAP interface with a good fit, such as very small infants or those with craniofacial differences. A 2013 randomized controlled trial compared the efficacy of HFNC to nasal CPAP among 432 infants in a neonatal intensive care unit who were candidates for PAP.[17] They found that infants randomized to the HFNC arm of the trial were no more likely to require intubation or supplemental oxygen compared to those randomized to CPAP. Specific to OSA, it has been previously demonstrated that HFNC can result in a significant reduction in obstructive events and can help alleviate symptoms. A recent 2020 retrospective study of 22 infants with OSA found that HFNC led to a significant reduction in obstructive events (28.9 events/hour versus 2.6 events/hour, $P < 0.001$).[18] Overall, it appears that HFNC might be an alternative treatment modality for infants who would otherwise be candidates for PAP.

SUPPLEMENTAL OXYGEN

Low-flow supplemental oxygen has previously been used to treat OSA in adult populations, and its use in children has also been documented. In a limited number of pediatric studies, low-flow supplemental oxygen has been shown to improve oxyhemoglobin saturation and decrease obstructive events primarily by decreasing desaturation needed to score hypopnea, without necessarily a concomitant decrease in ventilatory drive.[19,20] While the literature is scarce, there may be utility in using low-flow supplemental oxygen in the treatment of OSA in infants. One recent study evaluated polysomnography data in a cohort of infants who underwent two sequential sleep studies, initially without and then with supplemental oxygen.[21] This study found that the use of low-flow supplemental oxygen was associated with improved oxygenation and fewer obstructive events. Importantly, there was no significant difference in alveolar ventilation as measured by both end-tidal CO_2 or transcutaneous CO_2 monitoring. While additional studies may be needed to evaluate long-term outcomes, there appears to be some preliminary data to support the use of low-flow supplemental oxygen in this age group.

ORAL AND NASAL APPLIANCES

Primarily studied in patients with Robin sequence (RS), who classically present with micrognathia and/or retrognathia with glossoptosis, oral appliances may result in some improvement to OSA due to relief of tongue-based obstruction.[22] OSA in patients with RS results from posterior movement of the tongue base toward the posterior pharyngeal wall, which can be accompanied by inward collapse of the lateral pharyngeal walls. Treatment should focus on both shifting the tongue forward and stabilizing the pharynx. Unlike strategies which are more invasive, including tongue-lip adhesion, mandibular distraction osteogenesis, and tracheostomy, noninvasive alternatives that allow correction of tongue displacement and pharyngeal stability are needed. Oral appliances, including the pre-epiglottic baton plate (PEBP), consist of a hard acrylic plate made to fit the patient based on a silicone impression of the oropharynx, attached to a hard acrylic velar extension.[23] One case series with long-term follow-up showed a significant decrease in the mixed-obstructive-apnea index at time of discharge and near resolution 3 months later in a small cohort of infants with RS and OSA.[24] The PEBP, and a similar apparatus named the Tuebingen palatal place, have been used in other populations as well, including infants with femoral facial syndrome and Down syndrome.[25-27] In addition to OSA, these devices may also allow for both swallowing and phonation development.[23] These devices may not be widely available, and thus providers may need to consider alternative options.

Like an oral appliance, an oropharyngeal airway or nasopharyngeal airway (NPA) also has been used in children to bypass nasopharyngeal obstruction. Predominantly used in adults, it has also been studied in infants with syndromic craniosynostosis or glossoptosis with concurrent OSA. With midface hypoplasia known to be a contributing factor to OSA in patients with syndromic craniosynostosis, a study out of the United Kingdom looked at the efficacy of using an NPA to bypass midface obstruction in both infants and children with moderate-severe OSA.[28] In this study, 27 children aged 5 months through 48 months with syndromic craniosynostosis and moderate to severe OSA were treated with an NPA. Results showed an improvement in AHI in 96% of the cohort, in addition to oxyhemoglobin saturation, although most still had mild residual OSA. Risk of the NPA include mucosal irritation resulting in pain or bleeding and nasal ulcers/infections,[29] some of which can be mitigated by adjustments to NPA tube size, shape, and material. Most studies assessing its efficacy have done so in the postoperative period or for short-term use, and there is little data to support its long-term use, which may impact both its availability and its use in general.

POSITIONING

In some patients, prone positioning during sleep can reduce the effect of gravity on upper airway collapsibility, particularly related to tongue-based obstruction. Therefore, prone positioning may be used in infants, including those with glossoptosis, although its efficacy remains unclear. One case series of three infants with micrognathia and severe OSA found that there was a significant improvement in obstructive polysomnographic indices with prone positioning compared to supine positioning, with one having complete resolution and one other with mild residual OSA.[30] However, a recent study compared polysomnographic data in 11 infants with RS in the supine and prone positions who were turned halfway through a diagnostic sleep study.[31] In this small cohort, results showed that there was a significant decrease in the OAHI in some infants when turned prone versus supine, but significant OSA persisted in most cases. In a retrospective chart review of 23 infants with cleft palate who slept in both the supine and prone positions during a polysomnogram, there were no significant improvements in polysomnographic metrics, including apnea-hypopnea index and gas exchange data, between the two sleep positions.[32] Even in the setting of improved OSA, one must also consider the concurrent risk of sudden infant death syndrome in young infants who are turned prone while asleep. Overall, the data to support prone positioning is limited, and additional evidence is necessary to support its use in infancy. Polysomnography should be performed in infants in the prone position to evaluate for efficacy.

Surgical Management of Infant OSA

General indications for surgical management of OSA include moderate-to-severe OSA on polysomnography as well as overnight and daytime symptoms and failure or lack more conservative medical management.[3] Surgical options are targeted to the site of obstruction, which may include the nasal cavity, nasopharynx, oropharynx, and hypopharynx. In children, adenotonsillectomy is considered first-line treatment for children with obstructive sleep apnea who have adenotonsillar hypertrophy.[5] While some patients less than 2 years old with OSA do have adenotonsillar hypertrophy, there are a variety of additional anatomic factors specific to this age group which are important to address and will dictate surgical management. In this section, we will review the most common surgical treatments used in the treatment of infant OSA.

ADENOTONSILLAR HYPERTROPHY

Adenotonsillar hypertrophy is a major contributor to OSA in older children, and the definitive treatment for many children is adenotonsillectomy. In contrast, in neonates and infants, a smaller portion will have enlarged adenoids and tonsils, particularly as the peak age for adenoid and tonsillar hypertrophy with associated OSA may be between 3 and 6 years of age.[33,34] Though adenotonsillectomy can be performed in infants, particularly 12 to 24 months old, there is the potential for increased complications, so the procedure should be done with additional monitoring in place for complications such as oxyhemoglobin desaturation, laryngospasm, airway obstruction due to edema, and postobstructive pulmonary edema.[35,36]

The American Academy of Otolaryngology—Head and Neck Surgery clinical practice guidelines, most recently updated in 2019, provides evidence-based recommendations for pre-, intra-, and postoperative care for children 1 to 18 years of age undergoing tonsillectomy.[37] For children with sleep-disordered breathing, polysomnography is recommended for children less than 2 years old in addition to those who are obese, have Down syndrome, craniofacial abnormalities, and mucopolysaccharidoses, among others. With regards to postoperative monitoring, the 2019 guidelines recommend overnight, inpatient monitoring for children less than 3 years of age, or who have severe OSA (defined as an apnea-hypopnea index (AHI) ≥ 10 events per hour and/or an SpO_2 nadir $<80\%$).

Several studies have evaluated the safety and efficacy of adenotonsillectomy in infants. One recent study that compared adenoidectomy complications, including postoperative bleeding and hypoxemia, in infants under 1 year of age to those between 3 and 5 years old[38] found that the rates of complication were low and did not vary significantly across age groups. A separate case series looked at the efficacy of adenotonsillectomy in 25 infants with OSA younger than 1 year of age, of which 12 were otherwise healthy and 13 had significant comorbid conditions including Down syndrome, prematurity, hypoxic-ischemic encephalopathy, and heart disease.[39] They found that adenotonsillectomy was successful in treating OSA through a combination of subjective improvement in symptomatology and postoperative polysomnography; however, the success rate was higher in those who were otherwise healthy compared to infants with comorbid conditions. Postoperative complications, including dehydration, persistent hypoxemia, and bleeding, occurred in 25% and 33% of healthy patients and those with comorbid conditions, respectively.

While the use of adenotonsillectomy in infants remains more complex than in older children, studies have demonstrated usefulness in treating OSA. As explored below, other etiologies for OSA, including some comorbid conditions, can drastically have an impact on management options.

ROBIN SEQUENCE/MICROGNATHIA

RS results from maldevelopment of the mandible resulting in micrognathia, subsequent glossoptosis, and ultimately upper airway obstruction.[40] While some infants with RS have an identified syndrome such as Stickler syndrome or Treacher Collins syndrome, others have micrognathia as an isolated finding. The severity of OSA in infants with RS is high variable, and management includes both nonsurgical and surgical modalities.[41] While in more mild cases, conservative methods may be used (see above), those with severe obstruction often require surgical therapy during the neonatal period.

Tongue-lip adhesion (TLA) is a procedure that dates to the 1940s when it was popularized as a treatment for airway obstruction in RS and has since gone through various iterations.[42] The procedure itself involves surgical fixation between the lip and tongue, a form of glossopexy, to prevent posterior displacement of the tongue resulting in obstruction.[43] While reports of this procedure include improvements in OSA among infants, the cohorts of patients being studied are small, and to our knowledge, there is little longitudinal follow-up to support its efficacy. Furthermore, some patients have been found to require either repeat TLA or secondary surgery such as mandibular distraction or tracheostomy.[44-46] In one 2009 study of 22 patients who underwent TLA for RS, 55% of the cohort developed a complication, with the 2 most common being wound dehiscence and chin abscess formation.[44] While TLA might be an effective treatment modality for some, there are few studies that have included polysomnography and other objective outcomes of OSA improvement.

Mandibular distraction osteogenesis (MDO) is another option for surgical management of micrognathia in infants with severe OSA. MDO involves bilateral osteotomies of the mandibular rami and distractor placement bilaterally, allowing for sequential lengthening of the hypoplastic mandible.[47] There have been several studies assessing the efficacy of MDO on OSA and feeding in the neonatal period. A longitudinal analysis of 31 neonates with RS and severe OSA who underwent MDO (median age at time of surgery of 23 days) found significant improvement in polysomnographic parameters, including a reduction in OAHI and improvements in both sleep efficiency and SpO_2 nadir.[48] Of note, though there was substantial improvement in the severity of OSA postoperatively, all patients had some degree of residual OSA. Some patients with RS and severe airway obstruction may need tracheostomy, particularly those with underlying neurologic disease, but MDO may be an alternative. One recent study showed successful treatment of severe OSA using MDO in a series of five infants with tongue-based obstruction without micrognathia, with all avoiding tracheostomy and two requiring respiratory support by either nasal cannula or CPAP postoperatively.[49] Complications of MDO may include tooth injury, nerve injury, infection, scarring, injury to the temporomandibular joint, and device failure.[50] Careful planning and proper surgical technique can help mitigate some of these occurrences, but these complications are important to keep in mind.

A recent 2018 review of 67 studies compared the effectiveness between TLA and MDO in children with RS.[51] They found that higher percentages of patients with MDO, as compared to TLA, avoided tracheostomy (95% versus 89%) and achieved full oral feeds (87% versus 70%). Additionally, rate of recurrent intervention due to residual obstruction was lower in the MDO group (4%–6%) as compared to the TLA group (22%–45%). There was too much variability between the study methodology to allow for metaanalysis. In a study of 1289 infants with micrognathia hospitalized in tertiary-care neonatal intensive care units who required surgical intervention, those undergoing MDO had significantly lower rates of secondary airway surgery and greater rates of exclusive oral feeding at hospital discharge compared to TLA.[52] Ultimately, both TLA and MDO appear to be viable surgical options for those with RS and OSA. Patient selection, like with other surgical procedures, appears to be crucial to ensure successful outcomes in this cohort. Additional studies are necessary to monitor the long-term outcomes of this procedure, as are studies looking at individual syndromes and clinical trials comparing different surgeries (or surgery versus nonsurgical management) to compare outcomes.

MACROGLOSSIA

Like mandibular hypoplasia, tongue-based airway obstruction in infants may occur because of macroglossia (Fig. 7.3), which may occur as part of an underlying syndrome, from a tumor, or in isolation. The degree of OSA in infants with macroglossia is related to the relative size of the tongue to the rest of the oral cavity as well as muscle tone and the presence of other airway abnormalities. The most common congenital syndrome resulting in macroglossia is Beckwith-Wiedemann syndrome (BWS), a pediatric overgrowth disorder characterized by hyperinsulinism, omphalocele, hemihypertrophy, distinct facial features, and increased risk for embryonal tumors.[53,54] As many as 50% of infants and children with BWS have OSA, and infants may be at the greatest risk due to more severe relative macroglossia.[54,55] In addition, macroglossia may be seen in infants with mucopolysaccharidoses, Down syndrome, and with hemangiomas and lymphangiomas.

Surgical tongue reduction, also called glossectomy, may be used to manage severe OSA in infants with macroglossia.[56] The surgical methods can vary depending on the bulk and shape of the tongue, as well as the degree of obstruction, and there are a variety of techniques. Likewise, the timing of this procedure is also highly variable. Some studies have cautioned against tongue reduction before 6 to 12 months of age due to the risk of surgical complications or tongue regrowth, while other studies recommend earlier intervention, as craniofacial deformities may progress with time.[57] Despite this uncertainty, tongue reduction surgery has been used successfully in infants with severe OSA and may allow infants to be able to avoid tracheostomy. As demonstrated in a recent retrospective review of infants with BWS who underwent tongue reduction surgery, there was a significant improvement in polysomnographic parameters (including OAHI and SpO_2 nadir).[57] There were few postoperative complications, but one patient did develop wound dehiscence and require surgical reclosure, while another did require additional tongue reduction. Long-term studies comparing outcomes of different infant populations who have had tongue reduction versus other therapies, at different ages, with varying sizes of debulked tongue are needed to evaluate the impacts on OSA as well as speech, feeding, and dental outcomes.

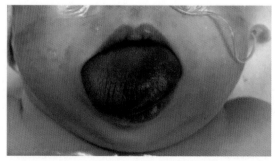

Fig. 7.3 Macroglossia in an infant who subsequently underwent tongue reduction surgery.

LARYNGOMALACIA

Laryngomalacia is a disorder characterized by supraglottic tissue collapse with resultant airflow obstruction, classically a cause of inspiratory stridor in infants.[58] While the prevalence of OSA in infants with laryngomalacia is unclear, OSA has been reported in nearly 100% of those who undergo surgical intervention for severe laryngomalacia.[59] Tracheostomy was previously considered the primary surgical treatment for laryngomalacia; however, newer techniques have evolved, including supraglottoplasty, improving symptoms and decreasing morbidity.[60] With a supraglottoplasty, an incision is made in the aryepiglottic folds, releasing the epiglottis, in addition to removing redundant tissues including the lateral edges of the epiglottis which result in collapse of the larynx on inspiration.[2]

Few studies have evaluated the utility of supraglottoplasty for the treatment of OSA. A 2011 study by Powitzky et al. retrospectively evaluated the clinical and polysomnographic effects of this procedure.[59] This study found improvements in the OAHI, SpO_2 nadir, and percentage of sleep spent with <90% O_2 saturation postsupraglottoplasty compared to presurgical values and that postoperative improvements were associated with improvements in symptoms. A more recent study from 2021 assessed sleep and respiratory parameters in infants with laryngomalacia and either OSA or central sleep apnea (CSA), comparing those who underwent supraglottoplasty to those who did not.[61] This study found that both OSA and CSA improved with age, regardless of whether they had undergone supraglottoplasty. While supraglottoplasty was associated with an earlier age for resolution of CSA, this was not the case for those with OSA, reflecting the impact that underlying genetic and neurologic disease has on those with OSA. While some infants with both laryngomalacia and OSA may benefit from supraglottoplasty, developmental changes, most notably airway growth and maturation of respiratory control, may mitigate the need for surgery. Additional studies in infants, particularly those evaluating long-term outcomes, are necessary to better understand which patients would benefit most from this procedure and the long-term impacts.

CONGENITAL NASAL OBSTRUCTION

Though uncommon, congenital nasal obstruction can cause upper airway obstruction, particularly as infants are obligate nasal breathers for the first several months of life.[62] Depending on the degree of obstruction, infants may present with tachypnea, nasal flaring, apnea, and cyanosis. These congenital airway abnormalities can cause increased upper airway resistance resulting in OSA and can become life-threatening if not addressed promptly. Choanal atresia is a congenital narrowing of the posterior nasal airway and can be unilateral or bilateral.[2] It can be associated with genetic conditions including CHARGE syndrome, Treacher Collins syndrome, and Crouzon syndrome, and whereas unilateral choanal atresia may be more insidious in presentation, bilateral choanal atresia presents immediately after birth with severe airway obstruction. A transnasal approach to repair with stenting is typically used to treat infants with choanal atresia, and in newborns with bilateral choanal atresia, this procedure is typically done as soon as possible.[63] Follow-up surgery may be necessary, as recurrent stenosis can occur, necessitating further dilation. A similar, but distinct, cause of upper airway obstruction is congenital nasal pyriform aperture stenosis. While its associated clinical features may mimic those of choanal atresia, pyriform aperture stenosis is described by the narrowing of the anterior bony nasal apertures, which anatomically represent the narrowest portion of the normal nasal airway.[64] Pyriform aperture stenosis can present in an isolated fashion or can present with other anomalies including midface dysostosis and central nervous system abnormalities. Initially, patients may require an oropharyngeal airway or other conservative measures for treatment; however, if more conservative methods fail or the stenosis is severe, surgical aims would include widening of the bony inlet at the stenosed segment using a sublabial approach.

SEVERE AIRWAY OBSTRUCTION

For some infants with OSA, surgical treatment options during the neonatal period may be limited, such as those with syndromic craniosynostoses (i.e., Apert syndrome), while others may have severe OSA which is refractory to surgical intervention. A definitive treatment for severe OSA, tracheostomy bypasses the anatomical obstruction. In adult populations, tracheostomy has improved symptoms associated with OSA, including daytime sleepiness and fatigue.[65] Studies evaluating outcomes from tracheostomy in infants and children with severe OSA are lacking. A recent multicenter review of a cohort of infants and children who underwent tracheostomy for severe OSA demonstrated that a vast majority of these patients had some form of underlying disease, including craniofacial conditions, Down syndrome, and hypotonia associated with neuromuscular disease.[65] Postoperatively, there were substantial improvements in clinical data, including a mean 89% decrease in AHI and a 29% increase in SpO_2 nadir. Of those patients followed beyond 2 years, only one patient (6%) was successfully decannulated at the 2-year mark.

These findings highlight an important difference between adults who require tracheostomy for OSA, who are often overweight or obese, and infants/children. For children, the most common risk factors for OSA, adenotonsillar hypertrophy and obesity, do not appear to be contributing factors for those who ultimately require tracheostomy.[65] There is limited data on the duration of tracheostomy for children with severe OSA, but typically decannulation would be an option after substantial growth or definitive surgical intervention, as with midface advancement in children with syndromic craniosynostosis. Though tracheostomy appears to be a viable treatment option, one must also consider the potential complications which may include tracheostomy tube occlusion or accidental decannulation, as well as prolonged hospitalizations immediately after tracheostomy placement and the need for continuous observation to monitor for airway emergency.[66] A 2016 retrospective review of 302 children who underwent tracheostomy at a mean age of 5 months[67] found that nearly 20% of children had a tracheostomy-related complication, most notably wound breakdown in 65% of those with complications. Accidental decannulation was rare, and there were no deaths reported. Ultimately, in severe cases patients may have limited options other than tracheostomy, and individualized care should be provided for those at risk. In all cases, continued assessment should aim to evaluate for options for decannulation with definitive surgical or medical management.

Special Considerations

REPEAT POLYSOMNOGRAPHY

Determining the optimal therapy for an individual infant with OSA is challenging and monitoring the efficacy of the chosen treatment modality can be equally so. In a recent statement from the European Respiratory Society (ERS),[68] it was suggested that in infants, polysomnography should be repeated every 2 to 4 months during the first year of life following initiation of CPAP and every 6 months thereafter.[68] One recent study retrospectively analyzed both infants and older children with OSA who underwent repeat PAP titration studies and found that repeat polysomnography did not result in significant changes in PAP modality, PAP pressure settings, or OAHI.[69] However, there may be greater changes in OSA severity in a short period of time for infants, so we recommend frequent reassessment to determine if PAP can be stopped or pressure adjustments need to be made. In addition to repeat polysomnography, the need to monitor growth, development, and response to illness are all potential markers to monitor treatment. For some infants, particularly in complex cases, multiple treatments may be required. This highlights the individualization required in each case and difficulties providers face in treating this age group. In many cases, a multidisciplinary approach that includes the parents, as well as medical and surgical specialists, may be needed to review potential treatment options in a stepwise approach.

WATCHFUL WAITING

Watchful waiting involves repeat clinical assessment of disease progression without active treatment and assumes that many infants with OSA will improve as they grow, such that in mild cases, active treatment may not always be necessary. While some children may improve spontaneously, the natural history of OSA in this age group is not completely understood, and thus the benefit of treating milder OSA versus watchful waiting is unclear. The childhood adenotonsillectomy trial (CHAT), which assessed the effectiveness of adenotonsillectomy in children ages 5 to 9 years old, found that data based on behavior, quality of life, and polysomnographic parameters supported early adenotonsillectomy as compared to watchful waiting.[70] A smaller randomized controlled trial evaluated the effectiveness of early adenotonsillectomy versus watchful waiting in 60 children with mild-moderate OSA between 2 and 4 years of age.[71] While there were small differences between both groups on repeat polysomnography, there was a much greater improvement in quality of life using the OSA-18 questionnaire in the adenotonsillectomy group compared to watchful waiting. To our knowledge, no such trials exist specifically evaluating the outcomes of watchful waiting versus either nonsurgical or surgical management in infants.

Future Directions

When considering the management options for infant OSA, there remains a bevy of unanswered questions and the need to address a number of key areas. There is a need for longitudinal studies to better understand the natural history of OSA in infants with a variety of underlying conditions mentioned above. While there may be a role for conservative management for mild OSA in infants, depending on the underlying cause of obstruction in these patients, this might obviate the need for more aggressive intervention, and longitudinal studies or comparative effectiveness trials could evaluate different approaches. Better understanding of the expected prognosis could have serious implications on both diagnostic and therapeutic management. Secondly, there is a need for infant-specific outcomes in therapy studies, including biomarkers, PSG targets, and/or more traditional outcomes like cardiovascular or neurodevelopmental changes. Much of the literature discussing both nonsurgical and surgical outcomes of treatments for infant OSA are either single-center studies or case studies. Many of these studies are either small or are not exclusive to infants. There is a need for multicenter studies evaluating the efficacy of treatment approaches specifically targeting this age group, both for common and rare conditions, which might allow for evidence-based consensus to standardize care.

Conclusions

There are a variety of treatment options, including surgical and nonsurgical, available for infants with OSA. Given the lack of evidence-based guidelines in this age group, much of what we know about the management of infant OSA comes either from smaller studies of infants less than 2 years or extrapolation from older children. Despite this, infant OSA is a growing topic of discussion, particularly as objective treatment outcomes including polysomnography are increasingly being used clinically and in studies evaluating treatment of OSA in this age group. Depending on the underlying comorbidities, there may be a role for either nonsurgical or surgical management of their OSA, or in some cases both, and shared decision-making with input from families is critical in determining the best approach. As this field continues to develop, there will need to be both an increase in clinicians willing to treat these patients as well as the development of evidence-based guidelines to help guide management.

References

1. Cielo CM, Hernandez P, Ciampaglia AM, Xanthopoulos MS, Beck SE, Tapia IE. Positive airway pressure for the treatment of OSA in infants. *Chest.* 2021;159(2):810-817.
2. Katz ES, Mitchell RB, D'Ambrosio CM. Obstructive sleep apnea in infants. *Am J Respir Crit Care Med.* 2012;185(8):805-816.
3. Holty JE, Guilleminault C. Surgical options for the treatment of obstructive sleep apnea. *Med Clin North Am.* 2010;94(3):479-515.
4. Gordon P, Sanders MH. Sleep.7: Positive airway pressure therapy for obstructive sleep apnoea/hypopnoea syndrome. *Thorax.* 2005;60(1):68-75.
5. Section on Pediatric Pulmonology, Subcommittee on Obstructive Sleep Apnea Syndrome, American Academy of Pediatrics. Clinical practice guideline: diagnosis and management of childhood obstructive sleep apnea syndrome. *Pediatrics.* 2002;109(4):704-712.
6. Cielo CM, Gungor A. Treatment options for pediatric obstructive sleep apnea. *Curr Probl Pediatr Adolesc Health Care.* 2016;46(1):27-33.
7. Marcus CL, Rosen G, Ward SL, et al. Adherence to and effectiveness of positive airway pressure therapy in children with obstructive sleep apnea. *Pediatrics.* 2006;117(3):e442-e451.
8. Katz SL, MacLean JE, Barrowman N, et al. Long-term impact of sleep-disordered breathing on quality of life in children with obesity. *J Clin Sleep Med.* 2018;14(3):451-458.
9. Kirk VG, Edgell H, Joshi H, Constantin E, Katz SL, MacLean JE. Cardiovascular changes in children with obstructive sleep apnea and obesity after treatment with noninvasive ventilation. *J Clin Sleep Med.* 2020;16(12):2063-2071.
10. Singh N, McNally MJ, Darnall RA. Does the ram cannula provide continuous positive airway pressure as effectively as the Hudson prongs in preterm neonates? *Am J Perinatol.* 2019;36(8):849-854.
11. Guilleminault C, Pelayo R, Clerk A, Leger D, Bocian RC. Home nasal continuous positive airway pressure in infants with sleep-disordered breathing. *J Pediatr.* 1995;127(6):905-912.
12. McNamara F, Sullivan CE. Obstructive sleep apnea in infants and its management with nasal continuous positive airway pressure. *Chest.* 1999;116(1):10-16.
13. Xanthopoulos MS, Kim JY, Blechner M, et al. Self-efficacy and short-term adherence to continuous positive airway pressure treatment in children. *Sleep.* 2017;40(7). doi:10.1093/sleep/zsx096.
14. Marcus CL, Ward SL, Mallory GB, et al. Use of nasal continuous positive airway pressure as treatment of childhood obstructive sleep apnea. *J Pediatr.* 1995;127(1):88-94.
15. Kwon JW. High-flow nasal cannula oxygen therapy in children: a clinical review. *Clin Exp Pediatr.* 2020;63(1):3-7.
16. Joseph L, Goldberg S, Shitrit M, Picard E. High-flow nasal cannula therapy for obstructive sleep apnea in children. *J Clin Sleep Med.* 2015;11(9):1007-1010.
17. Yoder BA, Stoddard RA, Li M, King J, Dirnberger DR, Abbasi S. Heated, humidified high-flow nasal cannula versus nasal CPAP for respiratory support in neonates. *Pediatrics.* 2013;131(5):e1482-e1490.
18. Ignatiuk D, Schaer B, McGinley B. High flow nasal cannula treatment for obstructive sleep apnea in infants and young children. *Pediatr Pulmonol.* 2020;55(10):2791-2798.
19. Marcus CL, Carroll JL, Bamford O, Pyzik P, Loughlin GM. Supplemental oxygen during sleep in children with sleep-disordered breathing. *Am J Respir Crit Care Med.* 1995;152(4 Pt 1):1297-1301.
20. Aljadeff G, Gozal D, Bailey-Wahl SL, Burrell B, Keens TG, Ward SL. Effects of overnight supplemental oxygen in obstructive sleep apnea in children. *Am J Respir Crit Care Med.* 1996;153(1):51-55.
21. Brockbank J, Astudillo CL, Che D, et al. Supplemental oxygen for treatment of infants with obstructive sleep apnea. *J Clin Sleep Med.* 2019;15(8):1115-1123.
22. Kukkola HK, Vuola P, Seppa-Moilanen M, Salminen P, Kirjavainen T. Pierre Robin sequence causes position-dependent obstructive sleep apnoea in infants. *Arch Dis Child.* 2021;106(10):954-960.
23. Schmidt G, Hirschfelder A, Heiland M, Matuschek C. Customized pre-epiglottic baton plate-a practical guide for successful, patient-specific, noninvasive treatment of neonates with robin sequence. *Cleft Palate Craniofac J.* 2021;58(8):1063-1069.
24. Bacher M, Sautermeister J, Urschitz MS, Buchenau W, Arand J, Poets CF. An oral appliance with velar extension for treatment of obstructive sleep apnea in infants with Pierre Robin sequence. *Cleft Palate Craniofac J.* 2011;48(3):331-336.
25. Muller-Hagedorn S, Arand J, Scholz T, Poets CF, Wiechers C. An innovative method for manufacturing the Tuebingen palatal plate for infants with robin sequence. *BMC Pediatr.* 2020;20(1):103.

26. Pang SL, Ho CHA, Law CML, Yang Y, Leung YY. Pre-epiglottic baton plate in the management of upper airway obstruction in an infant with femoral facial syndrome: a case report. *Cleft Palate Craniofac J.* 2023;60(3):367-375.
27. Linz A, Urschitz MS, Bacher M, Brockmann PE, Buchenau W, Poets CF. Treatment of obstructive sleep apnea in infants with trisomy 21 using oral appliances. *Cleft Palate Craniofac J.* 2013;50(6):648-654.
28. Ahmed J, Marucci D, Cochrane L, Heywood RL, Wyatt ME, Leighton SE. The role of the nasopharyngeal airway for obstructive sleep apnea in syndromic craniosynostosis. *J Craniofac Surg.* 2008;19(3):659-663.
29. Yau T, Bansal R, Hardin K, Senders C, Nandalike K. Nasal trumpet as a long-term remedy for obstructive sleep apnea syndrome in a child. *SAGE Open Med Case Rep.* 2021;9:2050313X211055303.
30. Kimple AJ, Baldassari CM, Cohen AP, Landry A, Ishman SL. Polysomnographic results of prone versus supine positioning in micrognathia. *Int J Pediatr Otorhinolaryngol.* 2014;78(12):2056-2059.
31. Hong H, Wee CP, Haynes K, Urata M, Hammoudeh J, Ward SLD. Evaluation of obstructive sleep apnea in prone versus nonprone body positioning with polysomnography in infants with robin sequence. *Cleft Palate Craniofac J.* 2020;57(2):141-147.
32. Greenlee CJ, Scholes MA, Gao D, Friedman NR. Obstructive sleep apnea and sleep position: does it matter for infants with a cleft palate? *Cleft Palate Craniofac J.* 2019;56(7):890-895.
33. Brigance JS, Miyamoto RC, Schilt P, et al. Surgical management of obstructive sleep apnea in infants and young toddlers. *Otolaryngol Head Neck Surg.* 2009;140(6):912-916.
34. Greenfeld M, Tauman R, DeRowe A, Sivan Y. Obstructive sleep apnea syndrome due to adenotonsillar hypertrophy in infants. *Int J Pediatr Otorhinolaryngol.* 2003;67(10):1055-1060.
35. Mitchell RB, Kelly J. Outcome of adenotonsillectomy for obstructive sleep apnea in children under 3 years. *Otolaryngol Head Neck Surg.* 2005;132(5):681-684.
36. Postic WP, Shah UK. Nonsurgical and surgical management of infants and children with obstructive sleep apnea syndrome. *Otolaryngol Clin North Am.* 1998;31(6):969-977.
37. Mitchell RB, Archer SM, Ishman SL, et al. Clinical practice guideline: tonsillectomy in children (update)-executive summary. *Otolaryngol Head Neck Surg.* 2019;160(2):187-205.
38. Stahl A, Dagan O, Nageris B, Ebner Y. Outcomes and safety of adenoidectomy in infants up to 12 months of age compared to older children. *Eur Arch Otorhinolaryngol.* 2020;277(9):2611-2617.
39. Cheng J, Elden L. Outcomes in children under 12 months of age undergoing adenotonsillectomy for sleep-disordered breathing. *Laryngoscope.* 2013;123(9):2281-2284.
40. Sahoo NK, Roy ID, Dalal S, Bhandari A. Distraction osteogenesis for management of severe OSA in Pierre Robin sequence: an approach to elude tracheostomy in infants. *J Maxillofac Oral Surg.* 2016;15(4):501-505.
41. Dauria D, Marsh JL. Mandibular distraction osteogenesis for Pierre Robin sequence: What percentage of neonates need it? *J Craniofac Surg.* 2008;19(5):1237-1243.
42. Singh V, Sinha C, Sahay N, Haq A, Sharma S, Payal S. Tongue-lip adhesion in Pierre-Robin sequence: role redefined. *Natl J Maxillofac Surg.* 2020;11(1):124-126.
43. Randall RS, Kian A, Chin K, French B. Resolution of obstructive sleep apnea after mandibular distraction osteogenesis in setting of delayed tongue-lip adhesion takedown: a case report. *Medicine (Baltimore).* 2018;97(42):e12853.
44. Bijnen CL, Don Griot PJ, Mulder WJ, Haumann TJ, Van Hagen AJ. Tongue-lip adhesion in the treatment of Pierre Robin sequence. *J Craniofac Surg.* 2009;20(2):315-320.
45. Sedaghat AR, Anderson IC, McGinley BM, Rossberg MI, Redett RJ, Ishman SL. Characterization of obstructive sleep apnea before and after tongue-lip adhesion in children with micrognathia. *Cleft Palate Craniofac J.* 2012;49(1):21-26.
46. Denny AD, Amm CA, Schaefer RB. Outcomes of tongue-lip adhesion for neonatal respiratory distress caused by Pierre Robin sequence. *J Craniofac Surg.* 2004;15(5):819-823.
47. Denny A, Amm C. New technique for airway correction in neonates with severe Pierre Robin sequence. *J Pediatr.* 2005;147(1):97-101.
48. Ehsan Z, Weaver KN, Pan BS, Huang G, Hossain MM, Simakajornboon N. Sleep outcomes in neonates with Pierre Robin sequence undergoing external mandibular distraction: a longitudinal analysis. *Plast Reconstr Surg.* 2020;146(5):1103-1115.
49. Kosyk MS, Carlson AR, Zapatero ZD, et al. Mandibular distraction osteogenesis for tongue-based airway obstruction without micrognathia. *Ann Plast Surg.* 2022;88(1):54-58.
50. Master DL, Hanson PR, Gosain AK. Complications of mandibular distraction osteogenesis. *J Craniofac Surg.* 2010;21(5):1565-1570.

51. Zhang RS, Hoppe IC, Taylor JA, Bartlett SP. Surgical management and outcomes of Pierre Robin sequence: A comparison of mandibular distraction osteogenesis and tongue-lip adhesion. *Plast Reconstr Surg*. 2018;142(2):480-509.

52. Resnick CM, Rottgers SA, Wright JM, et al. Surgical outcome and treatment trends in 1289 infants with micrognathia: a multicenter cohort. *Plast Reconstr Surg*. 2023.

53. Duffy KA, Cielo CM, Cohen JL, et al. Characterization of the Beckwith-Wiedemann spectrum: diagnosis and management. *Am J Med Genet C Semin Med Genet*. 2019;181(4):693-708.

54. Cielo CM, Duffy KA, Taylor JA, Marcus CL, Kalish JM. Obstructive sleep apnea in children with Beckwith-Wiedemann syndrome. *J Clin Sleep Med*. 2019;15(3):375-381.

55. Follmar A, Dentino K, Abramowicz S, Padwa BL. Prevalence of sleep-disordered breathing in patients with Beckwith-Wiedemann syndrome. *J Craniofac Surg*. 2014;25(5):1814-1817.

56. Cielo CM, Duffy KA, Vyas A, Taylor JA, Kalish JM. Obstructive sleep apnoea and the role of tongue reduction surgery in children with Beckwith-Wiedemann syndrome. *Paediatr Respir Rev*. 2018;25:58-63.

57. Cohen JL, Cielo CM, Kupa J, et al. The utility of early tongue reduction surgery for macroglossia in Beckwith-Wiedemann syndrome. *Plast Reconstr Surg*. 2020;145(4):803e-813e.

58. Camacho M, Dunn B, Torre C, et al. Supraglottoplasty for laryngomalacia with obstructive sleep apnea: a systematic review and meta-analysis. *Laryngoscope*. 2016;126(5):1246-1255.

59. Powitzky R, Stoner J, Fisher T, Digoy GP. Changes in sleep apnea after supraglottoplasty in infants with laryngomalacia. *Int J Pediatr Otorhinolaryngol*. 2011;75(10):1234-1239.

60. Pu S, Xu H, Li X. Supraglottoplasty in neonates and infants: a radiofrequency ablation approach. *Medicine (Baltimore)*. 2018;97(7):e9850.

61. Ratanakorn W, Brockbank J, Ishman S, Tadesse DG, Hossain MM, Simakajornboon N. The maturation changes of sleep-related respiratory abnormalities in infants with laryngomalacia. *J Clin Sleep Med*. 2021;17(4):767-777.

62. Patel VA, Carr MM. Congenital nasal obstruction in infants: a retrospective study and literature review. *Int J Pediatr Otorhinolaryngol*. 2017;99:78-84.

63. Samadi DS, Shah UK, Handler SD. Choanal atresia: a twenty-year review of medical comorbidities and surgical outcomes. *Laryngoscope*. 2003;113(2):254-258.

64. Thomas EM, Gibikote S, Panwar JS, Mathew J. Congenital nasal pyriform aperture stenosis: A rare cause of nasal airway obstruction in a neonate. *Indian J Radiol Imaging*. 2010;20(4):266-268.

65. Rizzi CJ, Amin JD, Isaiah A, et al. Tracheostomy for severe pediatric obstructive sleep apnea: indications and outcomes. *Otolaryngol Head Neck Surg*. 2017;157(2):309-313.

66. Carr MM, Poje CP, Kingston L, Kielma D, Heard C. Complications in pediatric tracheostomies. *Laryngoscope*. 2001;111(11 Pt 1):1925-1928.

67. D'Souza JN, Levi JR, Park D, Shah UK. Complications following pediatric tracheotomy. *JAMA Otolaryngol Head Neck Surg*. 2016;142(5):484-488.

68. Kaditis AG, Alonso Alvarez ML, Boudewyns A, et al. Ers statement on obstructive sleep disordered breathing in 1- to 23-month-old children. *Eur Respir J*. 2017;50(6):1700985.

69. Yendur O, Feld L, Miranda-Schaeubinger M, et al. Clinical utility of repeated positive airway pressure titrations in children with obstructive sleep apnea syndrome. *J Clin Sleep Med*. 2022;18(4):1021-1026.

70. Marcus CL, Moore RH, Rosen CL, et al. A randomized trial of adenotonsillectomy for childhood sleep apnea. *N Engl J Med*. 2013;368(25):2366-2376.

71. Fehrm J, Nerfeldt P, Browaldh N, Friberg D. Effectiveness of adenotonsillectomy vs watchful waiting in young children with mild to moderate obstructive sleep apnea: a randomized clinical trial. *JAMA Otolaryngol Head Neck Surg*. 2020;146(7):647-654.

Congenital Central Hypoventilation Syndromes and Other Disorders of Ventilation

Ambika Gnanam Chidambaram ▩ Olufunke Afolabi-Brown

Introduction

Hypoventilation refers to an elevated level of arterial carbon dioxide (CO_2), typically resulting from ineffective gas exchange.[1] Sleep-related hypoventilation based on pediatric polysomnographic scoring is defined by the arterial partial pressure of CO_2 (PCO_2) or surrogate higher than 50 mmHg for greater than 25% of the total sleep time.[2] Since arterial PCO_2 monitoring is an invasive test, the most commonly used surrogates are end-tidal or transcutaneous CO_2 monitoring.

Ventilatory control through the central nervous system ensures adequate gas exchange throughout the day and night, including wakefulness, sleep, and various activity levels. Disorders of ventilation can result from an ineffective respiratory drive and range from hypoventilation occurring only during sleep to the inability to maintain spontaneous ventilation both awake and asleep. As a result of increased diagnostic modalities with technologies that can rapidly detect these abnormalities, we can better care for patients with these disorders. Their management, however, often requires a multidisciplinary approach.

The International Classification of Sleep Disorders—Third Edition (ICSD-3) has classified sleep-related hypoventilation as the following[3]:

a. Congenital central hypoventilation syndrome (CCHS)
b. Obesity hypoventilation syndrome
c. Rapid-onset obesity with hypothalamic dysfunction, hypoventilation, and autonomic dysregulation (ROHHAD)
d. Idiopathic central alveolar hypoventilation
e. Sleep-related hypoventilation due to a medication or substance
f. Sleep-related hypoventilation due to a medical disorder
 i. Chest wall disorders
 ii. Neurologic and neuromuscular diseases (e.g., spinal muscular atrophy, Duchenne muscular dystrophy)
 iii. Airway or parenchymal disease (altered lung volume, abnormal ventilation-perfusion relationships)

This chapter will briefly describe normal control of breathing and review hypoventilation disorders in infants and children less than 24 months. Specifically, we will discuss CCHS, ROHHAD, Arnold Chiari malformation, Prader-Willi syndrome (PWS), achondroplasia, and neuromuscular disorders commonly seen in infants. Early identification of the above diseases is vital to ensure appropriate management strategies and improve patient outcomes.

Control of Breathing

Usually, the depth and frequency of our breathing are dictated by our brain, primarily by two mechanisms: metabolic/automatic control and voluntary/behavioral control. The metabolic system maintains a tight regulation of Partial pressure of oxygen (PO_2) and PCO_2. In normal individuals (Fig. 8.1), the central chemoreceptors sense changes in PCO_2, pH, and PO_2. These receptors are located in the retrotrapezoid nucleus, medullary raphe, caudal medulla, nucleus tractus solitarius, locus coeruleus, fastigial nucleus, rostral ventral respiratory group/pre-Botzinger complex.[4] In the cerebrospinal fluid, CO_2 forms carbonic acid combined with water (H_2O), causing increased hydrogen ion (H^+) concentration and stimulating increased minute ventilation. In addition, the presence of hypoxia also stimulates the central chemoreceptor ventilatory response. The peripheral chemoreceptors, located in the carotid and aortic bodies, are primarily involved in hypoxic ventilatory responses and stimulate breathing when PO_2 is low. The central and peripheral chemoreceptors send signals to the ventilatory controllers located in the medulla and pons. These signals are then sent to the respiratory muscles to respond appropriately by increasing or decreasing ventilation. Other receptors such as stretch receptors and irritant receptors in the lungs, chest wall receptors, and mechanoreceptors also play a role in controlling breathing.

To a certain extent, voluntary control of breathing can override central control through the cortex (premotor and primary motor area) and cerebellum. An example of this is being able to hold one's breath on command or to hyperventilate voluntarily. However, ventilatory control by this voluntary system causes significant fluctuations in PCO_2 and PO_2.

Central hypoventilation syndromes are characterized by absent chemoreceptor function, with absent or blunted response to hypoxia and/or hypercapnia.

Congenital Central Hypoventilation Syndrome

CCHS is a rare genetic syndrome of autonomic nervous system dysfunction and abnormal central control of breathing due to paired-like homeobox 2B (*PHOX-2B*) mutation on chromosome 4p12.[5] It is characterized by alveolar hypoventilation, resulting in hypercapnia and hypoxemia, most notable during sleep, and unexplained by a primary lung pathology, neuromuscular disease, cardiac disease, or brainstem lesion.[6] Presentation is seen typically in early infancy but can occur later in childhood and early adulthood.

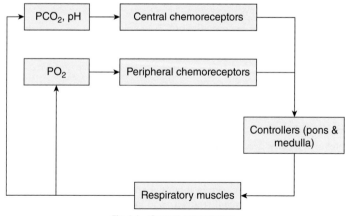

Fig. 8.1 Control of ventilation.

The term "Ondine's curse" was previously used to describe CCHS, but the terminology has been discouraged due to the inaccurate description of the clinical syndrome.

HISTORY

Mellins and colleagues (Fig. 8.2) first reported CCHS as a case of congenital alveolar hypoventilation in 1970[7] providing a comprehensive summary of the evaluation and management of a patient with the disorder. Initially, CCHS was attributed to an injury to the medullary chemoreceptors.[8] It was not until the early 1990s that larger cohorts were published. The American Thoracic Society (ATS) released its first statement in 1999, and at that time, there were about 160 to 180 children estimated to have CCHS. This led to a better understanding of the clinical presentation, associated conditions related to autonomic nervous system dysfunction, complications, and various treatment strategies applied in children with CCHS; however, an etiology was still unknown. In 2003, Amiel et al. discovered frameshift mutations and polyalanine repeats in the *PHOX-2B* gene in children with CCHS.[9] They also demonstrated that *PHOX-2B* was expressed in the central and peripheral autonomic nervous system in human embryonic development.[9] This was an essential milestone in the history of children with CCHS as it led to an opportunity for early diagnosis and optimization of ventilation and phenotyping of patients based on their mutations. In 2009, the ATS released its second statement providing a comprehensive summary of the role of *PHOX-2B*, diagnosis, and management strategies for individuals with CCHS. Based on the report, about 1000 patients with CCHS were diagnosed worldwide by then.[6] In 2013, the first international CCHS Research database was created.[10]

Prevalence of CCHS

To date, there has been no prospective study on the incidence of CCHS. However, in 2005, Trang et al. estimated the incidence of CCHS as about 1 per 200,000 live births based on the French CCHS registry.[11] At present, there are estimated to be about 1000 to 1200 cases worldwide.[12] The prevalence is likely underestimated due to the broad spectrum of presentations, variable severity, and late-onset CCHS.

Genetics

PHOX-2B, located on chromosome 4p12, is identified as the CCHS disease-causing gene. Amiel and colleagues described that the *PHOX-2B* gene encodes a highly conserved homeobox transcription factor of 314 amino acids with two short and stable polyalanine repeats of 9 and 20

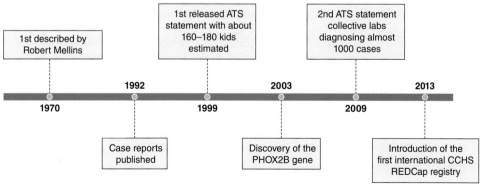

Fig. 8.2 History of CCHS.

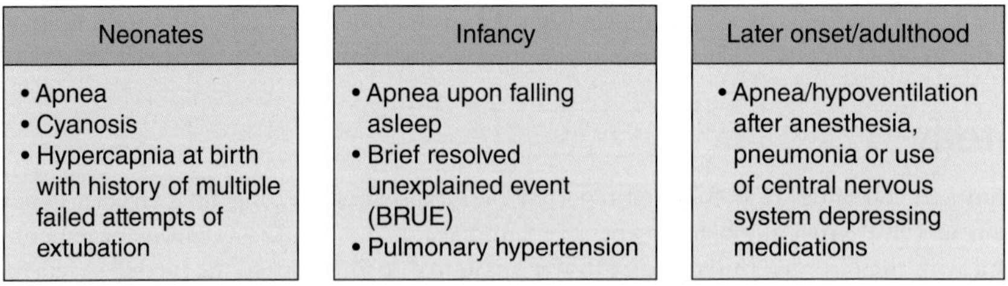

Neonates	Infancy	Later onset/adulthood
• Apnea • Cyanosis • Hypercapnia at birth with history of multiple failed attempts of extubation	• Apnea upon falling asleep • Brief resolved unexplained event (BRUE) • Pulmonary hypertension	• Apnea/hypoventilation after anesthesia, pneumonia or use of central nervous system depressing medications

Fig. 8.3   Clinical manifestations of CCHS.

residues, respectively. They also demonstrated the expression of *PHOX-2B* in the central and peripheral autonomic nervous systems in human embryonic development, which further supports the presence of various clinical manifestations (Fig. 8.3) of dysfunction of the autonomic nervous system.[9] Inheritance is typically autosomal dominant with variable penetrance; however, some mutations are *de novo*.[6] Once a patient is diagnosed with CCHS, the parents should undergo genetic counseling and testing, as this would inform their health risks if they carry mosaicism in their *PHOX-2B* gene and plan future pregnancies.[7]

Typically, healthy individuals have a repeat sequence of 20 alanines in exon 3 (normal genotype 20/20). The majority (~90%) of individuals with CCHS are heterozygous for a polyalanine repeat expansion mutations (PARM) mutation, and this can range from an additional 4 to 13 alanines added to the typical sequence of 20 alanine repeats. Hence, 20/24 to 20/33 are the genotypes produced by the PARMs mutation. Other patients with CCHS (~9%–10%) are heterozygous for a nonpolyalanine repeat mutation (NPARM), including nonsense, frameshift, missense splice-site, or stop codon mutations.[7] Genotypes 20/25, 20/26, and 20/27 are the most common.[13]

Genotype-phenotype relationships have been described and published in the literature.[7] For example, individuals with higher polyalanine repeats (genotypes 20/26, 20/27) and NPARMs are more likely to require day and night ventilation. In comparison, those with fewer polyalanine repeats (genotypes 20/24, 20/25) may only need nocturnal support.[13] Also, patients with NPARMs mutation are at a higher risk of developing tumors of neural crest origin and severe intestinal aganglionosis.[13] Sinus pauses (longest R-R interval ≥3 seconds) are more common in individuals with the 20/27 genotype, with some requiring a cardiac pacemaker.[13] Identifying a specific genotype is crucial as it has implications on evaluation and management of CCHS.

Despite the relationships noted between the genotype and phenotype of CCHS, individuals with NPARMs mutation present with differing severity due to variable penetrance and expressivity.[5] This has been described in a three-generational family of four with NPARM (c.245C > T) genotype. The affected family members had a milder phenotype of CCHS; two of them were ventilator-dependent at night and did not have neural crest tumors or Hirschsprung disease, while the remaining two were asymptomatic. One of the asymptomatic individuals eventually developed systemic hypertension as an adult.[14]

There have also been reports of non-*PHOX-2B* mutations, such as *MYO1H* and *LBX1*, in patients with CCHS born with consanguineous families, suggesting an autosomal recessive inheritance.[15,16]

Hence, further research is required to define further the relationships between the rare genotypes with variable penetrance and expressivity.

Clinical Presentation

Presentation in individuals with CCHS varies depending on the age of presentation and genotype. Newborns may present with apnea, cyanosis, respiratory failure at birth, or a history of multiple failed attempts of extubation. Some may be diagnosed with perinatal asphyxia; however, they do not show evidence of central nervous system depression. Infants can present with apnea at sleep onset and have brief apneic episodes diagnosed as brief resolved unexplained events (BRUE). Infants and older children can present with pulmonary hypertension depending on the severity of hypoxemia/hypercarbia.[5,17,18] Todd and colleagues also observed box-shaped facies in children with CCHS independent of those requiring chronic noninvasive ventilation mask use.[19]

CCHS can present in older children and adults with apnea or hypoventilation following anesthesia, respiratory tract infections, pneumonia, or use of central nervous system depressing agents. This form is known as the late-onset form of CCHS.[7] With the widespread availability of genetic testing for the *PHOX-2B* gene, milder phenotypes are most often diagnosed in older children and adults. This has also enabled the retrospective diagnosis of CCHS in individuals diagnosed with the associated conditions, such as Hirschsprung disease.

A better understanding of the role of *PHOX-2B* in various physiologic functions of the body and the resultant multisystem involvement is described in detail below.

Hypoventilation

The primary presenting feature for CCHS is hypoventilation, characterized by hypercapnia and/or hypoxemia during sleep or wakefulness due to abnormal control of breathing.[7] Patients have low tidal volumes with variable minute ventilation. They also lack the perception of dyspnea/asphyxia with or without exertion.[20] In polysomnograms of patients with CCHS, hypoventilation appears to be notably worse during nonrapid eye movement (NREM) sleep than rapid eye movement (REM) sleep. The phenomenon is attributed to ventilatory control driven by metabolic input during NREM sleep.[20] Central apneas can be present, but the predominant pattern includes low tidal volume or reduced flow.[20]

Studies have demonstrated a lack of arousal or increased minute ventilation in response to hypercarbia or hypoxemia, suggesting central and peripheral chemoreceptor abnormalities. On the other hand, Gozal et al. demonstrated decreased ventilatory drive in response to hyperoxia, suggesting that peripheral chemoreceptor function was intact.[21] A study by Marcus et al. showed that patients with CCHS have a higher arousal frequency than controls when challenged by a hypercarbic or hypoxic stimulus.[22] Thus, there is a strong suspicion of an abnormality in integrating the inputs from these chemoreceptors.[5,22] Furthermore, discovering the *PHOX-2B* gene and its presence in the central and peripheral autonomic system, including the brainstem where the respiratory controllers are present, further established the role of mutations in the *PHOX-2B* gene resulting in abnormal control of breathing. Many studies both in animal models and humans describe the role of the *PHOX-2B* gene in CCHS pathogenesis beyond the scope of this chapter.

Other Associated Conditions
NEUROCRISTOPATHY

Neurocristopathies, a spectrum of diseases related to abnormal migration of the neural crest cells, can be seen in children with CCHS. Common neurocristopathies seen in children with CCHS include Hirschsprung disease (partial or complete aganglionosis of the distal intestinal tract) and neural crest tumors, both of which have been observed in those with the NPARMs mutation. A subset of patients has less severe presentations, such as chronic constipation or esophageal dysmotility. The neural crest tumors, including ganglioneuroblastomas, neuroblastomas, and ganglioneuromas, have been described in CCHS. Neuroblastomas tend to present during infancy, and ganglioneuroblastoma and ganglioneuroma are often incidental findings. Death from neural crest tumors is rare.[23]

AUTONOMIC NERVOUS SYSTEM (ANS) DYSREGULATION

Cardiac abnormalities like sinus pauses and bradycardia, transient asystole, decreased heart rate variability, and blood pressure are seen. Some patients may require cardiac pacemakers.[23] Ophthalmologic manifestations such as anisocoria, altered response to light, strabismus, and convergent gaze may also be seen. Other signs of ANS dysregulation are temperature dysregulation (hypothermia), sporadic profuse sweating, poor pain perception, and anxiety.[5] Endocrinopathies have been described, such as hypoglycemia, hyperglycemia, and hyperinsulinism, suggesting possible hypothalamic dysfunction; however, the pathophysiology for this is not entirely understood.[23]

NEUROCOGNITIVE ABNORMALITIES

Reported neurological and neurocognitive deficits have been attributed to the possible direct result of a primary neurological problem, suboptimal ventilatory support, or dysfunction of cerebral autoregulation.[6] For example, a study by Zelko and colleagues demonstrated that parents reported that 30% of children with CCHS had a formal diagnosis of learning disabilities, and about half the children with CCHS had additional educational needs or were in supported classrooms.[24,25] Charnay and colleagues demonstrated significantly lower Bayley mental and motor scores in children with CCHS who had severe cyanotic breath-holding spells, required continuous ventilatory support, and had a history of prolonged sinus pauses. They also demonstrated that Bayley motor scores alone were significantly lower for children with seizures.[26] The degree of cognitive impairment may correlate with disease severity; however, this needs to be further explored.[26]

DIAGNOSTIC EVALUATION

A diagnosis of CCHS should be considered in a child with evidence of sleep-related hypoventilation without any known cardiopulmonary, neuromuscular, metabolic, or brainstem dysfunction. According to the ICSD-3, a diagnosis of CCHS is made based on the presence of sleep-related hypoventilation and an identified mutation in the *PHOX-2B* gene.[3]

A *PHOX-2B* screening test is initially recommended in patients with suspected CCHS to identify known PARM (genotypes 20/24 to 20/33), frameshift NPARM, and somatic mosaicism. The fragment analysis involves the polymerase chain reaction amplification of the 20 repeat polyalanine expansion region of exon three and determines the polyalanine repeat length, identifying 95% of patients with CCHS. If no mutations have been detected, with an ongoing strong suspicion for CCHS, a *PHOX-2B* sequencing test is recommended as this additionally identifies missense and nonsense mutations. As a final step, a *PHOX-2B* deletion/duplication analysis by multiplex ligation-dependent probe amplification (MLPA) test can also be performed. This would identify the whole gene or exon deletions and duplications and would be needed to identify asymptomatic or mildly symptomatic individuals with CCHS.[5]

Evaluation of Gas Exchange

A baseline polysomnogram characterizes the degree of hypoventilation and should include continuous CO_2 monitoring (via surrogates transcutaneous and end-tidal CO_2 monitoring). In addition, some centers measure the response to hypercarbia or hypoxemia challenges during wakefulness and sleep.

Other etiologies of sleep-related hypoventilation should be ruled out. This workup should include imaging for lung parenchymal abnormalities, neurologic or neuromuscular disease, and evaluation for cardiac anomalies.[5] Based on the clinical presentation, further testing may be required to evaluate for abnormalities on a case-by-case basis.

Evaluation of Other Associated Conditions

Once a diagnosis of CCHS has been established, comprehensive testing of the other associated conditions should be performed. For example, a 72-hour Holter monitor and echocardiogram are recommended to screen for cardiac arrhythmias and pulmonary hypertension, respectively.[23] Evaluation of the autonomic system can be considered when available or appropriate such as orthostatic testing, head-up tilt testing, ambulatory blood pressure, heart rate monitoring, thermoregulatory chamber sweat testing, Q-sweat testing, Valsalva maneuver, and measures of cerebral regional blood flow.[23] For those with suspected Hirschsprung disease, rectal biopsy should be obtained.[23] Depending on the age of diagnosis, appropriate neurocognitive evaluation is essential to implement early intervention.[23]

MANAGEMENT OF CENTRAL HYPOVENTILATION SYNDROMES

Respiratory Support

Since hypoventilation is the hallmark of CCHS, optimized ventilation is critical to reduce the deleterious effects of hypoventilation and improve growth and neurocognitive outcomes.[6] Four primary ventilatory support modalities include positive pressure ventilation provided via a tracheostomy or noninvasively via a mask, negative pressure ventilation, and diaphragm pacing.[18] Supplemental oxygen is insufficient to treat hypoventilation and may inadvertently blunt the hypoxic respiratory drive. Negative pressure ventilation has been used in the past; however, it is less preferred as an option now as it is not portable due to lack of battery support.[6,18]

Continuous ventilatory support via tracheostomy is strongly recommended in the first few years of life, given their unpredictable sleep-wake cycle and frequent naps. Older children and adults requiring only nocturnal ventilatory support via tracheostomy may be successfully decannulated and transitioned to noninvasive ventilation.[6]

Diaphragmatic pacing is an alternative option in ambulatory patients who require 24-hour ventilatory support. It is, however, performed in only a few centers worldwide. These patients can be liberated from the ventilator during waking hours to participate in activities of daily living. It supports ventilation by externally stimulating the phrenic nerve, stimulating diaphragmatic contraction.[5,6] Eligibility for diaphragm pacing is quite selective and can be considered in individuals who are not obese/overweight and have minimal or no intrinsic lung disease, normal diaphragm function, and an intact phrenic nerve. In addition, there is the risk for obstructive sleep apnea in individuals without a tracheostomy, as the stimulation of the diaphragm may be asynchronous with the contraction of the upper airway muscles.[5,6]

Regardless of the ventilation modality, behavioral issues may pose a challenge and limit adherence to therapies. For example, children may self-decannulate or resist wearing their masks. In these situations, behavior modification strategies are beneficial.[27] In some cases, patients may need to be monitored in a facility. Various ventilation modes have been reported in the literature; however, there are limited studies comparing their efficacy. Positive pressure ventilation modes include pressure control, timed, assist control, or spontaneous timed. Other, more recent alternatives include hybrid modes of ventilation providing targeted volumes via variable pressures and inspiratory times.[6] A goal of maintaining an end-tidal CO_2 ($ETCO_2$) level between 35 and 45 mmHg and oxyhemoglobin saturation above 94% is ideal.[18]

At a minimum, annual titration polysomnograms are recommended in children above 3 years of age and more frequently in younger children, as their ventilatory needs vary with growth.[6]

Management of Associated Conditions

A cardiac pacemaker may be needed to manage rhythm abnormalities, such as asystole. Appropriate pharmacotherapy may also be required for those who have developed pulmonary hypertension. Surgical treatment such as colectomy and reanastomosis is often required for gastrointestinal issues such as chronic constipation or Hirschsprung diseases. Close follow-up with oncology is required if neural crest tumors are detected, and treatment may include surgical interventions or chemotherapy if needed.[23]

As mentioned above, early intervention services are important to improve neurocognitive outcomes and other medical management strategies.

FOLLOW-UP

Close follow-up with a multidisciplinary team with expertise in CCHS is recommended, including parents/family members, pediatricians, pulmonologists, sleep medicine physicians, cardiologists, endocrinologists, gastroenterologists, ophthalmologists, neonatal and pediatric intensivists, psychologists, nursing support, respiratory therapists, speech therapists, occupational therapists, and social workers.

As patients with CCHS may not perceive dyspnea or manifest other signs of respiratory distress, careful monitoring of their respiratory status and gas exchange at home is required. Families should be informed about avoiding high-risk activities such as breath-holding, unsupervised swimming, and use of CNS depressants, alcohol, or other recreational drugs. Additionally, close cardiorespiratory monitoring during and after anesthesia with adequate respiratory support is vital to prevent acute respiratory failure.[18]

Families should be provided with resources to help with home management, including home nursing, parent support groups, durable medical companies to provide adequate supplies, and a sick plan. In addition, in case of natural disasters, it is helpful for the local emergency services, such as the fire department and police department, to be aware of the patient's medical needs.

Prognosis

With early diagnosis and optimized ventilation, more children with CCHS are living into adulthood. However, adults with CCHS face challenges related to independent living, such as responding to alarms during sleep.[18] Some patients live independently, whereas some may wish to live in communities with other adults with varying disabilities. Other accommodations include a trained partner, nursing aide, or therapy pets.

Pregnancy is possible in patients with CCHS but requires preplanning and genetic counseling. During pregnancy, labor, and delivery, patients require closer surveillance and may need higher respiratory support. Delivery should be conducted in a hospital with close collaboration with a CCHS referral center.[18]

Other Conditions With Hypoventilation Presenting During Infancy

RAPID-ONSET OBESITY WITH HYPOVENTILATION, HYPOTHALAMIC DYSFUNCTION, AUTONOMIC DYSREGULATION

ROHHAD is a rare disorder of central hypoventilation that was first described as a case report in 1965 by Fishman and colleagues from Southern California.[28] Based on the onset of hypoventilation during childhood and the association with hypothalamic endocrinopathies, it was initially referred to as "late-onset central hypoventilation syndrome with hypothalamic dysfunction" and later renamed in 2007 as ROHHAD.[29] Late-onset CCHS has been considered an important differential for ROHHAD but is now clinically distinguished based on the absence of the *PHOX-2B* gene.

The clinical presentation of ROHHAD is usually during early childhood, between 2 and 4 years of age, and most children are typically healthy until the onset of disease.[29] The clinical syndrome is characterized by rapid onset of excessive weight gain, other hypothalamic endocrinopathies (diabetes insipidus, syndrome of inappropriate antidiuretic hormone secretion, hyperprolactinemia, hypothyroidism, growth hormone deficiency, hypogonadism, or precocious puberty), followed by autonomic dysregulation, and alveolar hypoventilation. Manifestations of autonomic dysfunction include ophthalmologic findings (pupillary dysfunction and strabismus), cardiac arrhythmias, gastrointestinal dysmotility, and temperature dysregulation.[29] Sleep-related hypoventilation is variable in presentation and can occur at any point of the disease spectrum. Hypoventilation can also occur during wakefulness.[29] Patients may have a blunted hypoxic-hypercapnic ventilatory response suggesting central chemoreceptor dysfunction.[30] Given their obesity, these patients are also at risk for obstructive sleep apnea. In addition, a subset of patients with ROHHAD may present with neuroendocrine tumors, in which case their condition is referred to as ROHHAD-NET.[31] Behavioral issues may be seen and can be quite debilitating, with presentations varying from irritability and aggression to psychosis.[32] Other associated conditions such as autism, self-injurious behavior, oppositional-defiant disorder, major depressive disorder, anxiety, and hyperactivity have been reported.

The diagnosis of ROHHAD is based on the clinical findings and a negative *PHOX-2B* genetic test.[29] Despite evaluating several candidate genes, the genetic etiology for ROHHAD remains undetermined. Current theories include an unknown epigenetic etiology and/or an autoimmune process.[32] There have been case reports of improvement in neuropsychological comorbidities following treatment with immunosuppressants such as cyclophosphamide.[33] While pharmacotherapies are being investigated as potential forms of treatment, management of each comorbidity is essential to reduce morbidity and mortality.

Since central control of breathing in children with ROHHAD may progressively worsen, the outcome can be deleterious, including respiratory failure, pulmonary hypertension, and cardiac arrest. Therefore, prompt diagnosis and treatment, including aggressive ventilatory support, are needed.[29]

PRADER-WILLI SYNDROME

PWS is a rare genetic disorder that presents with hypotonia and failure to thrive in early infancy. It is due to the absence of paternal expression of imprinted genes on chromosome 15 (15q11.2-q13).[34] Later in childhood, hyperphagia, obesity, and behavioral issues may present. In addition, children with PWS are at risk for various sleep-disordered breathing, including central sleep apnea earlier in infancy, as well as OSA and hypoventilation. These are due to a combination of craniofacial factors, hypotonia, obesity hypothalamic dysfunction.[34] CSA is frequently seen in infants and children with PWS less than 2 years old, while OSA is more common in those older than 2 years.

While ventilation may be normal during wakefulness, patients with PWS have demonstrated hypoxic, hypercapnic, and hyperoxic response abnormalities, suggesting a dysfunction in the central and peripheral chemoreceptors. Gozal and colleagues demonstrated a paradoxical response to hyperoxia with an increase in minute ventilation compared to controls, suggestive of a peripheral chemoreceptor dysfunction and/or abnormalities in the afferent pathways to the central control of breathing.[35] Arens and colleagues observed a blunted hypercapnic ventilatory response in obese children with PWS compared to obese controls. They also demonstrated a higher threshold of PCO_2 for appropriate hypercapnic ventilatory response in obese PWS subjects, suggesting a central cause for hypoventilation.[36] Hypoxic ventilatory response was also evaluated, and most patients with PWS either had an absent or a decreased response, suggesting additional peripheral chemoreceptor dysfunction.[36]

Infants and young children with PWS may be at risk of developing severe respiratory failure during acute respiratory illness and initiation of growth hormone.[37] As a result, a screening polysomnogram should be obtained to evaluate for sleep-disordered breathing before starting growth hormone therapy and periodically afterward. Identifying sleep-disordered breathing in children with PWS and implementing prompt treatment may improve a variety of outcomes and reduce the likelihood of acute respiratory failure. Respiratory support depends on the primary etiology of sleep-disordered breathing and can include surgical intervention with adenotonsillectomy, supplemental oxygen, and noninvasive ventilation.

CHIAR II MALFORMATION

Chiari malformation type 2 (CM-2), often associated with myelomeningocele, is characterized by herniation of the cerebellum, fourth ventricle, and caudal brainstem through the foramen magnum into the cervical spinal cord. This herniation can obstruct the cerebrospinal fluid with resultant hydrocephalus.[38] Variable degrees of central apnea and hypoventilation can occur due to the involvement of the respiratory centers in the brainstem as a result of dysgenesis or damage of the neural tissues from traction and herniation into the spinal cord.[39] Ventilatory challenge testing in this population has shown blunted hypercapnic responses, suggesting impaired central chemoreceptor function.

Affected patients can present in the newborn period with apnea, dysphagia, aspiration, stridor, and vocal cord paralysis.[40] During sleep, patients with CM-2 may have OSA, CSA, or hypoventilation. Evaluation for sleep-disordered breathing should include a polysomnogram with CO_2 monitoring. The presence of these findings may suggest worsening hydrocephalus and should prompt further evaluation for this as a surgical intervention with posterior fossa decompression may be warranted. If the congenital dysgenesis of the neural structures of the brainstem dominates the clinical pathology, then hypoventilation may not resolve and increase the risk for mortality.[41] Patients with CM-2 and sleep-disordered breathing have been treated with oxygen, noninvasive or invasive mechanical ventilation long term.

NEUROMUSCULAR DISORDERS OF INFANCY

Diseases affecting the structure and function of the neuromuscular system can result in hypoventilation of varying degrees and are typically less likely a central etiology, depending on the disease process. Neuromuscular disorders frequently cause weakness and hypotonia, which may be generalized or focal. As these disorders may arise from the brain or spinal cord, history, physical examination, and diagnostic testing are essential for a definitive diagnosis. Common neuromuscular disorders present during the newborn period and infancy include spinal muscular atrophy, mitochondrial cytopathies, congenital myasthenic syndromes, and congenital myotonic dystrophy. Depending on the extent of neuromuscular involvement, respiratory manifestations could range from minimal to severe respiratory failure. During infancy, there should be a low threshold for polysomnogram if sleep-related hypoventilation is suspected, as these findings may be subtle. If hypoventilation is present, appropriate mechanical ventilatory support needs to be initiated to optimize gas exchange.[42]

ACHONDROPLASIA

Achondroplasia, skeletal dysplasia, is an autosomal dominant condition caused by a fibroblast growth factor receptor type 3 (*FGFR3*) gene mutation present on chromosome 4p26.3. While inheritance is autosomal dominant, most of the mutations are de novo.[43] FGFR3 is responsible for the formation of bones through endochondral ossification, and a mutation in this gene results in abnormal bone formation through cartilage, affecting longitudinal growth. Most of the bones in the base of the skull and the vertebral bodies are formed through this process and therefore are affected, resulting in foramen magnum and spinal canal stenosis, which can cause compression of the spine and sudden death in infants. Affected infants also have characteristic features, including macrocephaly, mid-face hypoplasia, short limbs, and brachydactyly.[43] These infants are at risk for various sleep-disordered breathing disorders, including hypoventilation in varying degrees. Studies have shown hypoxemia as the most frequent finding noted on polysomnograms, which may be related to a decreased pulmonary reserve from restrictive lung disease. Patients may also have central and obstructive sleep apnea and hypoventilation in varying degrees, some of which have been attributed to compression of the spinal cord or brainstem.[44] There have also been reports of significant respiratory compromise, including apnea and sudden death in infancy. Hence, neuroimaging studies are recommended in affected infants and children with achondroplasia who present with hypoventilation as a timely intervention with mechanical ventilation, and possibly surgical decompression of the spinal canal stenosis can be a life-saving measure.

FAMILIAL DYSAUTONOMIA

Familial dysautonomia (FD) is a rare disorder of the autonomic nervous system due to a mutation in the gene located on chromosome 9q31 encoding for IκB kinase complex-associated protein (IKAP).[45] IKAP is responsible for neuronal development in embryogenesis, and deficiency of IKAP mainly affects the primary sensory afferent neurons.[46] It is predominantly seen in the Ashkenazi Jewish population.[1] Clinical features include hypoventilation, hypoxemia, temperature dysregulation, altered pain perception, dysphagia, and ataxia. Cardiovascular manifestations such as episodic elevated blood pressure resulting in autonomic crises and postural hypotension without reflex tachycardia are more prominent in children and adults with FD. Patients also experience episodes of "autonomic crises" characterized by vomiting, hypertension, tachycardia, and red blotching of skin, typically triggered by stressors. Asystole is typically the cause of sudden death in affected individuals.[47]

Affected children and adults with FD have a blunted ventilatory response to hypoxia and hypercapnia independently. They also lack reflex tachycardia, sympathetic response to hypoxia, and have profound apnea with moderate hypercapnia challenge.[48] Carroll and colleagues demonstrated increased respiratory rate and increased respiratory variability during sleep in children with FD compared to age-, sex- and race-matched controls, indicating a disorder of respiratory control.[47] Hypoventilation has not been consistently demonstrated but is presumably due to profound hypoxemia and blunted ventilatory response to hypercapnia.[49]

Treatment of FD is primarily supportive, and if hypoventilation is present, appropriate mechanical ventilatory support will need to be initiated. This can potentially prevent the morbidity and mortality associated with cardiorespiratory depression from hypoxemia and presumed hypoventilation.

Conclusion

Central hypoventilation disorders, which often present during infancy, are rare in children but result in a significant impact on the lives of children and families affected. As specific mechanisms for some of these conditions have not been well elucidated, there is a need for ongoing research in this field. The primary treatment of central hypoventilation disorders focuses on optimizing gas exchange by mechanical ventilation. Given the deleterious effects of chronic hypoventilation on cardiopulmonary, neurocognitive, and developmental outcomes, prompt identification and management of these disorders are crucial to improving their overall health and quality of life.

References

1. Cielo C, Marcus CL. Central hypoventilation syndromes. *Sleep Med Clin.* 2014;9(1):105-118. doi:10.1016/j.jsmc.2013.10.005. Accessed December 13, 2021.
2. Berry RB, Quan SF, Abreu AR, et al. *The AASM Manual for The Scoring of Sleep and Associated Events: Rules, Terminology and Technical Specifications.* 2.6th ed. Darien, IL: American Academy of Sleep Medicine; 2020.
3. American Academy of Sleep Medicine. *International Classification of Sleep Disorders.* 3rd ed. Darien, IL: American Academy of Sleep Medicine; 2014.
4. Nattie E, Li A. Central chemoreceptors: locations and functions. *Compr Physiol.* 2012;2(1):221-254. doi:10.1002/cphy.c100083. Available at: https://www.ncbi.nlm.nih.gov/pmc/articles/PMC4802370/. Accessed December 19, 2021.
5. Bishara J, Keens TG, Perez IA. The genetics of congenital central hypoventilation syndrome: Clinical implications. *Appl Clin Genet.* 2018;11:135-144. doi:10.2147/TACG.S140629. Available at: https://www.ncbi.nlm.nih.gov/pubmed/30532577.
6. Weese-Mayer DE, Berry-Kravis EM, Ceccherini I, Keens TG, Loghmanee DA, Trang H. An official ATS clinical policy statement: Congenital central hypoventilation syndrome: genetic basis, diagnosis, and management. *Am J Respir Crit Care Med.* 2010;181(6):626-644. doi:10.1164/rccm.200807-1069ST. Accessed December 13, 2021.
7. Weese-Mayer DE, Rand CM, Zhou A, Carroll MS, Hunt CE. Congenital central hypoventilation syndrome: A bedside-to-bench success story for advancing early diagnosis and treatment and improved survival and quality of life. *Pediatr Res.* 2017;81(1-2):192-201. doi:10.1038/pr.2016.196. Accessed December 13, 2021.
8. Mellins RB, Balfour HH, Turino GM, Winters RW. Failure of automatic control of ventilation (Ondine's curse). report of an infant born with this syndrome and review of the literature. *Medicine (Baltimore).* 1970;49(6):487-504. Accessed December 15, 2021.
9. Amiel J, Laudier B, Attié-Bitach T, et al. Polyalanine expansion and frameshift mutations of the paired-like homeobox gene *PHOX2B* in congenital central hypoventilation syndrome. *Nat Genet.* 2003;33(4):459-461. doi:10.1038/ng1130. Accessed December 15, 2021.
10. Weese-Mayer D. *International congenital central hypoventilation syndrome (CCHS) REDCap Registry.* 021. Available at: https://clinicaltrials.gov/ct2/show/NCT03088020. Accessed December 15, 2021.
11. Trang H, Dehan M, Beaufils F, Zaccaria I, Amiel J, Gaultier C. The French congenital central hypoventilation syndrome registry: General data, phenotype, and genotype. *Chest.* 2005;127(1):72-79. doi:10.1378/chest.127.1.72. Accessed December 18, 2021.
12. *Congenital Central Hypoventilation Syndrome.* Available at: https://rarediseases.org/rare-diseases/congenital-central-hypoventilation-syndrome/. Accessed December 18, 2021.
13. Gronli JO, Santucci BA, Leurgans SE, Berry-Kravis EM, Weese-Mayer DE. Congenital central hypoventilation syndrome: *PHOX2B* genotype determines risk for sudden death. *Pediatr Pulmonol.* 2008;43(1):77-86. doi:10.1002/ppul.20744. Available at: https://onlinelibrary.wiley.com/doi/abs/10.1002/ppul.20744. Accessed December 19, 2021.
14. Kasi AS, Jurgensen TJ, Yen S, Kun SS, Keens TG, Perez IA. Three-generation family with congenital central hypoventilation syndrome and novel *PHOX2B* gene non-polyalanine repeat mutation. *J Clin Sleep Med.* 2017;13(7):925-927. doi:10.5664/jcsm.6670. Accessed January 7, 2022.
15. Hernandez-Miranda LR, Ibrahim DM, Ruffault P, et al. Mutation in *LBX1/Lbx1* precludes transcription factor cooperativity and causes congenital hypoventilation in humans and mice. *Proc Natl Acad Sci U S A.* 2018;115(51):13021-13026. doi:10.1073/pnas.1813520115. Accessed December 19, 2021.
16. Spielmann M, Hernandez-Miranda LR, Ceccherini I, et al. Mutations in MYO1H cause a recessive form of central hypoventilation with autonomic dysfunction. *J Med Genet.* 2017;54(11):754-761. doi:10.1136/jmedgenet-2017-104765. Accessed December 19, 2021.
17. Weese-Mayer DE, Silvestri JM, Menzies LJ, Morrow-Kenny AS, Hunt CE, Hauptman SA. Congenital central hypoventilation syndrome: Diagnosis, management, and long-term outcome in thirty-two children. *J Pediatr.* 1992;120(3):381-387. doi:10.1016/s0022-3476(05)80901-1. Accessed December 15, 2021.
18. Trang H, Samuels M, Ceccherini I, et al. Guidelines for diagnosis and management of congenital central hypoventilation syndrome. *Orphanet J Rare Dis.* 2020;15(1):252. doi:10.1186/s13023-020-01460-2. Accessed December 13, 2021.

19. Todd ES, Weinberg SM, Berry-Kravis EM, et al. Facial phenotype in children and young adults with *PHOX2B*-determined congenital central hypoventilation syndrome: quantitative pattern of dysmorphology. *Pediatr Res.* 2006;59(1):39-45. doi:10.1203/01.pdr.0000191814.73340.1d. Available at: https://www.ncbi.nlm.nih.gov/pubmed/16327002.
20. Marcus CL. Sleep-disordered breathing in children. *Am J Respir Crit Care Med.* 2001;164(1):16-30. doi:10.1164/ajrccm.164.1.2008171. Available at: https://www.atsjournals.org/doi/10.1164/ajrccm.164.1.2008171. Accessed January 7, 2022.
21. Gozal D, Marcus CL, Shoseyov D, Keens TG. Peripheral chemoreceptor function in children with the congenital central hypoventilation syndrome. *J Appl Physiol.* 1993;74(1):379-387. doi:10.1152/jappl.1993.74.1.379. Available at: https://journals.physiology.org/doi/abs/10.1152/jappl.1993.74.1.379. Accessed January 7, 2022.
22. Marcus CL, Bautista DB, Amihyia A, Ward SL, Keens TG. Hypercapneic arousal responses in children with congenital central hypoventilation syndrome. *Pediatrics.* 1991;88(5):993-998. doi:10.1542/peds.88.5.993. Available at: https://doi.org/10.1542/peds.88.5.993. Accessed December 19, 2021.
23. Weese-Mayer DE, Rand CM, Khaytin I, et al. Congenital central hypoventilation syndrome. In: Adam MP, Ardinger HH, Pagon RA, et al., eds. *GeneReviews®.* Seattle, WA: University of Washington, Seattle; 1993. Available at: http://www.ncbi.nlm.nih.gov/books/NBK1427/. Accessed December 15, 2021.
24. Zelko FA, Stewart TM, Brogadir CD, Rand CM, Weese-Mayer DE. Congenital central hypoventilation syndrome: broader cognitive deficits revealed by parent controls. *Pediatr Pulmonol.* 2018;53(4):492-497. doi:10.1002/ppul.23939. Accessed December 24, 2021.
25. Trang H, Bourgeois P, Cheliout-Heraut F. Neurocognition in congenital central hypoventilation syndrome: influence of genotype and ventilation method. *Orphanet J Rare Dis.* 2020;15(1):322. doi:10.1186/s13023-020-01601-7. Accessed December 24, 2021.
26. Charnay AJ, Antisdel-Lomaglio JE, Zelko FA, et al. Congenital central hypoventilation syndrome: neurocognition already reduced in preschool-aged children. *Chest.* 2016;149(3):809-815. doi:10.1378/chest.15-0402. Accessed January 7, 2022.
27. Marcus CL. *ROHHAD: Rapid-Onset Obesity, Breathing and Behavioral Issues Indicate a Very Sick Patient.* Updated 2016. Available at: https://www.chop.edu/news/rohhad-rapid-onset-obesity-breathing-and-behavioral-issues-indicate-very-sick-patient. Accessed January 4, 2022.
28. Fishman LS, Samson JH, Sperling DR. Primary alveolar hypoventilation syndrome (Ondine's curse). *Am J Dis Child.* 1965;110:155-161. doi:10.1001/archpedi.1965.02090030165011. Accessed December 15, 2021.
29. Ize-Ludlow D, Gray JA, Sperling MA, et al. Rapid-onset obesity with hypothalamic dysfunction, hypoventilation, and autonomic dysregulation presenting in childhood. *Pediatrics.* 2007;120(1):179. doi:10.1542/peds.2006-3324. Accessed January 7, 2022.
30. Carroll MS, Patwari PP, Kenny AS, Brogadir CD, Stewart TM, Weese-Mayer DE. Rapid-onset obesity with hypothalamic dysfunction, hypoventilation, and autonomic dysregulation (ROHHAD): response to ventilatory challenges. *Pediatr Pulmonol.* 2015;50(12):1336-1345. doi:10.1002/ppul.23164. Accessed January 4, 2022.
31. Abaci A, Catli G, Bayram E, et al. A case of rapid-onset obesity with hypothalamic dysfunction, hypoventilation, autonomic dysregulation, and neural crest tumor: Rohhadnet syndrome. *Endocr Pract.* 2013;19(1):e12-e16. doi:10.4158/EP12140.CR. Available at: https://www.sciencedirect.com/science/article/pii/S1530891X20412200. Accessed January 7, 2022.
32. Lazea C, Sur L, Florea M. ROHHAD (rapid-onset obesity with hypoventilation, hypothalamic dysfunction, autonomic dysregulation) syndrome—What every pediatrician should know about the etiopathogenesis, diagnosis and treatment: a review. *Int J Gen Med.* 2021;14:319-326. doi:10.2147/IJGM.S293377. Available at: https://www.ncbi.nlm.nih.gov/pmc/articles/PMC7853626/. Accessed Jan 4, 2022.
33. Jacobson LA, Rane S, McReynolds LJ, Steppan DA, Chen AR, Paz-Priel I. Improved behavior and neuropsychological function in children with ROHHAD after high-dose cyclophosphamide. *Pediatrics.* 2016;138(1):e20151080. doi:10.1542/peds.2015-1080. Accessed January 4, 2022.
34. Driscoll DJ, Miller JL, Schwartz S, Cassidy SB. *Prader-Willi Syndrome.* University of Washington, Seattle; 2017. Available at: https://www.ncbi.nlm.nih.gov/sites/books/NBK1330/. Accessed January 6, 2022.
35. Gozal D, Arens R, Omlin KJ, Ward SL, Keens TG. Absent peripheral chemosensitivity in Prader-Willi syndrome. *J Appl Physiol (1985).* 1994;77(5):2231-2236. doi:10.1152/jappl.1994.77.5.2231. Accessed January 6, 2022.

36. Arens R, Gozal D, Omlin KJ, et al. Hypoxic and hypercapnic ventilatory responses in Prader-Willi syndrome. *J Appl Physiol (1985)*. 1994;77(5):2224-2230. doi:10.1152/jappl.1994.77.5.2224. Accessed January 6, 2022.
37. Tauber M, Diene G, Molinas C, Hébert M. Review of 64 cases of death in children with Prader-Willi syndrome (PWS). *Am J Med Genet A*. 2008;146A(7):881-887. doi:10.1002/ajmg.a.32131. Accessed January 12, 2022.
38. Adzick NS, Walsh DS. Myelomeningocele: Prenatal diagnosis, pathophysiology and management. *Semin Pediatr Surg*. 2003;12(3):168-174. doi:10.1016/S1055-8586(03)00029-5. Available at: https://www.sciencedirect.com/science/article/pii/S1055858603000295. Accessed January 6, 2022.
39. Gilbert J, Jones K, Rorke L, Chernoff G, James H. Central nervous system anomalies associated with meningomyelocele, hydrocephalus, and the Arnold-Chiari malformation: Reappraisal of theories regarding the pathogenesis of posterior neural tube closure defects. *Neurosurgery*. 1986;18(5):559-564. doi:10.1227/00006123-198605000-00008. Accessed January 6, 2022.
40. Hidalgo JA, Tork CA, Varacallo M. Arnold Chiari malformation. In: *StatPearls*. Treasure Island, FL: StatPearls Publishing; 2021. Available at: http://www.ncbi.nlm.nih.gov/books/NBK431076/. Accessed January 6, 2022.
41. Hays RM, Jordan RA, McLaughlin JF, Nickel RE, Fisher LD. Central ventilatory dysfunction in myelodysplasia: An independent determinant of survival. *Dev Med Child Neurol*. 1989;31(3):366-370. doi:10.1111/j.1469-8749.1989.tb04005.x. Accessed January 6, 2022.
42. Darras BT. Neuromuscular disorders in the newborn. *Clin Perinatol*. 1997;24(4):827-844. Accessed January 7, 2022.
43. Kubota T, Adachi M, Kitaoka T, et al. Clinical practice guidelines for achondroplasia. *Clin Pediatr Endocrinol*. 2020;29(1):25-42. doi:10.1297/cpe.29.25. Accessed January 12, 2022.
44. Mogayzel PJ, Carroll JL, Loughlin GM, Hurko O, Francomano CA, Marcus CL. Sleep-disordered breathing in children with achondroplasia. *J Pediatr*. 1998;132(4):667-671. doi:10.1016/s0022-3476(98)70358-0. Accessed January 7, 2022.
45. Norcliffe-Kaufmann L, Kaufmann H. Familial dysautonomia (Riley–Day syndrome): When baroreceptor feedback fails. *Auton Neurosci*. 2012;172(1):26-30. doi:10.1016/j.autneu.2012.10.012. Available at: https://www.sciencedirect.com/science/article/pii/S1566070212001804. Accessed January 7, 2022.
46. Lee G, Papapetrou EP, Kim H, et al. Modelling pathogenesis and treatment of familial dysautonomia using patient-specific iPSCs. *Nature*. 2009;461(7262):402-406. doi:10.1038/nature08320. Accessed January 7, 2022.
47. Carroll MS, Kenny AS, Patwari PP, Ramirez J, Weese-Mayer DE. Respiratory and cardiovascular indicators of autonomic nervous system dysregulation in familial dysautonomia. *Pediatr Pulmonol*. 2012;47(7):682-691. doi:10.1002/ppul.21600. Available at: https://onlinelibrary-wiley-com.proxy.library.upenn.edu/doi/full/10.1002/ppul.21600. Accessed January 7, 2022.
48. Bernardi L, Hilz M, Stemper B, Passino C, Welsch G, Axelrod FB. Respiratory and cerebrovascular responses to hypoxia and hypercapnia in familial dysautonomia. *Am J Respir Crit Care Med*. 2003;167(2):141-149. doi:10.1164/rccm.200207-677OC. Available at: https://www.atsjournals.org/doi/full/10.1164/rccm.200207-677OC. Accessed January 7, 2022.
49. Weese-Mayer DE, Kenny AS, Bennett HL, Ramirez J, Leurgans SE. Familial dysautonomia: frequent, prolonged and severe hypoxemia during wakefulness and sleep. *Pediatr Pulmonol*. 2008;43(3):251-260. doi:10.1002/ppul.20764. Accessed January 7, 2022.

CHAPTER 9

Impact of Chronic Disease or Early Birth Complications on Sleep in Infancy

Courtney R.J. Kaar ▓ James S. Kemp ▓ Michael E. McLeland

Introduction

This chapter addresses problems with sleep, and primarily breathing during sleep, among several groups of infants with potentially chronic diseases that can be identified at birth or that appear and cause concern during the first months of life. The discussion focuses on issues of diagnosis and prognosis up to age 2 years. Suggestions for treatment are more often than not based on apparent consensus and clinical experience in those situations where something should be done, but the evidence for exactly what is not clear.

Some complex entities, for example, the spectrum of problems addressed under the rubric Pierre-Robin Sequence,[1] have been so variably described and treated that they cannot be addressed adequately in a chapter given over to many entities. Studies that are multicenter, with clear inclusion criteria based both on anatomic and pathophysiologic hypotheses, are scarce, and we need to do better.

Children at High Risk for Sleep-Disordered Breathing: Technical Concerns for Polysomnography

With a few well-known caveats, polysomnography technicians familiar with performing sleep studies in infants should be adept at obtaining reliable data in infants at much risk for sleep-disordered breathing (SDB) because of anatomic anomalies.

Infants with mid-face hypoplasia (e.g., Apert syndrome, Crouzon syndrome, trisomy 21, achondroplasia) can present particular challenges in obtaining measurements and estimates of flow, whether by thermistor or pressure transducer, or derived from respiratory inductance plethysmography (RIP). Both nasal and oral flow signals must be sought. RIP-derived flow calculations may be difficult to obtain during REM sleep.

Reliable, semiquantitative estimates of tidal volumes may be hard to acquire from infants with complex chest wall mechanics (those, for example, with myelomeningocele, achondroplasia, scoliosis, spinal muscular atrophy (SMA)). The assumption underlying conventional rib cage and abdominal belts for inductance plethysmography is that the respiratory system moves with essentially two "degrees of freedom,"[2] an assumption that may not be met when there is marked rib cage narrowing or deformation. Rib cage and abdominal dyssynchrony will be extreme in SMA1 (at least in times past!) and variable in most high-risk infants, especially during REM sleep. Because of much dyssynchrony at baseline, with even more variability depending on sleep state, the conventional, computerized autocalibration of RIP used to describe changes in tidal volume will be challenged.[2]

113

Perhaps both more challenging and more important is obtaining reliable noninvasive estimates of $PaCO_2$,[3,4] among infants at no small risk for hypoventilation during sleep (e.g., infants with myelomeningocele with a high spine defect and higher-grade Chiari malformation). Infants breathing rapidly often do not have acceptable plateaus on exhaled capnometric curves, so that the agreement between $P_{ET}CO_2$ and $PaCO_2$ can only be guessed. In our experience, transcutaneous capnometers often seem to "go out of cal," and require membrane replacement and repeat calibration, steps that can disrupt sleep.

Much vigilance and a high index of suspicion are needed for infants at higher risk for hypoventilation. Inspection of capnometry tracing and $P_{ET}CO_2$ during the long exhalation after a sigh breath may give a more or less accurate snapshot of actual $PaCO_2$. Increased serum HCO_3^- may also point to hypoventilation, albeit with marginal sensitivity.

Sleep and Sleep-Disordered Breathing Among Infants Born Prematurely

In the United States each year, 10,000 to 15,000 infants born prematurely are assigned the diagnosis of bronchopulmonary dysplasia (BPD). For this discussion, we will use a newer label, postprematurity respiratory disease (PPRD), to describe infants born before 37 weeks postmenstrual age (PMA), whether or not they were assigned the diagnosis of BPD.[5,6] We will focus on those with relatively long NICU stays.

There is nearly a three-fold increase in risk for SDB during childhood for infants born prematurely (7.2%).[7] Increased risk for SDB appears to extend into adulthood with more than twofold increase extending into the 5th decade of life.[8]

The prevalence and risk calculations are based on polysomnography (PSG) and questionnaire criteria for the diagnosis of SDB that have been validated in children older than 2 years and in adults, not for a population ≤2 years of age. The implications from PSG studies done before nursery or NICU discharge are not clear. When evaluated using PSG, the infants often seem to improve over several weeks without specific interventions, or their frequency of events seems to "respond" to supplemental O_2.[9-11]

Defined thresholds for the diagnosis of SDB among newborns during the first 28 days of life, or for infants recovering from premature birth, are not established. Findings in full-term newborns only seem to obscure any potential threshold at which intervention based on PSG might be recommended. One group of healthy term-born infants near 1 month of age had apnea-hypopnea indices (AHI) of 14.9 ± 9.1 (range 1.0–37.7)[12] Among older children, this frequency of events might be associated with excessive daytime sleepiness and usually lead to early adenotonsillectomy. However, in the absence of marked hypoxemia during sleep and suspected pulmonary hypertension, criteria for expected morbidity with thresholds for intervention are not clear for children ≤2 years of age.[13]

PREDISPOSING FACTORS AND MANIFESTATIONS OF SDB AMONG INFANTS WITH PPRD

Stertorous breathing and failure to thrive are classic findings of severe SDB in infants. When loud breathing and poor growth occur together among convalescing premature infants, airway endoscopy, at least limited PSG, and specific interventions are certainly indicated. How to proceed is much less clear when infants have quiet breathing, intermittent brief falls in SpO_2%, varying frequencies of central or obstructive apneas or hypopneas, and varying severity of chronic lung disease.[6,14] Often, without antecedent PSG or inspection of continuously recorded respiratory impedance data, supplemental O_2 is prescribed in the NICU and weaned slowly. It is likely, however, that infants thus treated have some combination of more or less mild lung disease, subtle upper airway narrowing, and abnormal maturation of ventilatory control, the effect of each hidden or ameliorated by preventing desaturations with supplemental O_2.[15,16]

LUNG DISEASE PER SE MAKES THE DIAGNOSIS OF SDB MORE LIKELY

Particularly while breathing ambient room air, preterm infants with smaller functional residual capacities are more likely to have greater desaturations with even short pauses in respiratory effort.[17] That is, reduced effective lung volumes for postinspiratory gas exchange, due to chronic lung disease, make desaturations per second of pause greater. In the PROP study (Prematurity and Respiratory Outcomes Program) of infants born between 24 and 28 weeks PMA, 17.7% had falls in SpO_2% by 2% or more per second of central apnea.[18] Even in the absence of long pauses and obvious upper airway obstruction, then, recovering premature infants are more likely to have events that are "scoreable" for SDB.

PROPOSED ANATOMIC FACTORS IN SDB AMONG INFANTS BORN PREMATURELY

Laryngeal injury and acquired subglottic stenosis typically cause soft cries or stertorous breathing and are usually suspected on clinical grounds. The prevalence and impact of adenotonsillar hypertrophy in the first 2 years of life among infants born prematurely are not known.

For most premature infants with intermittent desaturations during sleep, factors are likely in play that are more subtle and not associated with the turbulence giving rise to obvious stertorous breathing.

Pharyngeal hypotonia, acquired dolichocephaly, and similar difficult-to-quantify factors are postulated to cause subtle SDB, but they have only rarely been quantified in more detail.[19] One exception is the following: clinicians have long recognized that recovering premature infants may have narrow "arched" or "vaulted" hard palates, with the implicit assumption that the deformation is a complication of long-term placement of an orotracheal tube. It has been suggested, however, that some infants are predisposed to narrower palates because they were born very early. In a study of 244 premature infants, none of whom had "long-term intubation," the presence of a narrower hard palate at birth and at 6 months postnatal age was associated with higher apnea-hypopnea indices at 6 and 24 months of age.[20] The authors speculate that interruption by preterm birth of normal fetal sucking and chewing actions might predispose to palatal narrowing that persists and causes "more subtle forms of SDB such as abnormal amounts of flow limitation."

VENTILATORY CONTROL FACTORS: POTENTIAL CONTRIBUTION TO SDB

It appears that long central apneas (15–20 seconds or longer) as a complication of apnea of prematurity can be limited by the use of caffeine and resolve by 43 to 44 weeks PMA.[21-23] However, it is not clear when the abnormal ventilatory control maturation that readily gives rise to periodic breathing actually resolves.[24] Some aspects of periodic breathing among premature infants, with higher system "loop gain,"[25] resemble the pattern of breathing during severe obstructive SDB in adults. This "obstructive cycling" is a phenomenon that is periodic and often explained by high loop gain.[26,27]

Desaturations during periodic apnea that is part of periodic breathing patterns may not be benign (Fig. 9.1). Furthermore, it is not widely recognized that during periodic breathing spells, the rate of falls in SpO_2 is faster during the latter periodic apneas compared to those occurring earlier in the periodic breathing spell.[28,29]

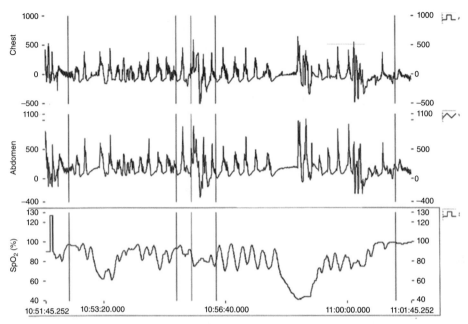

Fig. 9.1   Ten-minute tracing from preterm infant at 36 weeks PMA. Upper two tracings of respiratory impedance plethysmography show periodic breathing with 38 seconds central apnea. Bottom tracing shows pulse
oximetry (SpO$_2$%) with oscillations accompanying periodic apneas. Depth of oscillations during periodic
breathing/apneas likely increased by some measure of unresolved chronic lung disease. NadirSpO$_2$% = 46%
during long central apnea. *PMA*, Postmenstrual age.

In addition, among premature infants, it has long been known that hypopneas can also be
"periodic."[30] Indeed, the two tracings in Fig. 9.2 show that periodic apnea and periodic hypopnea
can take place in one child within minutes. The periodic hypopneas were scored as obstructive
hypopneas, as they would be in most sleep laboratories. It is clear that this infant has not "out-
grown" her propensity for periodic breathing.

It is generally accepted that a high CO$_2$ apnea threshold underlies the oscillatory breathing
pattern among some infants. Demonstrating this by manipulating and estimating PCO$_2$ by exhaled capnometry has been difficult because infants breathe too rapidly to be confident that alveolar gas is being sampled.[31] Perhaps the clearest depiction of the role of CO$_2$ thresholds is from
a study of 10 infants born at 28 weeks PMA and studied at 40 weeks PMA.[32] The infants were
intubated and EMG recordings were made from the diaphragm, alae nasi, genioglossus, and
posterior cricoarytenoideus muscles. Reliable P$_{ET}$CO$_2$ could be recorded, and protocol-guided
increases and decreases in the ventilator rate showed that the EMGs from the upper airway sites
were silenced at higher P$_{ET}$CO$_2$ ($\sim$42–47 mmHg) than the diaphragm ($\sim$39 mmHg) (Fig. 9.3).
The authors surmised that continued diaphragm activity when upper airway EMG signals were
reduced would set the stage for obstructive SDB. When and if these discrepant activation thresholds become more synchronous in infants born prematurely is not known.

NEUROCOGNITIVE AND BEHAVIORAL IMPACT OF SDB DURING THE FIRST 2 YEARS OF LIFE

It is not surprising that sleep disruption among former premature infants is associated in later
childhood with increased daytime sleepiness, hyperactivity, inattention, and emotional problems.

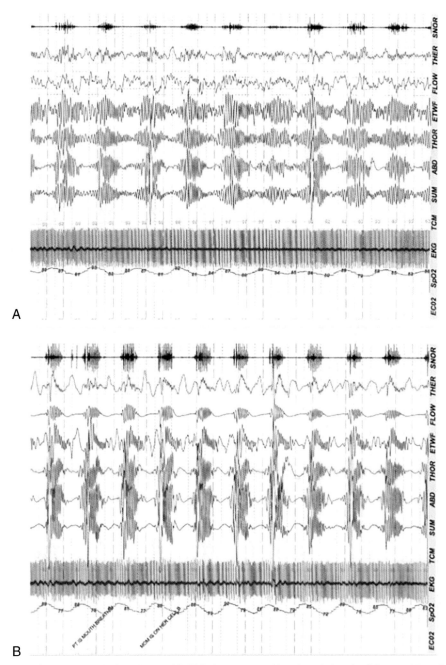

Fig. 9.2 Polysomnography from 3-year-old child who snores and is a "mouth breather." Born at 27 weeks PMA. Both screens are 4 minutes. (A) Early in study. Periodic breathing with periodic hypopnea and fluctuations in SpO$_2$%. (B) 20 minutes later. Periodicity persists but with periodic hyperpnea and periodic relative apnea and continued and more extreme fluctuations in SpO$_2$%. Snor is snore monitor. Ther nasal thermistor. Flow nasal/oral pressure sensor. ETWF capnometry tracing. Thor Abd Sum Inductance plethysmography from chest and abdomen and their sum. *PMA,* Postmenstrual age. *(From Mammel D, Kemp J. Prematurity, the diagnosis of bronchopulmonary dysplasia, and maturation of ventilatory control.* Pediatr Pulmonol. *2021;56(11):3533–3545.)*

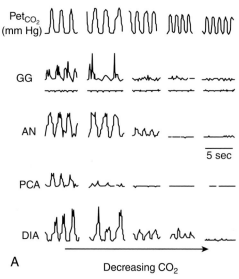

Fig. 9.3a Response of GG, AN, PCA, and DIA moving time averages during decreases in $PETCO_2$ in one infant. Initially, all EMGs showed phasic inspiratory activity. With hyperventilation and consequent reduction in $PETCO_2$, gradual decreases and ultimate disappearance of each EMG occurred. During this study, $PETCO_2$ decreased from 60 to 42 Torr. Usually, PCA had the lowest CO_2 threshold of all upper airway muscles, although in this infant, CO_2 threshold for PCA was higher than that of AN.

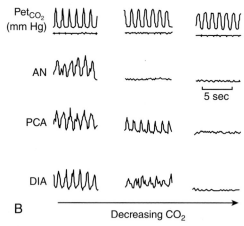

Fig. 9.3b Response of AN, PCA, and DIA moving time average during decreases in $PETCO_2$ in an infant who did not have GG recruitment. With hyperventilation there was reduction and finally disappearance of all EMGs.

In a study from the UK comparing 165 children born prematurely to 121 term-born, SDB worsened sleep disruption and increased the prevalence of neurocognitive and behavioral challenges.[13]

How SDB with its associated baggage affects infants in the first 2 years of life is not clear. Relevant studies are rare. Infants who received caffeine as newborns, as part of the Caffeine for Apnea of Prematurity trial, had higher performances on the Bayley Mental Development Index at 18 to 21 months,[33] and did better than the control group in fine motor coordination and tests of visual learning skills at age ~11 years.[34]

Whether neurocognitive and behavioral problems due to SDB in later childhood might be better addressed if diagnosed in infancy and treated earlier is not clear.[5]

SUMMARY

Premature infants who breathe quietly but have intermittent falls in SpO_2% while asleep, large enough to be "scored" as events on PSG, require thoughtful clinical approaches that consider lung disease, upper airway functional patency, and ventilatory control. Pulmonary and sleep practitioners should know that incompletely resolved lung disease makes "scoreable" events more likely. Neonatologists should be aware that incompletely resolved susceptibility to unstable, oscillatory breathing patterns can persist until at least 6 months postterm-corrected age.[24,35]

Polysomnographic thresholds for intervention are not clear; the cost-benefit calculations for treatment are likely not favorable when there are fewer than, for example, 2 to 5 events per hour.

Judicious use of supplemental O_2, timely follow-up studies, and perhaps more attention paid to the impact of sleep disruption caused by SDB may constitute the most prudent approach when the majority of evidence is of "very low certainty."[5]

Gastroesophageal Reflux

This section on gastroesophageal reflux [GER] and the next on Laryngomalacia address possible causes of SDB that are often considered as comorbidities in infants with SDB, particularly among infants with known neurologic disease. Their roles as a primary cause for SDB will also be considered.

Reflux of gastric contents into the esophagus and hypopharynx is cited as a common comorbidity among infants evaluated for SDB.[36] When GER is shown or postulated to exacerbate poor feeding, cough, irritability, frequent awakenings, and SDB, it is called GER disease. What is usually debated is the importance of GER in causing or exacerbating these problems. Despite published thresholds defining abnormal versus normal amounts of GER, a causal association with symptoms often remains unclear.

Although the comorbidity "GER" is often applied to infants with SDB, the presumed diagnosis is not more frequent than among the general population of infants without SDB.[36] Treatment of GER, particularly acidic GER, though often effective for esophagitis, does not predictably lead to resolution of other symptoms for which GERD is the putative explanation.[37-47]

SELECTED ANATOMIC AND PHYSIOLOGIC FACTS

The lower esophageal sphincter (LES), along with "sling" fibers from the crural diaphragm, forms the gastroesophageal (GE) junction.[48,49] Low resting tone of the LES is a risk factor for GERD, but the more important mechanism in infants is transient LES relaxation, particularly during and after swallowing. With maturation, the amount and duration of LES relaxation with swallowing are less.

Reflux may be acidic or nonacidic. Infants' esophagi average only 6.5 cm in length[50] and reflux often extends up to the pharynx.[51] In preterm infants, apnea can be so frequent that linking events temporally to antecedent reflux is challenging.[42,51-53]

HOW GER MIGHT DISRUPT BREATHING

Central apnea due to the laryngeal chemoreflex is a well-established and potent cause for interruption of breathing in young infants, particularly those born prematurely.[54,55] In experimental protocols, dripping as little as 1 mL of milk or water on to the larynx can elicit vocal cord adduction and central apnea, and, as swallowing begins to clear fluid from the cords, a few obstructed breaths.[56] With maturation, the more effective and brisk cough reflex supervenes to clear the larynx, with much briefer apnea. Studies in newborn lambs both sleeping and awake show that apnea as part of the laryngeal chemoreflex is prolonged during sleep.[57]

Thus, there is an established mechanism when GER is laryngopharyngeal that can explain its role in SDB in the youngest infants. It should be remembered, however, that the laryngeal chemoreflex can be elicited even without the involvement of gastric contents or acidic fluid. Rather, infants with exaggerated laryngeal chemoreflex do not require gastric contents to return to the esophagus or pharynx to become symptomatic during, for example, feedings or RSV infections.

Indeed, in very young infants RSV has been shown to elicit mixed apneas that resemble those seen with laryngeal chemoreflex apnea (LCRA)[58] and postulating GER as a cause for SDB during acute RSV infections may be superfluous (Fig. 9.4).

Endoscopic evaluation of infants with laryngomalacia often shows a puffy, inflamed supraglottis and larynx.[59] Whether or not acid reflux is an important or sole cause in a particular infant with laryngomalacia and this endoscopic picture is not clear. Nevertheless, GER is often implied to be a causal comorbidity, when laryngomalacia causes SDB.

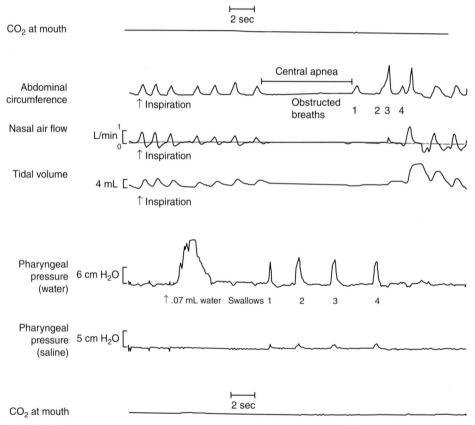

Fig. 9.4 The sequence of responses represents laryngeal chemoreflex apnea; in an infant. Upward deflections on pharyngeal pressure tracing reflect swallows. Application of less than 0.1 mL of water onto the larynx leads to swallows and central apnea, followed by obstructive apnea and restoration of eupnea after the water has been cleared by swallows. *(From Davies AM, Koenig JS, Thach BT. Upper airway chemoreflex responses to saline and water in preterm infants. J Appl physiol. 1988:64:1412–1420.)*

Whether acidic or not, mechanisms whereby reflux that does not reach the cervical esophagus might elicit pauses in breathing are less robust and difficult to define. In infants and in lambs, behavioral and electrocortical arousals, sometimes with sleep disruption, are the most consistent effects of stimulation of the mid-esophagus.[60-62] Though apnea has been described in lambs with esophageal stimulation and slower breathing in infants,[63] if and when there are responses to mid-esophageal stimulation they are often arousal, coughing, and swallowing, responses that favor airway protection.[64] These "vigilance mechanisms" are often accompanied by "respiratory arousals" with augmented breaths and more rapid breathing.[60]

TREATMENT

Treatment strategies when GER(D) is thought to exacerbate SDB should reflect hypotheses regarding how breathing is disrupted. For example, an exaggerated laryngeal chemoreflex with apnea has been shown to occur during acute RSV infections[58] and SDB in convalescing infants should not only be attributed to GER. Most events once labeled acute life-threatening events (ALTE), now more often called brief, resolved unexplained events (BRUE), resemble "choking"[65] and are consistent with laryngeal chemoreflex apnea, which, as we have explained, does not require either acidic fluid or GER to be elicited.

Feeding should be careful and slow for infants with exaggerated laryngeal chemoreflexes and with problematic GER because of transient relaxation of the LES that occurs with swallowing.

Unfortunately, the opportunity for better understanding of complex causes for SDB is missed when GERD is postulated to explain SDB and other breathing problems, with little consideration given to specific pathophysiologic mechanisms. In this regard, there are no clinical studies showing the effectiveness of acid suppression in reducing SDB. Furthermore, empiric use of proton pump inhibitors and other forms of acid suppression is not supported by studies addressing underlying mechanisms explaining how GER might cause SDB.[66]

SUMMARY

GERD is frequently cited as a comorbidity among infants with SDB, often with the implicit assumption that its role is also causative. The clearest mechanism for GERD's role in causing SDB is via apnea following the laryngeal chemoreflex, a reflex that can be elicited without either acidic fluid or GER.

Laryngomalacia

There have been several recent reports describing laryngomalacia, its symptoms, and the contribution of surgical supraglottoplasty (SGP) to its resolution.[67,68] Laryngomalacia is the most common cause for stridor in newborns and young infants, with symptoms often appearing in the first days or weeks of life.[69] While awake, short, high-pitched inspiratory stridor is common during vigorous feeding or crying. Our discussion will focus on sleep and SDB during sleep, although failure to thrive, due to difficulty in timing sucking, swallowing, and breathing[54,70] during awake feedings, is the most consistent reason for surgical SGP.

Nearly 80% of infants with the diagnosis of laryngomalacia by the ages of 7 to 17 months will have SDB as defined by conventional, though perhaps impractical, criteria: AHI >1.[12,67] Conversely, in large series of infants with SDB, 20% to 40% also have laryngomalacia.[67,71,72]

The functional "softness" ("malacia" = flaccidity due to softness) of the supraglottis and larynx can be seen by flexible laryngoscopy and, recently in some centers, by laryngeal ultrasound.[73] During spontaneous inspiration, there is prolapse of the supraglottis and/or the arytenoid mucosa and cartilages, often with an audible squeak.[74,75] Although findings of pathologic prolapse are often straightforward, care must be taken in interpreting laryngoscopic findings, because in the minimally sedated child, visualization may be difficult. And in the more deeply sedated child there may be relaxation of pharyngeal and hypopharyngeal structures, necessitating higher inspiratory pressures to accomplish breathing and causing more supraglottic and laryngeal prolapse.

Recent papers have not focused on isolated, structural softness of the supraglottis, or arytenoids.[76,77] Instead, laryngomalacia is more often reported as a comorbidity in infants with generalized hypotonia, e.g., infants with trisomy 21.[77] Unfortunately, the success rate of SGP in terms of symptom resolution is less among infants with known syndromes or neurologic disease causing hypotonia.[78] It is also speculated that otherwise healthy infants might have functionally significant but more or less isolated laryngeal hypotonia. The finding that as many as 44% of infants with laryngomalacia and OSA also have central sleep apnea (CAI >5)[79] that recedes over time also supports the notion that early, delayed maturation of ventilatory drive in some infants may underlie their laryngeal prolapse.[26,75]

Related brainstem and spinal cord sites that integrate laryngeal sensorimotor function and phrenic nerve output to the diaphragm are possible sites of delayed maturation.[75] In most children with SDB due to laryngomalacia, both the frequency and severity of respiratory events decrease without need for noninvasive ventilation or SGP. This may suggest improvement in delayed maturation of ventilatory drive and control that gave rise to laryngeal prolapse, and the spontaneous improvement with time is reminiscent of spontaneous maturation of other laryngeal reflexes, for example, exaggerated laryngeal chemoreflex with apnea.

Among infants with laryngomalacia, SDB can be mild (73%), moderate (11%), or severe (16%).[67] Published reports do not establish thresholds for AHI or SpO_2% nadir at which SGP is more strongly recommended. Refractory failure to thrive and recurrent apnea or cyanosis requiring stimulation or soothing are the accepted and reasonable clinical criteria for surgical intervention.[67,68]

A recent report on 102 infants examined retrospectively whether those who had SPG performed had earlier resolution of SDB than those infants who were observed and fed patiently.[68] PSG was repeated every 3 months until the AHI was <1. Initial PSG was done at ages ~70 to 108 days (2.3–3.6 months). Infants were analyzed by groups according to when the subsequent PSG was "normal" (0–6 months of age, 6–12, and >12 months). With increasing age, there were decreases in AHI, obstructive index (OI), and central apnea index in both groups. Children receiving SGP were more likely to have a reduction in OI between 6 and 12 months of age, but there were no differences in frequency of normalizing at <6 months or >12 months of age. Findings such as these have led some to suggest[69] that randomized, clinical trials can be done evaluating SGP versus observation and careful feeding among infants without additional comorbid factors.

In general, improvement in SDB is unpredictable after adenotonsillectomy among children with hypotonia and adenotonsillar hypertrophy.[78] Add laryngeal prolapse to generalized hypotonia and adenotonsillar hypertrophy, and it is even more unclear how to predict which infants will improve with SGP, or whether observation alone is ever acceptable.[26,80] It is furthermore unclear whether adenotonsillectomy that removes a "fixed" obstruction might expose the laryngeal structures to less inspiratory pressure and allow them not to collapse.[68]

Myelomeningocele and SDB

Despite reductions in incidence with folic acid fortification during pregnancy, spina bifida with myelomeningocele (MMC) occurs in 1 per 2000 live born infants in the United States.[81] Most (63%) children with MMC have been shown to have some measure of SDB and 20% have moderate-to-severe SDB when tested in later childhood (AHI >5).[82] Of those with moderate-to-severe, 34% had central sleep apnea, 41% obstructive SDB, and 16% central hypoventilation.[83] Some children, ~8% in one series, have hypoxemia without discrete respiratory events ("sleep-exacerbated restrictive lung disease.") This last group has pulmonary function tests showing forced vital capacity <50% predicted. All four types have been described among infants <2 years of age—central apnea, obstructive SDB, central hypoventilation, and sleep-exacerbated restrictive lung disease.[82-84] SDB can be quite severe in the youngest children with MMC, and as many as 15% of children between 3 and 30 months of age can have a syndrome of lower cranial nerve palsies, dysphagia, and severe central apnea, with unpredictable responses to posterior fossa decompression.[83]

A preliminary study in the first week of life has shown that infants with MMC have significantly more frequent respiratory events during PSG than a postmenstrual age (37.5 weeks) matched comparison group (AHI 34.2 + 21.9 versus 19.3 + 11.1).[84] Infants with MMC had significantly more hypopnea events than the comparison group (21.2/hour versus 12.4/hour). The comparison group had fewer central and obstructive apneas, but the difference was not significant. Eleven of 19 comparison group infants but only 3 of 19 infants with MMC had fewer than 20 events per hour. None of the infants with MMC in this series had apneas longer than 20 seconds, a typical duration threshold for apnea alarms in newborn intensive care units (NICUs). As a result, what would be diagnosed as moderate-to-severe SDB may not be detected in busy NICUs.[85]

Detailed studies of ventilatory control responses have not been done among infants with MMC. Studies in older children and adolescents (11.3 + SEM 1.5 years),[86] including some requiring support for central hypoventilation, have shown a range of abnormalities in both central (CO_2 response) and peripheral chemoreception (responses to hypoxia and hyperoxia). Though central chemoreception was clearly blunted in many, the most frequent and marked abnormality was in peripheral chemoreception. Gozal et al.[86] speculate that the more diffuse distribution of central chemoreception, beyond the brain stem, would tend to limit marked alterations in central chemoreception to patients with the most severe hindbrain malformations, including those with central hypoventilation. Conversely, they speculate that what is more common is direct injury to peripheral chemoreceptor afferents and the more focal brainstem areas "mediating" peripheral chemoreceptor integration. As a result, the more common characteristics of SDB in children with MMC are frequent short central apneas, obstructive apneas, and hypopneas.

MAGNETIC RESONANCE IMAGING AND SLEEP-DISORDERED BREATHING IN PATIENTS WITH MMC

Among older children (~9 years old), two brain MRI findings have been associated with moderate-to-severe SDB[82]: reduction in the subarachnoid space surrounding the medulla and cervical spinal cord and severe and extensive Chiari malformations.[87] The time course of appearance and the potential prognostic significance of these or related imaging abnormalities for infants have not been evaluated.

MECHANICAL "BELLOWS" FUNCTION OF THE RESPIRATORY SYSTEM AND SLEEP-DISORDERED BREATHING IN PATIENTS WITH MMC

Scoliosis and abnormal chest wall mechanics, associated with thoracic and high lumbar defects, have been linked to the "thoracic insufficiency syndrome."[88] Among older children, adolescents, and young adults with MMC, this has been defined as spirometric forced vital capacity and CT estimates of lung volume <50% predicted for age and fingertip-to-fingertip length. In one study of 31 nonambulatory subjects, reduction in FVC and CT volumes to <50% predicted were associated with reduction in T1 to S1 "seated height" to 67.6% predicted. Also, for these 31 patients with MMC, mean maximal inspiratory pressure was only 43 + 22 cm H_2O, on average less than half of expected, suggesting that many had marked inspiratory weakness.[88]

Findings like these point to explanations for "sleep-exacerbated restrictive lung disease" that begins with lung bellows dysfunction rather than primary lung parenchymal disease. How much bellows inadequacy contributes to SDB in infants has not been studied but is of obvious potential importance for infants with thoracic or higher lumbar defects.[83] Studies of hypercapneic ventilatory responses in older children[86] suggested, however, that responses were not ventilatory-function limited. Similar studies in infants of, for example, minute volume responses to inhaling 5% CO_2, might be informative. Such studies in infants with higher defects might clarify whether improvements in respiratory system mechanical efficiency during the first year of life lessen SDB, particularly during REM sleep.

INTERVENTION FOR SDB IN INFANTS WITH MMC

As with most causes of SDB in infants, thresholds of AHI at which treatment is clearly beneficial do not exist for patients with MMC. To be sure, profound central hypoventilation and frequent and long central apneas require intervention, most often via a tracheostomy and mechanical ventilation. Because these patients often have problematic central apnea, it must be remembered that snoring may not be a primary manifestation of SDB.

Treatment of obstructive SDB by adenotonsillectomy should be used in select patients with MMC, but it is often ineffective.[83] CPAP, Bi-level PAP, and trans-nasal mechanical ventilation are used in children with MMC and SDB with considerable success. Supplemental oxygen alone may stabilize ventilatory pattern, as well as limit hypoxemia, in very young infants with moderate central and obstructive SDB, especially if there are frequent hypopneas. This intervention for infants with MMC, in particular, should be tested and adjusted in the sleep laboratory to be certain that there is little or no increase in $PaCO_2$.

Recently, it has become clear that normal, term infants have frequent respiratory events during sleep at ~3 weeks of age,[12] some nearly as frequent as in infants with MMC.[84] Maturation will, presumably, lessen event frequency in ostensibly normal infants. Whether a parallel, benevolent course due to maturation of ventilatory control and stabilization of respiratory mechanics plays out in infants with MME, who almost always have AHI >20, remains to be seen.[84]

Spinal Muscular Atrophy

Spinal muscular atrophy (SMA) is an autosomal recessive neuromuscular disorder characterized by degeneration of the anterior horn cells in the spinal cord and motor nuclei in the lower brainstem. Untreated, this degeneration results in progressive atrophy and muscle weakness. The leading cause of mortality and morbidity in progressive neuromuscular disorders is respiratory dysfunction.

The most common form of SMA is due to a defect in the survival motor neuron 1 (SMN1) gene which has been mapped to 5q13; specifically, 5q11.2-q13.3.[89-98] The absence of exons 7 and 8 of the SMN1 gene cause 96% of SMA cases.[99-103] The protein produced by SMN1 appears to be involved in mRNA synthesis in motor neurons.[104] Differences in expression of SMA are usually related to a modifying gene called survival motor neuron 2 (SMN2). Phenotypic severity is inversely related to the copy number of SMN2, with the presence of three or more copies resulting in milder severity.[105-107]

The potential impact of SMA on posture, ambulation, etc. is severe, but for the purpose of this chapter, we will focus on the effects of SMA and its treatments on respiratory function during sleep.

Recent, profound advances that are effective and lifesaving make early diagnosis imperative so treatment can be delivered during the first weeks of life after newborn screening.

The gold standard of genetic testing is an analysis of SMN1 and SMN2 using quantitative polymerase chain reaction (qPCR), next-generation sequencing (NGS), or multiplex ligation-dependent probe amplification (MLPA).[108-111] Knowing the number of copies for both SMN1 and SMN2 is important for identification of heterozygous deletions, establishing prognosis, and choosing possible therapies.

Guidelines (see Table 9.1) for the timing and types of supportive intervention have been based upon the functional status of individuals: are they nonsitters, sitters, or walkers? These traditional categories may still be generally useful, even when, hopefully, few children will be unable to sit.

Noninvasive ventilation (NIV) should be used in all symptomatic infants, and in nonsitters prior to signs of respiratory failure.[112-114] Advantages in early use of NIV include improvement in sleep architecture and sleep quality, minimizing and delaying respiratory failure, lessening chest wall deformity, and managing dyspnea.[114-122] Continuous positive airway pressure (CPAP) and related NIV should not be used for long-term treatment of respiratory failure but they may be necessary for several days, even around-the-clock, when infants who have received newer therapies have respiratory infections.

Other traditional therapies, such as insufflation-exsufflation ("cough assist"), suctioning, and chest physiotherapies, will remain essential in reducing airway resistance during respiratory infections and maintaining lung volumes.

Detailed measurement of respiratory system function and sleep polysomnography have not been done among infants and children who have received new therapies. It is clear that progression to respiratory failure or the need for many hours per day of mechanical ventilatory support is much less frequent with newer therapies. However, providers should be urged to obtain PSG, or some truncated study, with "even minimal (clinical) suspicion of symptoms of nocturnal hypoventilation" (Table 9.1).

Besides SDB, other sleep disorders and disturbances may be more common in patients with SMA. In a study in 2017, Pera et al. used the Sleep Disturbance Scale for Children (SDSC), a validated scale to evaluate the occurrence of sleep disorders in the 6 months prior to assessment, to compare the frequency of sleep disturbances in pediatric patients with SMA versus healthy individuals. This study found a higher occurrence (16.4%) of sleep disturbances (problems with maintaining sleep) in SMA patients versus the normal population (5%).[123]

More abnormalities in sleep architecture have been demonstrated in SMA type 2 patients versus a comparison group of normal children, with significant increases of awakenings per hour, wake after sleep onset, and percentage of stage N1 being the most pronounced changes found.[124] A study published in 2019 showed persistent changes in sleep architecture despite long-term noninvasive positive pressure ventilation.[125]

APPROACHES SINCE INTRODUCTION OF NOVEL THERAPIES

Since 2016, three novel therapies have been approved by the FDA for treatment of SMA, with dramatic benefits for SMA 1. Therapies have become available that enhance the function of SMN2 protein by increasing gene copies (intrathecal nusinersin, enteral risdiplam) or directly replacing the pathologic *SMN1* gene mutation (intravenous onasemnogene abeparvovec, Zolgensma[R]). As noted above, these interventions have dramatically altered expectations for progression to respiratory failure or need for noninvasive respiratory support. Clinicians caring for these patients should exercise considerable vigilance, however, because it is not clear how much more improvement in the function of muscles supporting breathing, coughing, and deglutition can be expected as these children grow and develop, and whether the improvement can be sustained, even as the children are able to stand and walk.

It is essential that clinicians ask about daytime sleepiness and inattentiveness and increased fatigue. It seems likely that at least a cross-sectional research study of sleep and breathing using PSG will be needed, for example, during preschool years, particularly if concerns remain regarding sleep quality. Truncated tests with high negative-predictive values may prove useful, as has been shown, for example, for overnight oximetry in children with myelomeningocele.[83] Though

TABLE 9.1 ■ Pulmonary Assessment, Intervention, and Management Recommendations

	Assessment	Intervention	Care Considerations
Nonsitters	Physical examination Assessment of hypoventilation (end-tidal CO_2) Sleep study or pneumograms in all symptomatic patients or to determine if a patient needs to initiate NIV Clinical assessment of gastroesophageal reflux	Support airway clearance Oral suctioning Physiotherapy/respiratory therapy should be implemented immediately: Manual chest therapy Cough insufflator exsufflator Support ventilation with bilevel NIV in symptomatic patients	Acursements should be performed at least every 1 month initially, then every 6 months. Supporting airway clearance with nasal suctioning, physiotherapy/respiratory therapy, and cough assist is critical to all nonsitters with ineffective cough. Ventilation should be started in all symptomatic patients. Some experts recommend using it before documented respiratory failure to palliate dyspnea. This should be judged on individual basis. NIV should be initiated in observing the patient clinically for adequate gas exchange or during a sleep study. NIV interfaces should be fitted by skilled physiotherapists selecting two interfaces with different skin contact points.
		Nebulized bronchodilators in patients with asthma or a positive bronchodilator response Customary immunizations, palivizumab through 24 months, influenza vaccination annually after 6 months of age	Mucolytics should not be used long term.
Sitters	Physical examination Spirometry (when possible depending on age and cooperation) Sleep study or pneumograms in all patients with even minimal suspicion of symptoms of nocturnal hypoventilation Assessment of gastroesophageal reflux	Supon airway clearance Physiotherapy/respiratory therapy should be implemented immediately Manual chest physiotherapy Cough insufflator/exsufflator Support ventilation with bilevel NIV in symptomatic patients	Assessments should be performed every 6 months. Supporting airway clearance is critical to all patients with ineffective cough. Ventilation should be started in all symptomatic patients. Some experts recommend using it during acute respiratory illnesses to facilitate discharge. NIV should be initiated during a sleep study or observing the patient clinically for adequate gas exchange. NIV interfaces should be fitted by skilled physiotherapists selecting two interfaces to alternate skin contact points.
		Nebulized bronchodilators in patients with suspicion of asthma Customary immunizations, annual influenza, and pneumococcal vaccination	Mucolytics should not be used long term.
Ambulant	Clinical examination with review of cough effectiveness and detailed search for signs of nocturnal hypoventilation	Supportive care when needed Customary immunizations, annual influenza, and pneumococcal vaccination	Evidence of weak cough or recurrent infections or suspicion of nocturnal hypoventilation should prompt referral to a pneumologist.

there are no specific recommendations for doing PSG, as pointed out above and in Table 9.1, symptoms that might be explained by SDB should be investigated further.

Achondroplasia

Achondroplasia (ACH) is the most frequent form of disproportionate short stature, occurring in 1:10,000 to 1:30,000 live births.[126] In ≥97% of cases it is the result of a gain-of-function mutation in a gene identified in 1994, *FGFR3*. Fibroblast growth factor receptor 3 is permanently activated, leading to impaired chondrocyte proliferation and limited chondrocyte function at all growth plates.[127] Eighty percent of cases are believed to arise from *de novo*, autosomal dominant mutations.[128] Among average-stature children, the majority of the bones that make up vertebral bodies and the base of the skull are formed by ossification of cartilage that is present in adequate amounts. The gain-of-function mutation in children with ACH leads to early ossification with premature closure of synchondroses (cartilaginous joints), including at the foramen magnum.

In terms of ventilation and ventilatory control, the most dramatic effect of the *FGFR3* mutation is foramen magnum stenosis, which is shown most reliably with magnetic resonance imaging of the brainstem. The foramen is often misshapen and smaller in both transverse and sagittal dimensions than in children of average stature. In some children with ACH, however, it appears that foramen diameters can increase with age. Thus, infants in the first year of life are at most risk for cervico-medullary constriction.[128]

Foramen magnum stenosis may be associated with central apnea and obstructive SDB, both of which are thought to contribute to a surprising six-fold increase in rate of sudden death in the first year of life among infants with ACH.[129] Blunted arousal responses during sleep may also contribute to both SDB and increased risk for sudden death.[130]

Other complications of ACH that can compromise breathing during sleep include thoracic hypoplasia, and enlarged cerebral ventricles, but hydrocephalus, when present, is rarely symptomatic hydrocephalus because hydrocephalus is usually communicating. In fact, most infants with ACH have some degree of enlargement of the ventricles, presumably because premature ossification impairs jugular venous flow and, thereby, cerebrospinal fluid flow. Despite the high prevalence of ventricular enlargement, shunting is required in the minority.[131]

Over their lifetimes, up to 75% of people with ACH will have SDB that can be primarily obstructive, primarily central, or mixed.[132] Constriction of the brain stem and proximal spinal cord by hypertrophy of the occipital rim can lead to centrally mediated apneas, reduction in ventilatory drive, and direct compromise of cranial nerve nuclei and associated lower-motor neurons supporting upper airway patency (especially cranial nerves IX and XII). Nearly 40% will have SDB that is "moderate" or "severe" by conventional criteria.[133] Although infants are most at risk for sleep complications from cervico-medullary constriction, prospective data describing the prevalence and severity of SDB in the first 2 years of life are not yet available.

Neurosurgical intervention to relieve cervico-medullary constriction is done for ~20% of infants with ACH, usually in the first 2 years of life.[133] This involves foramen magnum decompression, and sometimes in some centers, C_1 and C_2 laminectomy, and removal of an epidural fibrous band below the occipital cervical junction.[134,135]

There have been no randomized trials to evaluate the effect of foramen magnum decompression on SDB, though in most case series most infants have significant reduction in AHI. With marked SDB, foramen magnum decompression is strongly recommended when imaging also shows cervico-medullary constriction, though the evidence supporting a given beneficial effect size might best be described as "intermediate."[136]

In the minority (<5%) of children with ACH who also have thoracic hypoplasia, particularly in the side-to-side chest diameter, clinical decision-making can be particularly challenging.[137] In our experience with this subgroup of children with ACH, it is difficult to predict improvements in ventilation during sleep after foramen magnum decompression. Reduction in central apneas and improvements in upper airway tone during sleep may not be enough to compensate for inadequate gas exchange if thoracic hypoplasia is marked. Unfortunately, among infants' measurements of lung volume, or even simpler measurements of chest circumference, that might be associated with successful neurosurgical intervention are not readily available.

GUIDELINES FOR CLINICAL MANAGEMENT OF INFANTS WITH ACHONDROPLASIA

A multicenter retrospective summary of how over 1300 children with ACH were cared for in four US centers has recently been published.[133] Retrospective summaries such as this should lead to a template for prospective studies that can provide stronger evidence bases for future guidelines. For now, the American Academy of Pediatrics Committee on Genetics has proposed extensive and user-friendly guidelines for "Health Supervision."[126]

Sleep physicians might be confused by findings and guidelines in the two publications cited above. Confusion may arise when deciding how best to combine and use normal neurologic examination and near-normal physiologic (PSG) findings on the one hand and MR imaging findings deemed "severe" enough to lead to neurosurgical intervention in most cases (see below, Imaging and Physiology).

Most infants with ACH are reported to snore,[126] and guidelines proposed by the AAP recommend that the first PSG be done for all within the first month of life, and thereafter as needed for evaluation of symptoms or to measure the success of intervention. Imaging of the brain and brainstem is also recommended by 1 month of age, though interventions based on MR findings alone are not recommended by the AAP.

Surgical intervention is recommended when there are neurologic findings (hypotonia, weakness, hyperreflexia, sustained ankle clonus), but clearly abnormal neurologic findings are rare (5%, or fewer).[134] Unless it is severe (e.g., AHI >10/hour), thresholds for intervention for SDB are not established. Events have been primarily obstructive, occasionally mixed apneas, and infrequently, only central.[134,138] Perhaps surprisingly, there may be little association between pathologic frequency of central events (>5/hour) and apparent severity of cervico-medullary constriction by MRI.[139]

During the first 2 years of life, the response to foramen magnum decompression with or without vertebral laminectomy is generally believed to be beneficial, in terms of SDB, but published reports are not more specific.

Adenotonsillar hypertrophy is often suspected to worsen SDB in children with ACH. Over 50% will have had an adenotonsillectomy, but the percent done by 2 years of age has not been reported. Success rate for adenotonsillectomy is not clear, perhaps because of concomitant facial hypoplasia.[138] Noninvasive support (CPAP, HHHF) is also used for obstructive SDB, and its use in children younger than 2 years has been described.[140]

IMAGING AND PHYSIOLOGY

"There is no consensus on how best to evaluate the complications related to foramen magnum stenosis, or the optimal time for intervention."[136] Current practice is to strongly consider neurosurgical intervention if there are definite abnormalities on neurologic examination (Rare, 1 in 20,[134]), or, more commonly, if the cervico-medullary constriction appears "severe." Clear and practical systems have been used to quantify apparent cervico-medullary constriction. In a small series of 36 infants, using a system that scored cervico-medullary constriction by MRI based on loss of CSF space, spinal cord distortion, and MR signal change, all but two infants had evidence for foramen magnum stenosis, and 50% had "flattening" of the cervical spinal cord with or without signal changes. Of those with cord distortion, only one had an abnormal neurological examination. Ninety percent of children with total AHI >10 had flattening of the cord and/or signal change, but severe SDB was only ~60% sensitive for concomitant marked MRI abnormalities.

Nine of 36 infants in the case series subsequently had neurosurgical intervention at ~15 months of age[134]; according to an *a priori* protocol, any infant with cord distortion had foramen magnum decompression (8/9). Standard clinical practice in most centers is to intervene when cervico-medullary constriction is severe because of the real, though infrequent, possibilities of paralysis and sudden death (2%–5%[126]). Furthermore, very specific recommendations to lessen risk for acute cervico-medullary injury (e.g., avoid sleeping unattended in car seats) are made for the positioning and support of infants with ACH whose macrocephaly and axial hypotonia cause poor head control.

Unfortunately, "no standards for (foramen magnum) foraminal size by MRI are currently available." Some authors contend that dynamic cord compression seen by MRI that also alters CSF flow with neck flexion and extension is a more logical guide to the need for intervention.[126,141]

Finally, the usefulness of PSG is uncertain in clinical decision-making regarding surgical intervention when the MR imaging is less ominous. Perhaps the frequent improvement in postoperative SDB with reductions in AHI from severe to mild should make surgery an attractive option even when cervico-medullary constriction appears much less than "severe."

NEW HORIZONS FOR THE CARE OF INFANTS AND CHILDREN WITH ACHONDROPLASIA

Careful analysis of retrospective data on 1374 children—"the primary Achondroplasia cohort"—collected using a multicenter protocol[126] has produced a template for prospective studies. Stronger evidence for the timing of evaluations and the usefulness of interventions will be the welcome result.

There is also hope for pharmacologic interventions that counter the effects of the gain-of-function gene and its products.[142] Drugs are being developed that target steps in the molecular disease mechanism. Targets include growth factor ligands such as FGFR3 and its downstream protein kinase-signaling pathway. (MAPK). Treatment will likely need to be very early in life, or prenatal, to prevent premature closure of growth plates and fusion of ossification centers.

RSV

Respiratory syncytial virus (RSV) is a single-stranded, negative-sense ribonucleic acid virus, member of the *Pneumoviridae* family and primarily transmitted by aerosol droplets and hand contact. Almost all children have been infected by RSV by 2 years of age and reinfection is common,[143] so common, that in a study of active surveillance at three sites in the United States (2004 to 2009), approximately 20% of 3339 children <24 months of age seen for acute respiratory infection or fever who were tested for RSV tested positive.[144]

While RSV is typically a self-limited process, infants who wheeze with RSV infections have long been considered predisposed to the development of asthma, in an interaction that is likely "bidirectional."[145-149] Recent studies may point to a similar bidirectional relationship between wheezing with more severe RSV infections and obstructive SDB.[150,151]

In a study of 5-year-olds, using PSG results from 21 children who had RSV bronchiolitis in the first year of life and matched controls, those who had had RSV had slightly greater obstructive AHI (2.3 ± 1,9 vs. 0.6 ± 0.8).[151]

In a study from the Boston Medical Center using their electronic health record (EHR), a birth cohort of 3114 subjects was used to assess the relationship between the diagnosis of OSA by age 5 years and the occurrence of a lower respiratory tract infection during the first year of life.[150]

Having had a lower respiratory tract infection increased the hazard ratio to 1.53 for subsequently developing OSA. Infants and children who had severe RSV had twice the odds of having OSA mentioned in the EHR as a diagnosis by age 5. The epidemiologic tools used for the EHR analyses had been validated in adults, as a way to efficiently study large numbers of subjects with SDB.[152] The Boston Medical Center study had a lower bar for the EHR diagnosis of OSA (1 "mention" versus 2 in validation paper), and the authors of the validation paper suggest caution about applying their methods for identifying and counting patients in a "safety net" system like the Boston Medical Center.

Thus, there is only early epidemiologic evidence for an association between wheezing during a lower respiratory tract infection in the first year of life and eventual diagnosis of OSA.[153] Nevertheless, if an association is more clearly shown, there are multiple plausible, related biological mechanisms to support a causal association. RSV can trigger responses that would increase upper airway resistance, particularly inflammation and lymphoproliferation. There are preclinical data suggesting that RSV alters neuromotor tone of the upper airway and induces neural inflammation.[154,155] Viruses and evidence for viral infection are often found in hypertrophied tonsils removed because of OSA.[156-158]

Cystic Fibrosis

CYSTIC FIBROSIS AND SLEEP IN INFANTS

Children with cystic fibrosis (CF) and children with marked SDB both have reduced quality of life (QofL), and are at risk for neurocognitive impairment, inattentiveness, anxiety, and depression.[159-164] Because it exacerbates pro-inflammatory states, marked SDB has the potential to make CF respiratory system disease worse and exacerbate the QofL-related hardships of life with CF.[165] Small children with severe SDB, and small children with CF, are at risk for poor growth. Older children and adults with CF often develop CF-related diabetes mellitus, and SDB in subjects without CF increases risk for insulin resistance and metabolic syndrome.[166,167]

CF and significant SDB thus share potential morbidities, particularly perhaps those reducing QofL. Whether these morbidities interact in a given child with CF is unpredictable. Of course, a patient with CF who has marked SDB should be treated using conventional approaches, for example, adenotonsillectomy, PAP, etc. But why, at what age, and how often CF might increase risk for or worsen SDB are poorly understood and are subjects of relatively recent interest.[164,168] Presently, there are no established guidelines in CF patients for screening for SDB using questionnaires or abbreviated objective testing.

Also, and not surprisingly, published reports provide even less information regarding the potential importance of SDB, or sleep disruption, during the first 2 years of life. Most recent reports describe children with CF referred to sleep laboratories because of suspicion of SDB. In one study of 40 apparently unselected children with CF, ages 6 months to 11 years, 28 (70%) had AHI >2; 21 of 40 were ≤5 years of age, and the average AHI for these children was ~8. The number of subjects younger than 2 years old is not reported, but at an average age of 3.8 years one-fourth had adenotonsillar hypertrophy.[169] Across all ages, 40% to 60% of children with CF are reported to have an AHI >1.[164,168] "Oropharyngeal crowding" (Mallampati score ≥3) has not been seen to be more common in children with CF and SDB than children with isolated SBD, that is, similar rates of "oropharyngeal crowding."[164]

It is not clear from published reports of risk factors for SDB in older children with CF which factors might be retrospectively looked at in children <2 years old with CF. For example, in a study comparing patients both with or without CF referred for PSG because of suspicion for SDB, neither a history of snoring nor daytime sleepiness was associated with a higher AHI among subjects with CF.[168] This finding suggests a disassociation between two classic symptoms of SDB and worsening SDB, despite the fact that CF subjects had a nearly three-fold increase over the non-CF comparison group in risk for an AHI >5. Clinical studies, to avoid potential "type 2 error," involving larger numbers of patients with CF and comparison subjects will be needed to clarify these apparently "negative" or paradoxical results. Interestingly, however, as older CF patients have attained better nutritional status, overweight or obesity have the same increased risk for SDB for patients with CF as for those without CF.[168]

SDB and worsening lung function certainly have the potential to synergistically worsen QofL in patients with CF. Advanced CF lung disease in older children and adolescents has long been known to cause alveolar hypoventilation in REM sleep, even in the absence of apnea or hypopneas.[170] With even milder, progressive lung disease, a given reduction in inspiratory volume will cause greater falls in $SpO_2\%$, yielding more "scoreable" respiratory events. Fortunately, however, it is becoming much less common for infants with CF to have demonstrable severe lung disease.

Other features of CF that have the potential to increase SDB and sleep disruption[171,172] include nasal obstruction by polyps and chronic rhinosinusitis due to persistent inflammation of the respiratory mucosa of the upper airway.[173] Among infants with CF, the prevalence and significance of these potential predisposing factors for SDB are not known. Certainly, the fact that the most prominent paranasal sinuses (maxillary, frontal, ethmoid) do not appear and aerate until age 4 makes sinusitis unlikely in infants. And though published reports involving older subjects further suggest potential risks for chronic upper airway inflammation, they do little to clarify specific factors that should be investigated prospectively in infants with CF. If anything, poorly understood factors that lead to a modest increase in sleep disruption may be most important for infants.[169] Certainly obtaining adequate, restful sleep that leads to an improved QofL and attentiveness to learning, and reduced anxiety and depression should be a priority for all children with CF, beginning in early childhood.

References

1. Cielo CM, Taylor JA, Vossough A, et al. Evolution of obstructive sleep apnea in infants with cleft palate and micrognathia. *J Clin Sleep Med.* 2016;12(7):979-987.
2. Adams J. Respiratory inductive plethysmography. In: Stocks J, Tepper RS, Morgan WJ, eds. *Infant Respiratory Function Testing.* New York: Wiley-Liss Publication; 1996.
3. Kirk VG, Batuyong ED, Bohn SG. Transcutaneous carbon dioxide monitoring and capnography during pediatric polysomnography. *Sleep.* 2006;29(12):1601-1608.
4. Tobias JD. Transcutaneous carbon dioxide monitoring in infants and children. *Paediatr Anaesth.* 2009; 19(5):434-444.
5. Cristea AI, Ren CL, Amin R, et al. Outpatient respiratory management of infants, children, and adolescents with post-prematurity respiratory disease: An Official American Thoracic Society Clinical Practice Guideline. *Am J Respir Crit Care Med.* 2021;204(12):e115-e133.
6. Mammel D, Kemp J. Prematurity, the diagnosis of bronchopulmonary dysplasia, and maturation of ventilatory control. *Pediatr Pulmonol.* 2021;56(11):3533-3545.
7. Rosen CL, Larkin EK, Kirchner HL, et al. Prevalence and risk factors for sleep-disordered breathing in 8- to 11-year-old children: association with race and prematurity. *J Pediatr.* 2003;142(4):383-389.
8. Crump C, Friberg D, Li X, Sundquist J, Sundquist K. Preterm birth and risk of sleep-disordered breathing from childhood into mid-adulthood. *Int J Epidemiol.* 2019;48(6):2039-2049.
9. Kulkarni G, de Waal K, Grahame S, et al. Polysomnography for the management of oxygen supplementation therapy in infants with chronic lung disease of prematurity. *J Matern Fetal Neonatal Med.* 2019;32(21):3640-3646.
10. Sekar KC, Duke JC. Sleep apnea and hypoxemia in recently weaned premature infants with and without bronchopulmonary dysplasia. *Pediatr Pulmonol.* 1991;10(2):112-116.
11. Simakajornboon N, Beckerman RC, Mack C, et al. Effect of supplemental oxygen on sleep architecture and cardiorespiratory events in preterm infants. *Pediatrics.* 2002;110(5):884-888.

12. Daftary AS, Jalou HE, Shively L, Slaven JE, Davis SD. Polysomnography reference values in healthy newborns. *J Clin Sleep Med.* 2019;15(3):437-443.
13. Trickett J, Bernardi M, Fahy A, et al. Disturbed sleep in children born extremely preterm is associated with behavioural and emotional symptoms. *Sleep Med.* 2021;85:157-165.
14. Coste F, Ferkol T, Hamvas A, et al. Ventilatory control and supplemental oxygen in premature infants with apparent chronic lung disease. *Arch Dis Child Fetal Neonatal Ed.* 2015;100(3):F233-F237.
15. Bancalari EH, Jobe AH. The respiratory course of extremely preterm infants: a dilemma for diagnosis and terminology. *J Pediatr.* 2012;161(4):585-588.
16. McEvoy CT, Jain L, Schmidt B, et al. Bronchopulmonary dysplasia: NHLBI Workshop on the Primary Prevention of Chronic Lung Diseases. *Ann Am Thorac Soc.* 2014;11 suppl 3:S146-S153.
17. Tourneux P, Léké A, Kongolo G, et al. Relationship between functional residual capacity and oxygen desaturation during short central apneic events during sleep in "late preterm" infants. *Pediatr Res.* 2008;64(2):171-176.
18. Ren CL, Feng R, Davis SD, et al. Tidal breathing measurements at discharge and clinical outcomes in extremely low gestational age neonates. *Ann Am Thorac Soc.* 2018;15(11):1311-1319.
19. Sadras I, Reiter J, Fuchs N, et al. Prematurity as a risk factor of sleep-disordered breathing in children younger than two years: a retrospective case-control study. *J Clin Sleep Med.* 2019;15(12):1731-1736.
20. Huang YS, Hsu JF, Paiva T, et al. Sleep-disordered breathing, craniofacial development, and neurodevelopment in premature infants: a 2-year follow-up study. *Sleep Med.* 2019;60:20-25.
21. Eichenwald EC, Aina A, Stark AR. Apnea frequently persists beyond term gestation in infants delivered at 24 to 28 weeks. *Pediatrics.* 1997;100(3 Pt 1):354-359.
22. Jobe AH. What do home monitors contribute to the SIDS problem? *JAMA.* 2001;285(17):2244-2245.
23. Ramanathan R, Corwin MJ, Hunt CE, et al. Cardiorespiratory events recorded on home monitors: Comparison of healthy infants with those at increased risk for SIDS. *JAMA.* 2001;285(17):2199-2207.
24. Siriwardhana LS, Yee AK, Mann DL, et al. Ventilatory control instability as a predictor of persistent periodic breathing in preterm infants. *Pediatr Res.* 2022;92(2):513-519.
25. Edwards BA, Nava-Guerra L, Kemp JS, et al. Assessing ventilatory instability using the response to spontaneous sighs during sleep in preterm infants. *Sleep.* 2018;41(11):zsy161.
26. Katz ES, Mitchell RB, D'Ambrosio CM. Obstructive sleep apnea in infants. *Am J Respir Crit Care Med.* 2012;185(8):805-816.
27. Younes M. Role of arousals in the pathogenesis of obstructive sleep apnea. *Am J Respir Crit Care Med.* 2004;169(5):623-633.
28. Poets CF, Southall DP. Patterns of oxygenation during periodic breathing in preterm infants. *Early Hum Dev.* 1991;26(1):1-12.
29. Sands SA, Edwards BA, Kelly VJ, et al. Mechanism underlying accelerated arterial oxygen desaturation during recurrent apnea. *Am J Respir Crit Care Med.* 2010;182(7):961-969.
30. Shannon DC, Carley DW, Kelly DH. Periodic breathing: quantitative analysis and clinical description. *Pediatr Pulmonol.* 1988;4(2):98-102.
31. Rigatto H, Brady JP, de la Torre Verduzco R. Chemoreceptor reflexes in preterm infants: I. The effect of gestational and postnatal age on the ventilatory response to inhalation of 100% and 15% oxygen. *Pediatrics.* 1975;55(5):604-613.
32. Carlo WA, DiFiore JM. Respiratory muscle responses to changes in chemoreceptor drive in infants. *J Appl Physiol (1985).* 1990;68(3):1041-1047.
33. Schmidt B, Roberts RS, Davis P, et al. Long-term effects of caffeine therapy for apnea of prematurity. *N Engl J Med.* 2007;357(19):1893-1902.
34. Murner-Lavanchy IM, Doyle LW, Schmidt B, et al. Neurobehavioral outcomes 11 years after neonatal caffeine therapy for apnea of prematurity. *Pediatrics.* 2018;141(5):e20174047.
35. Rhein LM, Dobson NR, Darnall RA, et al. Effects of caffeine on intermittent hypoxia in infants born prematurely: a randomized clinical trial. *JAMA Pediatr.* 2014;168(3):250-257.
36. Ehsan Z, Glynn EF, Hoffman MA, et al. Small sleepers, big data: leveraging big data to explore sleep-disordered breathing in infants and young children. *Sleep.* 2021;44(2):zsaa176.
37. Corvaglia L, Zama D, Gualdi S, et al. Gastro-oesophageal reflux increases the number of apnoeas in very preterm infants. *Arch Dis Child Fetal Neonatal Ed.* 2009;94(3):F188-F192.
38. Corvaglia L, Zama D, Spizzichino M, et al. The frequency of apneas in very preterm infants is increased after non-acid gastro-esophageal reflux. *Neurogastroenterol Motil.* 2011;23(4):303-307, e152.

39. Cresi F, Martinelli D, Maggiora E, et al. Cardiorespiratory events in infants with gastroesophageal reflux symptoms: is there any association? *Neurogastroenterol Motil.* 2018;30(5):e13278.

40. Di Fiore J, Arko M, Herynk B, et al. Characterization of cardiorespiratory events following gastro-esophageal reflux in preterm infants. *J Perinatol.* 2010;30(10):683-687.

41. Funderburk A, Nawab U, Abraham S, et al. Temporal association between reflux-like behaviors and gastroesophageal reflux in preterm and term infants. *J Pediatr Gastroenterol Nutr.* 2016;62(4):556-561.

42. Hasenstab KA, Jadcherla SR. Respiratory events in infants presenting with apparent life threatening events: is there an explanation from esophageal motility? *J Pediatr.* 2014;165(2):250-255.e1.

43. Hasenstab KA, Jadcherla SR. Gastroesophageal reflux disease in the neonatal intensive care unit neonate: controversies, current understanding, and future directions. *Clin Perinatol.* 2020;47(2):243-263.

44. Kenigsberg K, Griswold PG, Buckley BJ, et al. Cardiac effects of esophageal stimulation: possible relationship between gastroesophageal reflux (GER) and sudden infant death syndrome (SIDS). *J Pediatr Surg.* 1983;18(5):542-545.

45. Nobile S, Marchionni P, Noviello C, et al. Correlation between cardiorespiratory events and gastroesophageal reflux in preterm and term infants: Analysis of predisposing factors. *Early Hum Dev.* 2019; 134:14-18.

46. Rossor T, Andradi G, Ali K, et al. Gastro-oesophageal reflux and apnoea: is there a temporal relationship? *Neonatology.* 2018;113(3):206-211.

47. Wheatley E, Kennedy KA. Cross-over trial of treatment for bradycardia attributed to gastroesophageal reflux in preterm infants. *J Pediatr.* 2009;155(4):516-521.

48. Mittal RK. The sphincter mechanism at the lower end of the esophagus: an overview. *Dysphagia.* 1993;8(4):347-350.

49. Mittal RK, Balaban DH. The esophagogastric junction. *N Engl J Med.* 1997;336(13):924-932.

50. Gupta A, Jadcherla SR. The relationship between somatic growth and in vivo esophageal segmental and sphincteric growth in human neonates. *J Pediatr Gastroenterol Nutr.* 2006;43(1):35-41.

51. Peter CS, Sprodowski N, Bohnhorst B, et al. Gastroesophageal reflux and apnea of prematurity: no temporal relationship. *Pediatrics.* 2002;109(1):8-11.

52. Di Fiore JM, Arko M, Whitehouse M, et al. Apnea is not prolonged by acid gastroesophageal reflux in preterm infants. *Pediatrics.* 2005;116(5):1059-1063.

53. Wenzl TG, Schenke S, Peschgens T, et al. Association of apnea and nonacid gastroesophageal reflux in infants: Investigations with the intraluminal impedance technique. *Pediatr Pulmonol.* 2001;31(2):144-149.

54. Koenig JS, Davies AM, Thach BT. Coordination of breathing, sucking, and swallowing during bottle feedings in human infants. *J Appl Physiol (1985).* 1990;69(5):1623-1629.

55. Menon AP, Schefft GL, Thach BT. Apnea associated with regurgitation in infants. *J Pediatr.* 1985;106(4):625-629.

56. Davies AM, Koenig JS, Thach BT. Upper airway chemoreflex responses to saline and water in preterm infants. *J Appl Physiol (1985).* 1988;64(4):1412-1420.

57. Marchal F, Corke BC, Sundell H. Reflex apnea from laryngeal chemo-stimulation in the sleeping premature newborn lamb. *Pediatr Res.* 1982;16(8):621-627.

58. Pickens DL, Schefft GL, Storch GA, Thach BT. Characterization of prolonged apneic episodes associated with respiratory syncytial virus infection. *Pediatr Pulmonol.* 1989;6(3):195-201.

59. May JG, Shah P, Lemonnier L, et al. Systematic review of endoscopic airway findings in children with gastroesophageal reflux disease. *Ann Otol Rhinol Laryngol.* 2011;120(2):116-122.

60. Jadcherla SR, Parks VN, Peng J, et al. Esophageal sensation in premature human neonates: temporal relationships and implications of aerodigestive reflexes and electrocortical arousals. *Am J Physiol Gastrointest Liver Physiol.* 2012;302(1):G134-G144.

61. Machado R, Woodley FW, Skaggs B, et al. Gastroesophageal reflux causing sleep interruptions in infants. *J Pediatr Gastroenterol Nutr.* 2013;56(4):431-435.

62. Nault S, Samson N, Nadeau C, et al. Reflex cardiorespiratory events from esophageal origin are heightened by preterm birth. *J Appl Physiol (1985).* 2017;123(2):489-497.

63. Ramet J, Praud JP, d'Allest AM, et al. Cardiac and respiratory responses to esophageal dilatation during REM sleep in human infants. *Biol Neonate.* 1990;58(4):181-187.

64. Lyons M, Cooper T, Cave D, et al. Pharyngeal dysfunction associated with early and late onset sleep disordered breathing in children. *Int J Pediatr Otorhinolaryngol.* 2019;127:109667.

65. Davies F, Gupta R. Apparent life threatening events in infants presenting to an emergency department. *Emerg Med J.* 2002;19(1):11-16.
66. Rosen R, Vandenplas Y, Singendonk M, et al. Pediatric Gastroesophageal Reflux Clinical Practice Guidelines: Joint Recommendations of the North American Society for Pediatric Gastroenterology, Hepatology, and Nutrition and the European Society for Pediatric Gastroenterology, Hepatology, and Nutrition. *J Pediatr Gastroenterol Nutr.* 2018;66(3):516-554.
67. Fard D, Rohlfing ML, Razak A, Cohen MB, Levi JR. Prevalence and natural history of obstructive sleep apnea in pediatric patients with laryngomalacia. *Int J Pediatr Otorhinolaryngol.* 2020;133:109967.
68. Ratanakorn W, Brockbank J, Ishman S, et al. The maturation changes of sleep-related respiratory abnormalities in infants with laryngomalacia. *J Clin Sleep Med.* 2021;17(4):767-777.
69. MacLean JE. Laryngomalacia in infancy improves with increasing age irrespective of treatment. *J Clin Sleep Med.* 2021;17(4):619-620.
70. Irace AL, Dombrowski ND, Kawai K, et al. Evaluation of aspiration in infants with laryngomalacia and recurrent respiratory and feeding difficulties. *JAMA Otolaryngol Head Neck Surg.* 2019;145(2):146-151.
71. Ramgopal S, Kothare SV, Rana M, et al. Obstructive sleep apnea in infancy: a 7-year experience at a pediatric sleep center. *Pediatr Pulmonol.* 2014;49(6):554-560.
72. Sarber KM, von Allmen DC, Tikhtman R, et al. Polysomnographic outcomes after observation for mild obstructive sleep apnea in children younger than 3 years. *Otolaryngol Head Neck Surg.* 2021;164(2):427-432.
73. Shirley F, Oshri W, Ari D, Gad F. The role of laryngeal ultrasound in the assessment of pediatric dysphonia and stridor. *Int J Pediatr Otorhinolaryngol.* 2019;122:175-179.
74. Garritano FG, Carr MM. Characteristics of patients undergoing supraglottoplasty for laryngomalacia. *Int J Pediatr Otorhinolaryngol.* 2014;78(7):1095-1100.
75. Thompson DM. Abnormal sensorimotor integrative function of the larynx in congenital laryngomalacia: a new theory of etiology. *Laryngoscope.* 2007;117(6 Pt 2 suppl 114):1-33.
76. Wailoo M, Emery JL. The trachea in children with respiratory diseases including children presenting as cot deaths. *Arch Dis Child.* 1980;55(3):199-203.
77. Qubty WF, Mrelashvili A, Kotagal S, Lloyd RM. Comorbidities in infants with obstructive sleep apnea. *J Clin Sleep Med.* 2014;10(11):1213-1216.
78. Goldberg S, Shatz A, Picard E, et al. Endoscopic findings in children with obstructive sleep apnea: effects of age and hypotonia. *Pediatr Pulmonol.* 2005;40(3):205-210.
79. Tanphaichitr A, Tanphaichitr P, Apiwattanasawee P, et al. Prevalence and risk factors for central sleep apnea in infants with laryngomalacia. *Otolaryngol Head Neck Surg.* 2014;150(4):677-683.
80. Love H, Slaven JE, Mitchell RM, et al. Outcomes of OSA in surgically naive young children with and without DISE identified laryngomalacia. *Int J Pediatr Otorhinolaryngol.* 2020;138:110351.
81. Boulet SL, Yang Q, Mai C, et al. Trends in the postfortification prevalence of spina bifida and anencephaly in the United States. *Birth Defects Res A Clin Mol Teratol.* 2008;82(7):527-532.
82. Waters KA, Forbes P, Morielli A, et al. Sleep-disordered breathing in children with myelomeningocele. *J Pediatr.* 1998;132(4):672-681.
83. Kirk VG, Morielli A, Gozal D, et al. Treatment of sleep-disordered breathing in children with myelomeningocele. *Pediatr Pulmonol.* 2000;30(6):445-452.
84. Shellhaas RA, Kenia PV, Hassan F, et al. Sleep-disordered breathing among newborns with myelomeningocele. *J Pediatr.* 2018;194:244-247.e1.
85. Shellhaas RA. Sleep in infants with myelomeningocele-an opportunity to improve outcomes? *J Perinatol.* 2019;39(10):1325-1326.
86. Gozal D, Arens R, Omlin KJ, et al. Peripheral chemoreceptor function in children with myelomeningocele and Arnold-Chiari malformation type 2. *Chest.* 1995;108(2):425-431.
87. Wolpert SM, Anderson M, Scott RM, et al. Chiari II malformation: MR imaging evaluation. *AJR Am J Roentgenol.* 1987;149(5):1033-1042.
88. Ramirez N, Valentín P, Mayer OH, et al. The spinal structure and lung function relationship in an untreated nonambulatory myelomeningocele group of patients. *J Am Acad Orthop Surg.* 2019;27(9):327-334.
89. Brzustowicz LM, Lehner T, Castilla LH, et al. Genetic mapping of chronic childhood-onset spinal muscular atrophy to chromosome 5q11.2-13.3. *Nature.* 1990;344(6266):540-541.
90. Clermont O, Burlet P, Burglen L, et al. Use of genetic and physical mapping to locate the spinal muscular atrophy locus between two new highly polymorphic DNA markers. *Am J Hum Genet.* 1994;54(4):687-694.

91. Gilliam TC, Brzustowicz LM, Castilla LH, et al. Genetic homogeneity between acute and chronic forms of spinal muscular atrophy. *Nature.* 1990;345(6278):823-825.
92. Lien LL, Boyce FM, Kleyn P, et al. Mapping of human microtubule-associated protein 1B in proximity to the spinal muscular atrophy locus at 5q13. *Proc Natl Acad Sci U S A.* 1991;88(17):7873-7876.
93. Melki J, Abdelhak S, Sheth P, et al. Gene for chronic proximal spinal muscular atrophies maps to chromosome 5q. *Nature.* 1990;344(6268):767-768.
94. Melki J, Burlet P, Clermont O, et al. Refined linkage map of chromosome 5 in the region of the spinal muscular atrophy gene. *Genomics.* 1993;15(3):521-524.
95. Melki J, Sheth P, Abdelhak S, et al. Mapping of acute (type I) spinal muscular atrophy to chromosome 5q12-q14. The French Spinal Muscular Atrophy Investigators. *Lancet.* 1990;336(8710):271-273.
96. Morrison KE, Daniels RJ, Suthers GK, et al. High-resolution genetic map around the spinal muscular atrophy (SMA) locus on chromosome 5. *Am J Hum Genet.* 1992;50(3):520-527.
97. Sheth P, Abdelhak S, Bachelot MF, et al. Linkage analysis in spinal muscular atrophy, by six closely flanking markers on chromosome 5. *Am J Hum Genet.* 1991;48(4):764-768.
98. Soares VM, Brzustowicz LM, Kleyn PW, et al. Refinement of the spinal muscular atrophy locus to the interval between D5S435 and MAP1B. *Genomics.* 1993;15(2):365-371.
99. Lefebvre S, Bürglen L, Reboullet S, et al. Identification and characterization of a spinal muscular atrophy-determining gene. *Cell.* 1995;80(1):155-165.
100. Rodrigues NR, Owen N, Talbot K, et al. Deletions in the survival motor neuron gene on 5q13 in autosomal recessive spinal muscular atrophy. *Hum Mol Genet.* 1995;4(4):631-634.
101. Simard LR, Rochette C, Semionov A, et al. SMN(T) and NAIP mutations in Canadian families with spinal muscular atrophy (SMA): genotype/phenotype correlations with disease severity. *Am J Med Genet.* 1997;72(1):51-58.
102. Velasco E, Valero C, Valero A, et al. Molecular analysis of the SMN and NAIP genes in Spanish spinal muscular atrophy (SMA) families and correlation between number of copies of cBCD541 and SMA phenotype. *Hum Mol Genet.* 1996;5(2):257-263.
103. Wirth B. An update of the mutation spectrum of the survival motor neuron gene (SMN1) in autosomal recessive spinal muscular atrophy (SMA). *Hum Mutat.* 2000;15(3):228-237.
104. Friesen WJ, Massenet S, Paushkin S, et al. SMN, the product of the spinal muscular atrophy gene, binds preferentially to dimethylarginine-containing protein targets. *Mol Cell.* 2001;7(5):1111-1117.
105. Hsieh-Li HM, Chang JG, Jong YJ, et al. A mouse model for spinal muscular atrophy. *Nat Genet.* 2000; 24(1):66-70.
106. Mailman MD, Heinz JW, Papp AC, et al. Molecular analysis of spinal muscular atrophy and modification of the phenotype by SMN2. *Genet Med.* 2002;4(1):20-26.
107. Prior TW, Leach ME, Finanger E. Spinal Muscular Atrophy. 2000 Feb 24 [Updated 2020 Dec 3]. In: Adam MP, Feldman J, Mirzaa GM, et al., editors. *GeneReviews®* [Internet]. Seattle (WA): University of Washington, Seattle; 1993-2023. Available from: https://www.ncbi.nlm.nih.gov/books/NBK1352/.
108. Arkblad E, Tulinius M, Kroksmark AK, et al. A population-based study of genotypic and phenotypic variability in children with spinal muscular atrophy. *Acta Paediatr.* 2009;98(5):865-872.
109. Feldkotter M, Schwarzer V, Wirth R, et al. Quantitative analyses of SMN1 and SMN2 based on real-time lightCycler PCR: fast and highly reliable carrier testing and prediction of severity of spinal muscular atrophy. *Am J Hum Genet.* 2002;70(2):358-368.
110. Feng Y, Ge X, Meng L, et al. The next generation of population-based spinal muscular atrophy carrier screening: comprehensive pan-ethnic SMN1 copy-number and sequence variant analysis by massively parallel sequencing. *Genet Med.* 2017;19(8):936-944.
111. Tiziano FD, Pinto AM, Fiori S, et al. SMN transcript levels in leukocytes of SMA patients determined by absolute real-time PCR. *Eur J Hum Genet.* 2010;18(1):52-58.
112. Amaddeo A, Frapin A, Fauroux B. Long-term non-invasive ventilation in children. *Lancet Respir Med.* 2016;4(12):999-1008.
113. Amaddeo A, Moreau J, Frapin A, et al. Long term continuous positive airway pressure (CPAP) and non-invasive ventilation (NIV) in children: Initiation criteria in real life. *Pediatr Pulmonol.* 2016;51(9):968-974.
114. Ward S, Chatwin M, Heather S, Simonds AK. Randomised controlled trial of non-invasive ventilation (NIV) for nocturnal hypoventilation in neuromuscular and chest wall disease patients with daytime normocapnia. *Thorax.* 2005;60(12):1019-1024.
115. Bach JR, Baird JS, Plosky D, Navado J, Weaver B. Spinal muscular atrophy type 1: management and outcomes. *Pediatr Pulmonol.* 2002;34(1):16-22.

116. Bach JR, Niranjan V, Weaver B. Spinal muscular atrophy type 1: a noninvasive respiratory management approach. *Chest*. 2000;117(4):1100-1105.

117. Bach JR, Saltstein K, Sinquee D, et al. Long-term survival in Werdnig-Hoffmann disease. *Am J Phys Med Rehabil*. 2007;86(5):339-345 quiz 346-348, 379.

118. Bach JR, Vega J, Majors J, Friedman A. Spinal muscular atrophy type 1 quality of life. *Am J Phys Med Rehabil*. 2003;82(2):137-142.

119. Mellies U, Dohna-Schwake C, Stehling F, Voit T. Sleep disordered breathing in spinal muscular atrophy. *Neuromuscul Disord*. 2004;14(12):797-803.

120. Oskoui M, Levy G, Garland CJ, et al. The changing natural history of spinal muscular atrophy type 1. *Neurology*. 2007;69(20):1931-1936.

121. Petrone A, Pavone M, Testa MB, et al. Noninvasive ventilation in children with spinal muscular atrophy types 1 and 2. *Am J Phys Med Rehabil*. 2007;86(3):216-221.

122. Schroth MK. Special considerations in the respiratory management of spinal muscular atrophy. *Pediatrics*. 2009;123 suppl 4:S245-S249.

123. Pera MC, Romeo DM, Graziano A, et al. Sleep disorders in spinal muscular atrophy. *Sleep Med*. 2017;30:160-163.

124. Verrillo E, Bruni O, Pavone M, et al. Sleep architecture in infants with spinal muscular atrophy type 1. *Sleep Med*. 2014;15(10):1246-1250.

125. Verrillo E, Pavone M, Bruni O, et al. Effects of long-term non-invasive ventilation on sleep structure in children with Spinal Muscular Atrophy type 2. *Sleep Med*. 2019;58:82-87.

126. Hoover-Fong J, Scott CI, Jones MC. Health supervision for people with achondroplasia. *Pediatrics*. 2020;145(6):e20201010.

127. Bellus GA, Hefferon TW, Ortiz de Luna RI, et al. Achondroplasia is defined by recurrent G380R mutations of FGFR3. *Am J Hum Genet*. 1995;56(2):368-373.

128. Pauli RM. Achondroplasia: a comprehensive clinical review. *Orphanet J Rare Dis*. 2019;14(1):1.

129. Brouwer PA, Lubout CM, van Dijk JM, et al. Cervical high-intensity intramedullary lesions in achondroplasia: aetiology, prevalence and clinical relevance. *Eur Radiol*. 2012;22(10):2264-2272.

130. Ednick M, Tinkle BT, Phromchairak J, et al. Sleep-related respiratory abnormalities and arousal pattern in achondroplasia during early infancy. *J Pediatr*. 2009;155(4):510-515.

131. Unger S, Bonafe L, Gouze E. Current care and investigational therapies in achondroplasia. *Curr Osteoporos Rep*. 2017;15(2):53-60.

132. Zucconi M, Weber G, Castronovo V, et al. Sleep and upper airway obstruction in children with achondroplasia. *J Pediatr*. 1996;129(5):743-749.

133. Hoover-Fong JE, Alade AY, Hashmi SS, et al. Achondroplasia Natural History Study (CLARITY): a multicenter retrospective cohort study of achondroplasia in the United States. *Genet Med*. 2021;23(8):1498-1505.

134. Cheung MS, Irving M, Cocca A, et al. Achondroplasia Foramen Magnum Score: screening infants for stenosis. *Arch Dis Child*. 2021;106(2):180-184.

135. Sano M, Takahashi N, Nagasaki K, et al. Polysomnography as an indicator for cervicomedullary decompression to treat foramen magnum stenosis in achondroplasia. *Childs Nerv Syst*. 2018;34(11):2275-2281.

136. Kubota T, Adachi M, Kitaoka T, et al. Clinical Practice Guidelines for Achondroplasia. *Clin Pediatr Endocrinol*. 2020;29(1):25-42.

137. Stokes DC, Phillips JA, Leonard CO, et al. Respiratory complications of achondroplasia. *J Pediatr*. 1983;102(4):534-541.

138. Mogayzel Jr PJ, Carroll JL, Loughlin GM, et al. Sleep-disordered breathing in children with achondroplasia. *J Pediatr*. 1998;132(4):667-671.

139. White KK, Parnell SE, Kifle Y, et al. Is there a correlation between sleep disordered breathing and foramen magnum stenosis in children with achondroplasia? *Am J Med Genet A*. 2016;170A(1):32-41.

140. Afsharpaiman S, Saburi A, Waters KA. Respiratory difficulties and breathing disorders in achondroplasia. *Paediatr Respir Rev*. 2013;14(4):250-255.

141. Mukherjee D, Pressman BD, Krakow D, et al. Dynamic cervicomedullary cord compression and alterations in cerebrospinal fluid dynamics in children with achondroplasia: review of an 11-year surgical case series. *J Neurosurg Pediatr*. 2014;14(3):238-244.

142. Hogler W, Ward LM. New developments in the management of achondroplasia. *Wien Med Wochenschr*. 2020;170(5-6):104-111.

143. Kimberlin DW, Barnett ED, Lynfield R, Sawyer MH. Respiratory syncytial virus. In: *Red Book: 2021–2024 Report of the Committee on Infectious Diseases*. 31 ed. Itasca, IL: American Academy of Pediatrics; 2021.

144. Lively JY, Curns AT, Weinberg GA, et al. Respiratory syncytial virus-associated outpatient visits among children younger than 24 months. *J Pediatric Infect Dis Soc*. 2019;8(3):284-286.

145. Fjaerli HO, Farstad T, Rød G, et al. Acute bronchiolitis in infancy as risk factor for wheezing and reduced pulmonary function by seven years in Akershus County, Norway. *BMC Pediatr*. 2005;5:31.

146. Kusel MM, de Klerk NH, Kebadze T, et al. Early-life respiratory viral infections, atopic sensitization, and risk of subsequent development of persistent asthma. *J Allergy Clin Immunol*. 2007;119(5):1105-1110.

147. Sigurs N, Bjarnason R, Sigurbergsson F, Kjellman B. Respiratory syncytial virus bronchiolitis in infancy is an important risk factor for asthma and allergy at age 7. *Am J Respir Crit Care Med*. 2000;161(5): 1501-1507.

148. Sigurs N, Gustafsson PM, Bjarnason R, et al. Severe respiratory syncytial virus bronchiolitis in infancy and asthma and allergy at age 13. *Am J Respir Crit Care Med*. 2005;171(2):137-141.

149. Stein RT, Sherrill D, Morgan WJ, et al. Respiratory syncytial virus in early life and risk of wheeze and allergy by age 13 years. *Lancet*. 1999;354(9178):541-545.

150. Gutierrez MJ, Nino G, Landeo-Gutierrez JS, et al. Lower respiratory tract infections in early life are associated with obstructive sleep apnea diagnosis during childhood in a large birth cohort. *Sleep*. 2021;44(12):zsab198.

151. Snow A, Dayyat E, Montgomery Downs HE, et al. Pediatric obstructive sleep apnea: a potential late consequence of respiratory syncitial virus bronchiolitis. *Pediatr Pulmonol*. 2009;44(12):1186-1191.

152. Keenan BT, Kirchner HL, Veatch OJ, et al. Multisite validation of a simple electronic health record algorithm for identifying diagnosed obstructive sleep apnea. *J Clin Sleep Med*. 2020;16(2):175-183.

153. Cielo CM, Tapia IE. More than just a wheeze: bronchiolitis and obstructive sleep apnea in children. *Sleep*. 2021;44(12):zsab227.

154. Dakhama A, Park JW, Taube C, et al. Alteration of airway neuropeptide expression and development of airway hyperresponsiveness following respiratory syncytial virus infection. *Am J Physiol Lung Cell Mol Physiol*. 2005;288(4):L761-L770.

155. Larsen GL, Colasurdo GN. Neural control mechanisms within airways: disruption by respiratory syncytial virus. *J Pediatr*. 1999;135(2 Pt 2):21-27.

156. Proenca-Modena JL, Buzatto GP, Paula FE, et al. Respiratory viruses are continuously detected in children with chronic tonsillitis throughout the year. *Int J Pediatr Otorhinolaryngol*. 2014;78(10): 1655-1661.

157. Proenca-Modena JL, Pereira Valera FC, Jacob MG, et al. High rates of detection of respiratory viruses in tonsillar tissues from children with chronic adenotonsillar disease. *PLoS One*. 2012;7(8):e42136.

158. Yeshuroon-Koffler K, Shemer-Avni Y, Keren-Naus A, Goldbart AD. Detection of common respiratory viruses in tonsillar tissue of children with obstructive sleep apnea. *Pediatr Pulmonol*. 2015;50(2):187-195.

159. Cepuch G, Gniadek A, Gustyn A, Tomaszek L. Emotional states and sleep disorders in adolescent and young adult cystic fibrosis patients. *Folia Med Cracov*. 2017;57(4):27-40.

160. Piasecki B, Stanisławska-Kubiak M, Strzelecki W, et al. Attention and memory impairments in pediatric patients with cystic fibrosis and inflammatory bowel disease in comparison to healthy controls. *J Investig Med*. 2017;65(7):1062-1067.

161. Piasecki B, Turska-Malińska R, Matthews-Brzozowska T, et al. Executive function in pediatric patients with cystic fibrosis, inflammatory bowel disease and in healthy controls. *Eur Rev Med Pharmacol Sci*. 2016;20(20):4299-4304.

162. Tomaszek L, Dębska G, Cepuch G, et al. Evaluation of quality of life predictors in adolescents and young adults with cystic fibrosis. *Heart Lung*. 2019;48(2):159-165.

163. Vandeleur M, Walter LM, Armstrong DS, et al. Quality of life and mood in children with cystic fibrosis: associations with sleep quality. *J Cyst Fibros*. 2018;17(6):811-820.

164. Shakkottai A, Irani S, Nasr SZ, et al. Risk factors for obstructive sleep apnea in cystic fibrosis. *Pediatr Pulmonol*. 2022;57(4):926-934.

165. Irwin MR. Why sleep is important for health: a psychoneuroimmunology perspective. *Annu Rev Psychol*. 2015;66:143-172.

166. Koren D, Gozal D, Philby MF, et al. Impact of obstructive sleep apnoea on insulin resistance in non-obese and obese children. *Eur Respir J*. 2016;47(4):1152-1161.

167. Suratwala D, Chan JS, Kelly A, et al. Nocturnal saturation and glucose tolerance in children with cystic fibrosis. *Thorax.* 2011;66(7):574-578.
168. Shakkottai A, Nasr SZ, Hassan F, et al. Sleep-disordered breathing in cystic fibrosis. *Sleep Med.* 2020;74:57-65.
169. Spicuzza L, Sciuto C, Leonardi S, La Rosa M. Early occurrence of obstructive sleep apnea in infants and children with cystic fibrosis. *Arch Pediatr Adolesc Med.* 2012;166(12):1165-1169.
170. Tepper RS, Skatrud JB, Dempsey JA. Ventilation and oxygenation changes during sleep in cystic fibrosis. *Chest.* 1983;84(4):388-393.
171. Jiang RS, Liang KL, Hsin CH, Su MC. The impact of chronic rhinosinusitis on sleep-disordered breathing. *Rhinology.* 2016;54(1):75-79.
172. Mahdavinia M, Schleimer RP, Keshavarzian A. Sleep disruption in chronic rhinosinusitis. *Expert Rev Anti Infect Ther.* 2017;15(5):457-465.
173. Ramos RT, Salles C, Gregório PB, et al. Evaluation of the upper airway in children and adolescents with cystic fibrosis and obstructive sleep apnea syndrome. *Int J Pediatr Otorhinolaryngol.* 2009;73(12): 1780-1785.

CHAPTER 10

Sleep Disorders in Neurological Disorders and Sleep-Related Movement Disorders in Children Less Than 2 Years of Age

Madeleine M. Grigg-Damberger ▨ Kathy M. Wolfe

Sleep in early life plays crucial roles in optimal neural and cognitive brain development, cortical maturation, and brain connectivity. Complex bidirectional relationships between sleep and development are observed in infants.[1-4] Sleep (or lack of it) in typically developing fetuses, infants, and toddlers has lasting effects on later neurocognition.[1,5,6] Sleep disturbances and disorders are highly prevalent in infants with particular neurogenetic syndromes; neurological and neurodevelopmental disorders (NDDs) contribute to worsening of their conditions.[7-9]

Studies show that sleep/wake disorders (SWDs) in children with NDDs compared to typically developing (TD) children are: (1) far more prevalent; (2) multifactorial; (3) caused by an interplay of genetic, neurobiological, environmental, and epigenetic factors; (4) associated with worse functioning, increased parental stress and worse parental health; (5) more often persist into adolescence and adulthood; and (6) but do vary across disorders and individuals, and are often treatable.[10,11] Although NDDs affect only 2% of the general population, they represent a third of children referred to tertiary pediatric sleep clinics.[12]

Here we will review what is known about SWDs in some of the most common neurogenetic, neurodevelopmental, and neurological disorders which present to pediatric sleep clinics or in-hospital in children <2 years of age. We will also review sleep-related movement disorders of infancy which are more often benign, remit, save again infants with NDDs.

Sleep Need for Optimal Brain Health and Development

In 2016, the American Academy of Sleep Medicine (AASM) published consensus recommendations based on a systematic review which thought children ages 4 to 12 months need 12 to 16 hours per 24; and children ages 1 to 2 years 12 to 16 hours for optimal health.[13] Two large prospective cohort studies found healthy infants between ages 4 and 12 months sleep slightly greater than 13 to slightly greater than 14 hours.[14,15] Forty percent of US infants aged 4 to 11 months sleep less than recommended amounts.[16] Persistent short sleepers followed until age 7 tended to have poorer physical, emotional, and social health-related quality of life (QoL) than typical sleepers.[15] TD children 12 to 35 months of age usually sleep 11 to 12 hours; sleeping <10 hours is associated with a greater risk for accidental injury.[17]

Impact of Premature Birth on Sleep, Brain Development, and Later Cognitive Performance

Premature birth alone is a major risk for later neurodevelopmental disorders. Infants born preterm often have lower cognitive performance and more developmental disorders than those born at term. A 2018 metaanalysis (74 studies, 64,061 children) found that children born preterm compared to those born at term had: (1) lower cognitive scores for full scale, performance and verbal intelligence quotients (FSIQ, PIQ, and VIQ, respectively); (2) lower scores motor skills, behavior, reading, math and spelling at primary school age; persisted secondary school (except for mathematics); and (3) a 1.6-fold greater risk for attention-deficit/hyperactivity disorder (ADHD) with a differential effect according to the severity of prematurity.[18]

Premature birth interrupts brain development preferentially occurring during sleep in the third trimester of pregnancy.[1] Studies using polysomnography (PSG), electroencephalography (EEG), functional neuroimaging, and later neurodevelopmental testing have shown that premature birth is associated with impaired sleep ontogenesis, aberrant functional neuronal network connectivity, and poorer neurodevelopmental outcomes.[19-21] Further, the Developing Human Connectome Project had showed that preterm birth is associated with disrupted formation of functional brain connectivity networks;[19] and reduced cerebral gray and white matter volumes and neurocognitive deficits in adults born preterm.[20,21]

ALTERED SLEEP ARCHITECTURE IN PRETERM NEWBORNS IMPACTS ON LATER COGNITIVE DEVELOPMENT

Premature infants sleep differently than infants born at term at similar postmenstrual age (PMA) with higher quiet/NREM sleep percentages, fewer arousals, fewer rapid eye movements, longer sleep cycle length, lower respiratory regularity, and lower beta EEG power.[22-24] Infants born premature who had less REM sleep time on PSG had poorer developmental outcomes on the Bayley II at 6 months; whereas better neurodevelopmental outcomes were observed in those who had longer periods of sustained sleep, more REM sleep time, and more periods of REM sleep with rapid eye movements.[23] Preterm born infants who slept poorly as neonates exhibited poorer attention and greater distractibility at 4 and 18 months than those who slept well.[24] Sleep/wake transitions from NREM to W were associated with greater neonatal neuromaturation, less negative emotionality, and better verbal, symbolic, and executive competences at age 5 in 143 infants born mean age 32 weeks postmenstrual age (wPMA), while REM sleep and cry, short episodes of REM and NREM sleep with poorer outcomes.[22]

Preterm Birth Increases Risk for Later Pediatric Obstructive Sleep Apnea

Premature birth also increases the risk for pediatric obstructive sleep apnea (OSA).[25-27] A 2019 study found gestational age (GA) was the only significant predictor of SDB in a cohort of 98 children <2 years of age; premature birth increased the risk for OSA four-fold.[26] Every additional week of gestation decreased the odds for SDB by 12.5%. SDB in those born preterm was associated with more severe nocturnal hypoxemia, increased frequency of central apnea, and altered sleep architecture. A recent study found premature birth was associated with a 2.97-fold higher likelihood of developing severe OSA, higher apnea-hypopnea index (AHI) and requiring more upper airway surgeries for OSA than children born at term.[25]

Sleep Disorders in Neurogenetic Syndromes Which Present in Infancy

Sleep disorders are so common in infants with particular neurogenetic syndromes that they are considered phenotypic of the particular syndrome.

DOWN (TRISOMY 21) SYNDROME

Down syndrome (DS) is the most common genetic cause of intellectual disability (ID) accounting for approximately 30% of all cases of moderate-to-severe ID. DS is caused by a partial or complete duplication in chromosome 21q22.3 and occurs in approximately 1 of 1200 live births worldwide.[28,29] Phenotypic expression of the trisomy 21 genotype shows great inter-individual variability modified by allelic variation, genomic imbalances, epigenetic, but also early intervention programs and parental nurturing.[30,31] ID in DS can vary from borderline to profound.

Obstructive Sleep Apnea Highly Prevalent in Infants and Toddlers With Down Syndrome

The most common sleep disorder in DS is OSA, highly prevalent in them across their life. A 2018 metaanalysis (18 studies, 1200 children with DS, mean age 7.7 years) found the prevalence of OSA based on AHI of 2, 5, and 10 events/hour were 75%, 50%, and 34%, respectively.[32] AHI >5/h correlated inversely with age.[32] OSA when present in infants with DS tends to be severe.[33,34] A study of 177 infants (≤6 months old) with DS attending a tertiary DS clinic suspected in 31%; PSG confirmed OSA in 95% of the severe in 71%.[34]

Multiple factors predispose infants with DS to OSA and begin with craniofacial and upper airway abnormalities are common among them: midface and mandibular hypoplasia; a relatively large and/or posteriorly placed tongue in relatively small oral cavity; glossoptosis; small nose with a low nasal bridge; hypoplastic trachea; pharyngeal collapse; and increased secretions.[35]

Hypotonia is a near universal finding in DS, most marked in infancy and affecting ligamentous laxity and gait. Poor tone in the airway predisposes them to glossoptosis, laryngomalacia, and hypopharyngeal collapse. When present, congenital heart disease, pulmonary arterial hypertension, hypothyroidism, and/or obesity further predispose them to OSA and often increase the severity of it found on PSG.[35,36] Risk factors for obesity in DS: increased leptin, decreased energy expenditure, subclinical hypothyroidism, and less favorable diets.[37]

DS is the most common genetic syndrome associated with immune dysregulation. Children with DS have a 12-fold greater risk for infections especially pneumonia due to impaired cellular immunity and a four- to six-fold higher risk for autoimmune diseases than.[38] Increased mortality from sepsis and increased oxidative stress are observed in people with DS.[39]

Given the prevalence and predisposition for OSA in DS, the American Academy of Pediatrics (AAP) recommends all caregivers of children with DS receive information about the symptoms of OSA by 6 months of age and PSG be performed by age 4 years.[40] Fig. 10.1 shows severe OSA recorded in an infant with DS.

Central Sleep Apnea Also Common in Down Syndrome Especially Those Younger Than Two

A retrospective review of 158 children with DS found: (1) central sleep apnea (CSA) was common in children with DS <2 years old but rare after age 10; (2) if CSA persisted beyond age 2, it was more likely to occur in females; and (3) CSA was usually associated with concomitant OSA and hypoxemia.[41] Another study of 60 infants and toddlers with DS (median age 1.5 years) found OSA in 61%, CSA 25%, and sleep-related central hypoventilation 32%.[42]

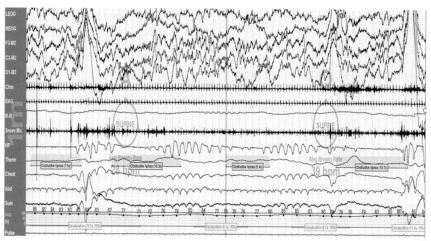

Fig. 10.1 60-second epoch of PSG recorded in an infant with Down Syndrome and severe obstructive sleep apnea.

Other Sleep/Wake Disturbances in Infants With Down Syndrome

Beyond SDB, infants with DS are at risk for other sleep problems. A large 2019 case-control study compared parent-reported sleep in 104 infants and toddlers with DS and 489 TD controls using the Brief Infant Sleep Questionnaire (BISQ).[43] They found more parent-reported sleep problems in the children with DS compared to TD controls (45% versus 19%) including snoring (19% versus 2%), roomsharing (37% versus 17%), less nighttime sleep (55 minutes), and total sleep over 24 hours (38 minutes). Parents of an infant/toddler with DS were 4.4 times more likely to report needing to be present when their child fell asleep. A complaint of snoring increased reports of problematic nighttime awakenings.

A cross-sectional study recording actigraphy in 66 children with DS (aged 5–67 months) and 43 TD controls found infants born with DS exhibited worse sleep fragmentation than TD controls, but sleep efficiency and consolidation increased with age.[44] Thirty-five percent of infants with DS showed a phase advance preference. Another study found more fragmented sleep and less leg movement activity when sleeping was observed in 3- to 6-months-old infants with DS compared to TD infants.[45]

Impact of Sleep Disorders on Development in Children With Down Syndrome

A 2020 study of 10 children with DS (mean age 33 months) compared with 10 TD children and found more frequent parent-reported sleep problems were associated with more forgetfulness in the children with DS relative to TD.[46] A prospective cross-sectional study found severity of SDB (AHI) correlated with more behavioral abnormalities (especially ADHD) and poorer development scores in 53 children with DS (ages 3–12).[47] Fewer children with DS had nocturnal dipping of heart rate and blood pressure compared to TD children.[48] A 2020 study found 30 children with DS had shorter nocturnal sleep duration and poorer sleep efficiency than 37 TD controls.[8] Nocturnal sleep duration predicted receptive vocabulary size in the children with DS: for every 2 minutes more of nocturnal sleep, language comprehension in them increased by one word.

AUTISM SPECTRUM DISORDERS

Autism spectrum disorder (ASD) is the most prevalent NDD in the United States with a prevalence in 2018 of 17 per 1000 (1 in 59) 4-year-old children.[5] ASD is a group of clinically heterogeneous neurological and NDDs associated with mild-to-severe impairments in socialization, communication, and/or reciprocal social interaction and often accompanied by restricted, ritualistic, and/or repetitive behaviors and interests.[49] The male-to-female prevalence ratio of ASD is 3.4 to 1 and 52% had ID (IQ ≤70).[5,50] Twenty percent of cases of ASD are familial. More than 100 copy variants and point mutations have been identified in subjects with ASD; most *de novo*, and more often involved in gene regulation or synaptic connectivity.[51]

Children with ASD often have: (1) difficulty understanding the intent of others; (2) decreased interactive eye contact; (3) atypical use and understanding of gesture; (4) atypical development of social communication, pretend play, and interest in other children; (5) repetitive behaviors or perseveration; and (6) sleep disturbances.[52]

Sleep Disturbances Highly Prevalent and Persistent in Children With Autism Spectrum Disorders

Sleep problems are reported in up to 86% of children with ASD,[53] still present in 50% in late adolescence.[54-56] Sleep problems are reported as the most agonizing symptom for parents of children with ASD.[57] Children with ASD often take longer than an hour to fall asleep, awakenings may last 2 to 3 hours and can begin with screaming or nightmares.[58] Difficulty falling asleep, frequent night waking, and reduced nocturnal sleep duration are the most common sleep problems in children with ASD, but SDB, periodic limb movements (PLMs), restless legs (RLS), and nightmares were reported.[59]

Problematic sleep in children with ASD is associated with repetitive ritualistic compulsive behaviors,[60] ASD severity, and greater impairments in functional performance (mobility, self-care, and social function).[61] Large cohort studies found sleep problems in ASD were associated with a higher prevalence of internalizing (anxiety, depression) and externalizing (aggression, defiance) daytime behaviors and lower overall intelligence, fewer verbal skills, less adaptive functioning, fewer daily living skills, communication, and socialization.[62,63] A study of 427 children with ASD admitted to psychiatric units found: (1) early morning awakening associated with higher autism symptom severity; (2) difficulty staying asleep/multiple insomnia symptoms scored low on adaptive behaviors (communication, self-care, socialization) and higher on maladaptive behaviors (irritability, hyperactivity, emotional reactivity, and dysphoria).[64]

Core neurobehavioral deficits in children with ASD may contribute to their difficulty falling asleep: (1) impaired emotional regular may limit their ability to calm themselves; (2) difficulty transitioning from preferred or stimulating daytime activities because of fixation on daytime events; (3) inability to understand parental expectations related to bedtime and sleep due to impaired communication skills; (4) anxiety or fear about falling asleep; and (5) sensory processing issues.[65] Abnormally low levels of melatonin and/or its urinary metabolic derivatives have been found in ASD and correlate with sleep problems and autistic behaviors.[66]

Recognizing Early Signs of Autism in Infants

Prospective studies show the diagnostic features of ASD typically appear during the latter part of the first and second years of life.[67] Earliest signs sometimes detected in infants <12 months old are: difficulties responding to name and/or attending to faces or social scenes; motor delay; and atypical visual orienting (Table 10.1). Delays in acquiring language or disengagement of visual attention are red flags for ASD in children 12 to 18 months old. Regression in language or social behavior occurs in approximately a third of children with ASD, most often between 18 and 24 months of age.[50] The Centers for Disease Control and Prevention (CDC) has a website which is useful for parents to identify symptoms and signs of ASD (www.cdc.gov/ncbddd/actearly). The Autism Navigator website provides a video glossary of early symptoms of ASD in toddlers (www.autismnavigator.com).

TABLE 10.1 ■ Early Warning Signs of Autism and Developmental Delay in Infants

Age	Warning Signs
6 months	No affection for caregivers; does not squeal or laugh; does not make vowel sounds (eh, ah, oh) or respond to sounds; does not reach, or unusually stiff or floppy.
9 months	Does not respond to name, babble, look where pointed, or recognize familiar people; does not sit with help, bear weight on legs with support, or transfer objects from one hand to other.
12 months	Does not point to things, say single words, crawl, search for hidden objects, or stand when supported; does not learn gestures like shaking head yes or no, or waving bye-bye; losing skills once had.
18 months	Does not point, imitate/copy others, notice/react when caregiver returns or leaves, walk, say at least six words, or know what familiar items are (phone, spoon, cup); losing skills once had.
24 months	Does not know what familiar items are (phone, spoon, cup), walk steadily, follow simple instruction, imitate words/actions; use two-word phrases; losing skills once had.

Sleep Problems in Infants and Toddlers Later Diagnosed With Autism Spectrum Disorder

Sleep patterns in children with ASD appear to diverge from typical development in the second or third year of life. One study found infants later diagnosed with ASD were much more likely to require ≥ two consult referrals for excessive crying, feeding, and sleeping problems compared to TD controls (44% versus 16%).[68] A large prospective longitudinal study in 5151 children followed from 1.5 to 9 years of age found: (1) sleep problems did not precede autistic behavior but cooccurred with the development of autistic traits in early childhood; (2) sleep problems in children with ASD increased in severity with increasing age; (3) unlike sleep problems in TD children which tend to decrease with increasing age.[54] A third study found toddlers with autistic features found they exhibited more bedtime resistance, abnormal circadian rhythms, and sleepiness outside of naptime than the TD toddlers.[69]

A 2020 longitudinal neuroimaging study of 432 infants at high or low risk for ASD found sleep onset problem scores (derived from an infant temperament measure) were more prevalent at 6 to 12 months among infants who later developed ASD.[70] Sleep onset difficulties at 6 to 12 months in infants at high risk for ASD were associated with weaker social communication skills by age 24 months and correlated with increased hippocampal volume trajectories from 6 to 24 months.[70]

Treatment strategies for difficulty sleeping in children with ASD discussed elsewhere in this book in greater detail include: (1) behavioral therapy[71]; (2) extended release melatonin, alpha agonists, and gabapentin;[72,73] (3) identifying and treating SDB, PLMS, RLS, ferritin/iron/vitamin deficiencies, and gastrointestinal disturbances; (4) increased daytime physical activity.[74] In-laboratory PSG should not be the first test for ASD unless symptoms of SDB, frequent atypical paroxysmal nocturnal behaviors, restless sleep disorder, and/or PLMs are suspected.[65]

Of note, pediatric prolonged-release melatonin (PedPRM) is the first drug licensed for insomnia in children with ASD.[75,76] PedPRM treatment improves sleep onset, duration and consolidation, and daytime externalizing behaviors in children and adolescents with ASD and subsequently caregivers' QoL and satisfaction with their children's sleep. The coated, odorless, and taste-free minitablets are well-accepted in this population who often have sensory hypersensitivity and problems swallowing standard tablet preparations. The most frequent long-term treatment-related adverse events were fatigue (6%), somnolence (6%), and mood swings (4%) and

---

BOX 10.1 ■ **Cognitive Behavioral and Behavioral Treatment Strategies Used to Treat Insomnia in Children With Autism Spectrum and Other Severe Neurodevelopmental Disorders**

Parents serve as active agents of change and are taught to:
- **Create a quality sleeping environment:**
  - Dark, quiet, nonstimulating and perceived as safe (dim nightlight if needed);
  - Eliminate visual and auditory stimuli (turn off electronics);
  - Adjust ambient temperature if necessary (cool better than warm);
  - Develop a successful bedtime routine which is consistently followed and tailored to the developmental age and abilities of the child;
  - Promote self-soothing skills which allow the child to fall and return to sleep on own.
- **Maintain a consistent sleep/wake schedule:**
  - Put to bed and get them up same time every day;
  - Difficulty falling asleep:
    - Temporarily delay child's bedtimes by calculating the average sleep onset time during baseline then adding 30 minutes (e.g., average sleep onset 9:30 p.m. during baseline, initial bedtime 10 p.m.).
    - Once child falls asleep within 15–20 minutes, gradually move the bedtime earlier in 30-minute increments as long as the child continues to fall asleep quickly until reaching a parent-determined goal bedtime (e.g., 8:30 p.m.).
    - Do not allow the child to make up for lost sleep by going to bed earlier or sleeping later.
- **Parent-child interactions:**
  - Parents avoid responding to the child's disruptive bedtime behaviors (crying, tantrums, calling out, or leaving the bedroom);
    - Parents who have difficulty ignoring the child can use the Excuse-Me Drill; parents periodically check on the child but only when the child is showing desire behaviors (calm, quiet, and in bed). This is repeated for nighttime awakenings.
    - A bedroom pass (allowing only one bedroom exit per night) is often useful.

---

with no evidence of delay in height, BMI, or pubertal development, or withdrawal effects.[76] The starting dose is 2 mg once daily, independent of age or weight, escalated to 5 to 10 mg/day if predefined treatment success criteria are unmet. Slow melatonin metabolizers (approximately 10% of children) may require lower doses. Cognitive behavioral and behavioral treatment strategies used to treat insomnia in children with ASD and other severe NDDs are summarized in Box 10.1.

PRADER-WILLI SYNDROME

Prader-Willi syndrome (PWS) is neurogenetic syndrome which occurs in approximately 1 of 15,000 births and most often due to a sporadic microdeletion in paternally derived chromosome 15q11-q13, less often when both copies of the chromosome are inherited from the mother (maternal uniparental disomy).

Recognizing Infants With Prader-Willi Syndrome

PWS is the most frequent cause of *secondary* obesity in children but the clinical presentation of PWS is striking different in infants.[77] The prenatal features of PWS include: decreased fetal activity; polyhydramnios, breech presentation; and an abnormal posture on ultrasound: elbows flexed; feet dorsiflexed. Infants with PWS typically present with: severe central hypotonia; weak cry and difficulty feeding due to poor suck; growth retardation; and dermal and ocular depigmentation; and genital hypoplasia. A 2020 study of 134 infants with PWS found that 99% had severe central axial hypotonia and feeding difficulties; 98% weak (or even no) cry; 95% failure to thrive (FTT) requiring feeding tubes in 66%.[78] This most often prompts genetic testing confirming the diagnosis.

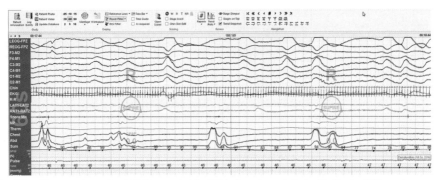

Fig. 10.2 60-second epoch of PSG recorded in REM sleep in an infant with Prader-Willi syndrome and central apneas lasting 10-12 seconds.

After infancy, children with untreated PWS often exhibit hyperphagia, obesity, short stature, pubertal delay, hypogonadism, and behavioral and learning problems.[79] Distinctive facial features in people with PWS: almond-shaped eyes, thin upper lip with down-turned corners of the mouth; and narrow nasal bridge. Hypothalamic dysfunction in PWS predisposes them to: temperature instability; high pain thresholds; and deficiencies in growth hormone, thyroid stimulating hormone, and central adrenal insufficiency. Mild-to-moderate ID, temper tantrums, resistance to change, manipulative tactics, food foraging, skin picking, and compulsiveness are common in them.[80-83]

Sleep Apnea More Often Central in Infants With Prader-Will Syndrome

CSA is the predominant type of SDB in children with PWS <2 years old, OSA >2 years.[84-88] CSA tends to remit with increasing age in PWS, often replaced by OSA and/or sleep alveolar hypoventilation.

CSA was initially present in 53% of 28 infants with PWS but at a median follow-up of 2 years only 4 had residual CSA, and 3 had developed OSA[87] CSA (but no OSA) on overnight PSG in 72% of children with PWS <2 years of age.[88]

Another study found: (1) CSA in 43% of 23 children with PWS who were <2 years old versus 5% of 21 who were >2 years old; (2) OSA alone in 17% < age 2 years; (3) OSA sole type of SDB in 53% >2 years old versus 5% <2 years.[86] CSA in infants with PWS often responds to supplemental oxygen.[85,86] Fig. 10.2 shows CSA recorded on a PSG in an infant with PWS.

Benefits of Exogenous Growth Hormone Therapy in Infants With Prader-Willi Syndrome

Infants diagnosed with PWS are typically offered exogenous growth hormone (GH) therapy. GH therapy in infants with PWS has many beneficial effects. One study found 21 children with PWS treated with GH for 6 years (beginning at age 13 ± 6 months) had lower body fat (mean 36% versus 45%), greater height (131 versus 114 cm), greater motor strength, and better lipid profiles compared to 27 children of a similar age (ages 5–9 years) prior to GH treatment.[89]

A prospective study showed starting GH in infants with median age of 9.6 months resulted in less fat/more muscle body composition and them walking earlier by 15 months of age.[90] Children with PWS who started GH during infancy (median age 1.4 years) had greater vocabularies and higher total intelligence quotient (IQ) than those who started GH later (median age 8.1 years).[91]

However, GH (especially at higher doses) can accelerate the growth of lymphoid tissue and tonsillar hypertrophy; this may be related to insulin-like growth factor 1 (IGF-1) levels and contribute to development of OSA. A 2020 longitudinal PSG study found OSA develops independently of GH therapy in PWS.[92] Pathological OSA increased significantly during the first 3 months of GH therapy but dropped below baseline after 1 year. A 2022 retrospective multicenter study of 112 patients with PWS followed from a mean age of 1.9 years found the mean obstructive AHI (oAHI) was 0.4/hour at baseline; 35% >1/hour.[93] After GH initiation, there was no change in central AHI. The median oAHI did not increase significantly, but 12 children (13%) developed moderate/severe OSA. The AAP recommends PSG be repeated 6 to 10 weeks after starting GH therapy.[94] Children with PWS treated with GH need regular follow-up screening for emergence of SDB.

Increased Risk for Sudden Death in Prader-Willi Syndrome

Individuals with PWS are at increased risk for sudden or premature death and have an annual all-cause death rate of 3%. Sudden death in PWS during infancy is more often secondary to milk aspiration; viral infections when sleeping in older children and adolescents; and respiratory failure, pulmonary embolism, cellulitis, or other complications of morbid obesity in the adults.[95] Initial reports raised great concern that exogenous GH therapy contributed to/caused sudden death in PWS. Subsequent studies by in large refute this.[96-98] A long-term study of 48 treated children suggests that the benefits of treatment with GH greatly exceed the risks.[99]

Central Hypersomnia Common in Prader-Willi Syndrome

Infants, children, and adults with PWS often have excessive daytime sleepiness (EDS) unrelated to SDB, attributed to hypothalamic dysfunction.[100,101] However, longer sleep needs in infants with PWS may not prompt complaints from caregivers.[8]

SMITH-MAGENIS SYNDROME

Smith-Magenis syndrome (SMS) is a neurogenetic complex multisystem disorder caused by a heterozygous deletion at chromosome 17p11.2 in the retinoic acid-induced 1 gene (*RAI1*) or a heterozygous RAI1 pathogenic variant.[102] The prevalence is estimated to be 1 in 15,000 to 25,000 live births.

SMS is characterized by developmental delay with ID, short stature, a deep hoarse voice, obesity, scoliosis, peripheral neuropathy, a distinctive neurobehavior syndrome and often severe sleep problems.[102] The particular neurobehavioral phenotype seen in SMS (usually not recognizable until 18 months of age or older) is characterized by: (1) severe maladaptive sleep behaviors with inverted circadian rhythm of melatonin secretion; (2) self-injury with low sensitivity to pain (hitting, biting, skin picking, inserting foreign objects into body orifices, yanking nails); (3) peculiar motor stereotypies (upper body self-hugging, compulsive finger licking, and book or magazine page flipping); (4) temper tantrums, oppositional defiant behaviors, and attention-deficit/hyperactivity disorder (ADHD); and (5) emotional maturity delayed beyond intellectual functioning.[103]

Recognizing Infants With Smith-Magenis Syndrome

Infants with SMS have feeding difficulties, FTT, hypotonia, hyporeflexia, prolonged napping (often need to be awakened to feed), generalized lethargy, relative insensitivity to pain and a mild 6 to 8 Hz intention tremor of the upper extremities. Crying in infancy is infrequent and often hoarse. The majority show markedly decreased babbling and vocalization for age with/without hearing loss. Head banging, which may begin as early as age 18 months is also frequent.[102,103]

Infants with SMS are often described as having a cherubic face with DS-like features: a characteristic downturned tent-shaped vermilion of the upper lip; up-slanting palpebral fissures, short upturned nose, broad forehead; mild micrognathia, brachycephaly, and a fair (hypopigmented) complexion with rosy pudgy cheeks. Childhood onset obesity and scoliosis predispose older children and adolescents to OSA when older.

Sleep Problems in Smith-Magenis Syndrome Are Often Severe and Persistent

Caregivers of children with SMS usually do not recognize significant sleep problems before age 12 to 18 months, although fragmented sleep with reduced total sleep time has been documented as early as age 6 months.[103] SWDs in children with SMS are characterized by fragmented and shortened sleep cycles with frequent nocturnal and early morning awakenings, daytime sleepiness, and sleep attacks.[104-106]

A 2020 actigraphy study of 20 children with SMS (mean age 8.7 ± 2.7) and 20 TD controls found children with SMS had shorter total sleep times, shorter total sleep time (TST), extended night waking, shorter sleep onset, more daytime naps, and earlier morning waking compared to the TD group.[104] In the SMS group, increased afternoon sleepiness was associated with increased irritability and hyperactivity.

Inverted Circadian Rhythm of Melatonin Secretion in Smith-Magenis Syndrome

The *RAI1* gene is a crucial transcriptional regulator gene of the mammalian circadian clock. The *RAI1* gene loss of function in SMS is thought to be a significant factor contributing to SWDs in them.[106] Seminal studies in children with SMS (20 ages 4–17 years) showed all had a phase shift of their circadian rhythm of melatonin with onset of melatonin secretion at 06:00 ± 2 hours, peaking at 12:00 ± 1 hours.[107] Sleep/wake complaints in these children improved by giving early morning oral acebutolol (a beta-blocker to suppress the daytime melatonin secretion) and evening melatonin (to replace the normal nighttime peak).[107,108] Another study showed the 24-hour circadian rhythm of body temperature was phase advanced by about three hours (not inverted) in patients with SMS relative to controls.[109]

Effective treatment of SWDs in SMS is best achieved by combination of behavior intervention techniques, oral extended release melatonin, and/or other medications including melatonin receptor agonists, beta1-adrenergic antagonists, and stimulant medications, to improve sleep outcomes.[105] A multicenter double-blinded randomized placebo-controlled crossover study showed tasimelteon modestly increased TST in people with SMS.[110]

WILLIAMS SYNDROME (7Q11.23 DUPLICATION SYNDROME)

Williams syndrome (WS) is a multisystem genetic disorder which occurs in one in 7500 births and is caused by a contiguous gene deletion of the Williams-Beuren syndrome critical region on chromosome 7q11.23 that includes the elastin gene (ELN).[111] WS is characterized by: usually mild ID (IQs in 60s and 70s), visual spatial deficits, relatively preserved expressive language, and a distinctive personality profile (social, friendly, gregarious, empathetic, loquacious, difficulty interpreting social cues, and prone to worries and fears). People with WS also have: cardiovascular diseases (elastin arteriopathy, peripheral pulmonic stenosis, supravalvular aortic stenosis, hypertension), endocrinopathies (hypercalcemia, hypothyroidism, hypercalciuria, early puberty), hypotonia, hyperextensible joints, and particular facial features (full cheeks and lips, broad nasal tip, widely spaced teeth).[111,112]

Recognizing Infants With Williams Syndrome

Infants with WS are often born postterm and small.[111] Impaired suck and swallow, textual aversion, GERD and vomiting often lead to failure to gain weight. Prolonged colic (>4 months) in infants with WS warrants consideration of GERD, chronic constipation, and/or hypercalcemia. Hypotonia and hyperextensible joints predispose to motor milestone delay; walking usually occurs by age 24 months. Other medical problems that often occur in the first year include: strabismus, chronic otitis media, rectal prolapse, umbilical and/or inguinal hernia, and cardiovascular disease. Speech delay and fine motor difficulties are common.

Sleep Problems in Infants and Toddlers With Williams Syndrome

Parents of 16 infants and toddlers with WS reported sleep problems in 31%.[113] Large case-control studies have shown that children with WS have: greater bedtime resistance; sleep anxiety; nighttime awakening; sleep-onset insomnia; enuresis; body pain; and decreased sleep efficiency, increased respiratory-related arousals, increased slow wave sleep, more difficulty falling asleep, greater restlessness, and more arousals from sleep.[114-116]

A 2020 study assessed sleep in 13 with WS and 25 TD controls at 18, 24, and 30 months of age.[117] Parents of children with WS reported they had more nighttime waking, longer settling times, and required higher levels of parental involvement. Sleep duration measured using actigraphy was shorter in WS at all ages. Sleep quality with age improved in the TD controls but persisted in those with WS. Infants and toddlers with WS are at increased risk for SDB. A 2020 case-control study of 96 2 year olds with WS found SDB in 16% and EDS in 30%.[118]

Children with WS children with SDB symptoms had significantly more behavior problems and those with EDS more attention/hyperactivity, stress, and externalizing problems. Shorter nighttime sleep duration correlated with language difficulties and internalizing problems; daytime sleepiness with externalizing problems. Another study found sleep problems correlated with a proportion of variance in language development scores in infants and toddlers with WS.[119] Behavioral treatment strategies are needed to treat insomnia in WS, often supplemented by extended release melatonin.[120] A less pronounced rise in nocturnal melatonin levels was found in children with WS compared with TD controls.[121]

ANGELMAN SYNDROME

Angelman syndrome (AS) is a neurogenetic disorder caused by loss of loss of function of the maternal copy of ubiquitin-protein ligase E3A (UBE3A) of chromosome 15q11-13.[122] AS occurs one in 12,000 to 20,000 live births. Clinical features characteristic of AS include: global developmental delay; severe ID; lack of speech; and a unique behavior of frequent inappropriate laughter, smiling easily, excitability, epilepsy, hand-flapping coupled with a peculiar ataxic gait prompting them to be called "happy puppets."[123] Medically refractory epilepsy is particularly common in AS and usually begins before age 3 years. Also observed are: hyperactive lower-extremity deep-tendon reflexes; wide-based gait with pronated/valgus positioned ankles and an uplifted flexed arm when walking; attraction/fascination with water, paper, and plastics. Abnormal EEG awake and asleep with characteristic very high amplitude rhythmic 2 to 4 Hz slow waves (sometimes intermixed with spikes) are characteristic of AS (Fig. 10.3).

Recognizing With Infants With Angelman Syndrome

Infants with AS have a normal prenatal and birth history, normal head circumference at birth and no major birth defects. Delay in developmental milestones first appear by age 6 to 12 months, eventually classified as severe without loss of skills. Feeding problems and/or hypotonia, tongue thrusting, suck/swallowing disorders, frequent drooling, excessive chewing/mouthing behaviors, and tremulousness and jerky limb movements should prompt consideration of the diagnosis and genetic testing. Delayed or disproportionately slow growth in head circumference usually results in absolute or relative microcephaly by age 2 years. Features which suggest AS in infants: minimal or no use of words; open mouth; tongue protrusion; ataxic gait and/or tremulous movements of limbs; frequent laughter/smiling, hand-flapping, hypermotor behavior, microcephaly; fair skin and hair; and problem sleeping.

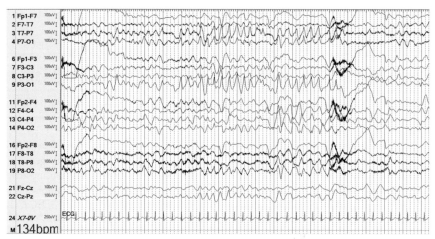

Fig. 10.3 20-second epoch of EEG recorded in NREM sleep in a 2-year-old showing almost continuous runs of very high amplitude rhythmic posterior 2-3 Hz delta activity which were sometimes intermixed with spikes characteristic of Angelman syndrome awake and asleep.

Sleep Problems So Pervasive in Angelman Syndrome to Be Considered Part of Clinical Phenotype

Sleep problems in children with AS are so common that they are regarded as part of the syndrome and include: difficulty falling and staying asleep; frequent nighttime and early morning awakenings; irregular sleep/wake cycles; reduced sleep duration with increased WASO; heightened sensitivity to their sleep environment, being easily aroused by noise; and a variety of disruptive nocturnal behaviors (including periods of laughing), sleepwalking/sleep terrors, bruxism, seizures, and PLMs.[124,125] A 2018 metaanalysis found daytime sleepiness, frequent arousals sleeping, and short sleep duration were the most common sleep/wake complaints in people with AS.[126] A recent study found low serum ferritin levels common in children with AS, often associated with periodic limb movements of sleep (PLMs) and sleep quality improved by iron supplementation.[127] Separation anxiety and aggressive behavior correlated with sleep difficulties in another study of children with AS.[128]

MUCOPOLYSACCHARIDOSES

Mucopolysaccharidoses (MPS) are a group of inherited autosomal recessive lysosomal storage disorders caused by the deficiency of hydrolases involved in the degradative pathway of glycosaminoglycans. MPS are progressive disorders in which the concentration of glycosaminoglycans in cells increase over time. The incidence of MPS in the United States was found to 0.98 per 100,000 live births (prevalence 2.67 per 1 million).[129]

Infants are usually born without the clinical features of MPS but progressively develop clinical signs. Symptom onset and severity vary between subtypes, but coarse facial features, organomegaly, skeletal and joint abnormalities, dysfunction in vision and hearing, and cardiorespiratory problems are common across all MPS subtypes.

People with MPS are at great risk for multifactorial upper airway obstruction and often severe obstructive SDB.[130,131] Risk factors for OSA in them: macroglossia, excessive glycosaminoglycans deposited in tracheobronchial mucosa, restrictive lung disease due to a small thoracic cage, and reduced abdominal dimension due to hepatosplenomegaly and lumbar hyperlordosis. OSA is most often severe in MPS I (also known as Hurler syndrome), II (Hunter), and IV-A (Morquio) and VI (Maroteaux-Lamy).[130,132] Chronic hypoxemia may result in polycythemia, pulmonary hypertension, cor pulmonale, chronic respiratory failure and premature death.

Guidelines for managing MPS VI were published in 2019 and recommend overnight PSG at diagnosis (and no later than 2 years of age) and every 3 years thereafter or when signs and symptoms of OSA are noted.[133] One study in 19 children with MPS found OSA in 95% and typically severe (AHI >10/hour 11; 5–9/hour 2; 1–4/hour 5; and normal in 1).[132] Snoring, witnessed apnea, pectus carinatum, and macroglossia were the main clinical findings. Pulmonary hypertension was present on cardiac echo in 68%. Another study found OSA in all 24 children with various MPS, moderate/severe in 20.[134]

Treatment strategies for OSA in MPS: AT, PAP, tracheotomy, supraglottoplasty, and bone marrow transplantation.[135] Guidelines for managing MPS VI were published in 2019 and recommend overnight PSG at diagnosis (and no later than 2 years of age) and every 3 years thereafter or when signs and symptoms of OSA are noted.[133] Sadly, OSA usually remains following enzyme replacement therapy and/or hematopoietic stem cell transplantation.[136-138]

Sleep Disorders Associated With Brainstem and Cervicomedullary Dysfunction

Particular neurological disorders (often with a genetic basis) are associated with SBD related to either brainstem respiratory dysfunction or compression of medullary respiratory centers. SDB in them prompt referrals to pediatric sleep specialists.

CHIARI MALFORMATIONS

Chiari malformations (CM) are various rhombencephalic anomalies of cerebellar tonsillar herniation of increasing severity which present with varying combinations of spina bifida, meningomyelocele, syringomyelia, bilateral abductor vocal cord paralysis, SDB, prolonged breath-holding spells, and sudden death due to cervicomedullary junction (CMJ) compression. CM are classified by severity: (1) Chiari 1 (CM1) characterized by caudal displacement of the cerebellar tonsils inferior to the plane of the foramen magnum by 3 to 5 mm; (2) Chiari 1.5 by tonsillar descent into the foramen magnum accompanied by brainstem descent[139]; (3) Chiari 2 by caudal herniation of the brain stem, caudal cerebellar vermis, and 4th ventricle through the foramen magnum into the cervical spinal canal; and (4) Chiari 3 by features of CM2 and occipital encephalocele.[140,141]

CM1 malformations occur in 1 in 1000 to 5000 births. The clinical presentation of symptomatic CM1 malformation (with/without syringomyelia) in children <3 years old is characterized by neck and cervical pain, short-lasting occipital "cough" headache, dizziness, gait impairment, feeding problems, signs of myelopathy, and sleep apnea.[142] Most infants with CM2 or CM3 are recognized at birth (many earlier by fetal ultrasound). Patients with CM2 are more likely than those with CM1 to have spina bifida, meningomyelocele, and spastic paraparesis with neurogenic bladder. Syringomyelia (central cavitation or tubular fluid-filled cavity in several spinal cord segments) is present in 40% to 75% of cases of CM1 (occurring as early as 12 months). Conversely, 90% of patients with syringomyelia have CM.

People With Chiari Malformations at Risk for Symptomatic Cervicomedullary Junction Compression

People with CM are at risk for cervical medullary junction (CMJ) compression. Symptoms and signs of CMJ compression include: (1) suboccipital headache may increase with coughing, sneezing, or bowel movement; (2) myelopathy can cause mono-, hemi-, para-, or quadriparesis which may develop acutely following a seemingly mild head or neck injury; (3) downbeat nystagmus, hearing loss or uni- or bilateral paralysis or dysfunction of soft palate or pharynx; (4) apneic episodes and often severe breath-holding spells awake when upset; and (5) sudden death in sleep.

Sleep Disordered Breathing Common in People With Chiari Malformations

SDB is common in individuals with CM and can be central and/or obstructive sleep apnea, bradypnea, sleep-related alveolar hypercapnic hypoventilation, or sleep-exacerbated restrictive lung disease causing sleep-related hypoxemia with apnea or hypercapnia.[143-148] SDB can be a sole or concomitant feature of CMC compression in CMs but is challenging to recognize in those unable to speak. A retrospective study of 16 infants and toddlers with CM1 diagnosed and surgically treated for CMJ compression found: (1) 75% presented with signs of headache with irritability, inconsolable crying, head grabbing, and/or arching back; (2) 63% presented with emesis, choking, gagging, snoring, sleep apnea, breathing pause, and/or vocal cord palsy.[149]

Sleep Disordered Breathing May Not Remit Following Posterior Fossa Decompression in Chiari Malformations

Varying degrees of symptomatic improvement occurred following decompression, second surgeries were needed in seven. Infants with myelomeningocele and symptomatic CM2 are at increased risk for death especially in the first 3 months of life, low APGAR scores, large myelomeningocele defects, large head circumference at birth, and early CSA.[150]

Overnight PSG with CO_2 monitoring is warranted to evaluate for CMJ compression and/or SDB in CM. Unexpectedly observing long runs of central apnea and/or marked bradypnea during NREM sleep in a PSG warrants ordering a brain MRI to exclude posterior fossa compression. Fig. 10.4 shows a PSG we recorded in an infant with Chiari 2 showing central apneas and bradypnea. Brain MRI is the initial best choice for neuroimaging (evaluates soft tissue structures, ligaments, and brain) to assess for the presence and severity of CMJ compression.

Treatment with CPAP, BPAP, BPAP-ST, and/or supplemental oxygen is often needed and tried depending upon the SDB found. Posterior fossa decompression in patients with symptomatic CM1 often improves or stabilizes symptoms including the SDB and headache. Syrinxes would usually stabilize (and sometimes decrease) in size. Acute hydrocephalus sometimes develops in the first week following surgery, heralded by worsening of the SDB.[151] PAP therapy is

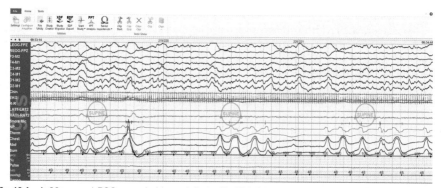

Fig. 10.4 A 90-second PSG recorded in an infant with Chiari 2 showing long-lasting central apneas and bradypnea during REM sleep.

often then needed or resumed. Better outcomes follow if decompression is performed while symptoms are present for less than 2 years. Another 2021 retrospective analysis of 15 children with symptomatic CM1 who underwent posterior fossa decompression for OSA and/or CSA found SDB improved but persistent SDB required PAP therapy in 47%.[144]

ACHONDROPLASIA

Achondroplasia (AC) is the most common cause of severe disproportionate short stature and short-limbed skeletal dysplasia (dwarfism) with an estimated birth incidence of 1 in 10,000 to 30,00 live births and affects >250,000 individuals worldwide.[152,153] The diagnosis of AC should be suspected in the newborn with proximal shortening of the arms, large head, narrow chest, and short stubby trident hands.[152]

The diagnosis of AC is based on clinical characteristics (short stature, macrocephaly, trident hand configuration, and a long near-normal length trunk) and specific radiographic findings (square pelvis, small sacroiliac notch, short vertebral pedicles with interpedicular narrowing from lower thoracic through the lumbar region, proximal shortening of long bones, proximal femoral radiolucency, and a characteristic chevron shape of the distal femoral epiphyses).[154] AC is suspected prenatally when fetal ultrasound shows macrocephaly, long bone foreshortening, and disproportionate small stature which is usually not noticeable until after 26 weeks' gestation.[154,155] Molecular confirmation of the *FGFR3* mutation can be done by droplet digital polymerase chain reaction (PCR) combined with mini-sequencing from maternal blood.[156]

AC is due to a heterozygous mutation in the *FGFR3* gene on chromosome 4p16.3 that codes for production of the FGFR3 (fibroblast growth receptor-3) protein.[157] FGFR3 (a membrane-spanning tyrosine kinase receptor) binds various fibroblast growth factors to regulate the normal endochondral bone growth. Gain of FGFR3 function in people with AC results in inhibition of endochondral ossification and which severely inhibits bone and cartilage growth. The gene mutation has 100% penetrance. Approximately 75% to 80% of AC are spontaneous new mutations of the *FGFR3* gene[153] but anyone with AC has a 50% chance of passing the mutation to their offspring given it has an autosomal dominant pattern of genetic transmission. *FGFR3* mutation testing should be considered in infants/children with atypical AC since some may have a second genetic condition and/or other *FGFR3* gene mutations (such as hypochondroplasia or thantophoric dysplasia.[154] Confirming these can be clinically important because GH therapy can be an effective treatment for hypochondroplasia (not AC). Thantophoric dysplasia is often lethal in the prenatal or early postnatal period and associated with severe thoracic and lung hypoplasia; survivors usually require significant respiratory support.

Recognizing Infants With Achondroplasia

Distinctive features of AC evident at birth: macrocephaly, frontal bossing, saddle nose, midfacial hypoplasia, short cranial base, short proximal limbs, and short squat long bones. Infants with AC also have: mild-to-moderate hypotonia which contributes to delayed motor development; thoracolumbar kyphoscoliosis; delayed self-feeding and fine motor development; and some may exhibit unusual patterns of motor development such as snowplowing (using head and feet to leverage movement). Infants with AC are usually able to hold up their heads by 4 to 7 months of age, sit by 9 to 10 months, and walk unassisted by 16 to 22 months. Respiratory problems in infants with AC can be due to chest deformity, upper airway obstruction, airway malacia, SDB, and craniocervical compression of lower brainstem and upper cervical spinal cord from foramen magnum stenosis and bony overgrowth in occipital skull regions. Compression of the spinal cord at the foramen magnum in AC occurs because of premature fusion of the four segments of the occiput.

Sleep Disordered Breathing and Respiratory Difficulties in Infants With Achondroplasia

Studies evaluating SDB in infants and children with AC have been few, all retrospective, and most have found that the most frequent SDB in AC is predominantly obstructive in type.[158-160] A 2020 retrospective chart review of 22 children with AC (median age 12 months) found that 73% had severe OSA on PSG (median preoperative OAHI 14/hour). Adenotonsillectomy was performed in 14, others required other upper airway surgeries. Following surgeries, OSA improved in 73% but only completely resolved in only 18%.[159] Moderate/severe OSA was found on overnight PSG in all nine toddlers with AC (mean age 21 months) with varying degrees of CMC due to FMS; four underwent cervicomedullary decompression and SDB improved in three.[161] SA was found on overnight PSG in 59% of 43 consecutive children with AC (mean age 3.9 ± 3.5 years) followed at a national referral center for skeletal dysplasia.[160] OSA was moderate (AHI 5–9/hour) in 9%, severe (AHI ≥10) in 16%.

Important to Evaluate for Symptomatic Foramen Magnum Stenosis in Infants With Achondroplasia

Overgrowth of bone in the occipital skull predisposes infants with AC to foramen to CMJ compression due to foramen magnum stenosis (FMS) and potentially sudden death. CMJ compression in AC often peaks around 12 months of age. Sudden death in infants with AC is now most uncommon. In 1987, the prevalence of sudden death in infants with AC was reported as 7.5%,[152] 0.3% in 2018 with proactive screening for symptomatic CMJ compression.[162] Nevertheless, the AAP 2020 revised clinical guidelines for managing the health of children with AC recommend neurological evaluation, craniocervical junction magnetic resonance imaging (MRI), and overnight PSG evaluating for symptomatic CMJ compression.[154]

When significant symptomatic CMJ compression is present, suboccipital decompression is performed. A 2020 longitudinal study of 114 people with AC found that 50% had craniocervical stenosis (involving the foramen magnum with/without cervical vertebrae C1 and/or C2) but only 6% had suboccipital decompressive surgeries.[163] Best predictors of need for suboccipital decompression include: (1) lower limb hyperreflexia and/or clonus; (2) radiographic evidence of CMJ compression/brainstem distortion at the level of the foramen magnum and/or T2-weighted signal abnormality with the cervical cord evident on MR; and (3) central hypopnea on PSG.[152,154,164,165] A 2020 longitudinal study of 114 people with AC found that 50% had craniocervical stenosis (involving the foramen magnum with/without cervical vertebrae C1 and/or C2) but only 6% had suboccipital decompressive surgeries.[163]

A 2021 study compared cervical spinal cord abnormalities on MRI and overnight PSG in 36 infants with AC.[166] They found: 6% had no FMS on MRI (graded AFMS-0); 36% had FMS but preserved cerebrospinal fluid (CSF) spaces (AFMS1); 8% loss of CSF space but no spinal cord distortion (AFMS2); 36% FMS flattening of the cervical cord without signal change (AFMS3); and 14% cervical cord signal change (AFMS4). Severity of total AHI on overnight PSG were 3.4, 6.4, 2.97, 10.5, and 25.8/hour for AFMS 0 to 5, respectively. Severe AHI had an 89% specificity but only 59% sensitivity for AFMS grades 3 or 4. The neurological examination was normal in 94%.

CENTRAL CONGENITAL HYPOVENTILATION SYNDROME

Central congenital hypoventilation syndrome (CCHS) is a neurogenetic disorder with an incidence of 1 in 50,000 to 200,000 live births which is almost always due to pathogenic variants in the transcriptional paired-like homeobox 2B (*PHOX2b*) gene.[167,168] The *PHOX2b* gene encodes a transcription factor crucial for the early development of the central autonomic nervous system (ANS).

More than 90% of patients with CCHS have in-frame tandem duplications of polyalanine repeat mutations (PARMs) in the exon 3 of *PHOX2B* gene producing genotypes of 20/24 to 20/33 (normal number of repeats is 20). CCHS. Remaining CCHS patients have frameshift, missense, or nonsense mutations in exons, 1, 2, or 3 of the *PHOX2B* gene (so-called non-PARMS). Two consanguineous CCHS families were recently found to have mutations in *MYO1H* and *LBX1* genes.

Infants with CCHS most often present in the first 30 days of life with duskiness or cyanosis upon falling asleep accompanied by progressive rise in carbon dioxide (CO_2) and fall in oxygen (O_2) which does not trigger breathlessness, an increase in respiratory rate, ventilatory effort, arousal or awakening.[169] Central hypoventilation in CCHS is typically most severe during NREM sleep but some hypoventilate awake and asleep, especially in the first few months of life.

Other infants with CCHS can present later (more often around age 3 months) with cyanosis, edema, and signs of right heart failure. At first these findings are mistaken for cyanotic congenital heart disease until only pulmonary hypertension found on cardiac catheterization.[170] A few other infants with CCHS (again most often around 3 months of age) present with: brief resolved unexplained events (BRUE); repeated oxygen desaturations; or episodes of tachycardia, diaphoresis, and/or cyanosis during sleep.[169,171] Another chapter in this text covers CCHS in detail and we encourage you to review it. Table 10.2 summarizes neurological disorders presenting as sleep-related central hypoventilation in infants.

Acquired Neurological Disorders With Sleep/Wake Disorders Which Present in Infancy

CEREBRAL PALSY

Cerebral palsy (CP) is the most common cause of motor abnormalities in infants and children with a prevalence of 1 in 500 live births. CP is a heterogenous group of complex motor and posture disorders that result from lesions, abnormalities, or nonprogressive interferences in developing fetal or immature brain.[172] Most CP insults occur in the pre- or perinatal period; the majority have no immediately identifiable risk factors for it; and only 8% can be attributed to postnatal causes.[172] Sleep problems were reported in 55% of 94 children with CP ages 4 to 14 years which resulted in poorer sleep quality and well-being reported by 71% of their caregivers.[173]

Recognizing Cerebral Palsy in Infants and Toddlers

Consider CP in any infant: (1) fisted hand(s), persistent head lag, or asymmetry of posture and movements after age 4 months; (2) unable to sit independently (without support) by age 9 months; (3) unable to bear weight on plantar surface of feet.[174] Diagnosing CP as early as possible in infants worthwhile because motor and cognitive gains are greater from diagnostic-specific early intervention.[174] Infants at high risk for CP include: term infants with neonatal encephalopathy who required resuscitation at birth and perinatal stroke; moderate risk factors are congenital disabilities, septicemia, meningitis, small for gestational age/growth restricted; and those who cannot sit by 9 months and who demonstrate early motor asymmetry.

Sleep Problems More Common in Children With More Severe Cerebral Palsy

Sleep problems are much more common in children with CP especially those who spastic quadriplegia or dyskinetic CP, more so those who also have epilepsy.[175,176] Sleep problems were present in 23% of one large cohort of children with different severities of CP. Active epilepsy increased the risk of a sleep disorder in them by 17-fold. The likelihood of difficulty falling and/or staying

TABLE 10.2 ■ Neurological Disorders Presenting as Sleep-Related Central Hypoventilation in Infants

Condition	Clinical Features	Diagnosis	Prognosis and Treatment Issues
Leigh disease (subacute necrotizing encephalopathy)	Usually presents before age 2 years with poor feeding, vomiting, sleep apnea, alveolar hypoventilation, bizarre eye movements, papillary changes, sleep/wake disturbances, hypotonia; later develops cerebellar ataxia, motor weakness, and developmental regression.	Mitochondrial disorder: order serum lactate and pyruvate. Brain MRI shows bilateral often asymmetric brainstem lesions which primarily involve gray matter.	Treat with vitamin B1 (thiamine), carnitine, lipoic acid. Consider a ketogenic diet to minimize lactate buildup. Prognosis is generally poor for patients with onset in infancy. Survival into adulthood is more likely for childhood onset, but morbidity is significant.
Carnitine deficiency	Progressive cardiomyopathy, encephalopathy caused by hypoketotic hypoglycemia, hypotonia, hepatomegaly.	Serum ammonia, urine ketones, blood glucose, liver enzymes, lactic acid, CK. Echocardiogram may show heart enlargement and left ventricular hypertrophy. Mutation in OCTN2 gene.	IV/oral carnitine for primary carnitine deficiency; good prognosis with prompt recognition and treatment. For secondary carnitine deficiency include riboflavin, glycine, or biotin in the diet to treat the primary metabolic defect.
Joubert syndrome	Presents at birth with recurring episodes of tachypnea (up to 100–200 breaths per minute) alternating with prolonged apneas awake and asleep accompanied by hypotonia, abnormal eye movements, and severe psychomotor retardation.	Brain MRI shows "molar tooth sign" due to agenesis of cerebellar vermis. Sleep study and visualization of vocal cords needed as they often have obstructive sleep apnea and/or vocal cord paralysis.	Prognosis varies among affected individuals. Treatment approach includes close monitoring of respiratory status and supportive care.
Congenital myasthenic syndromes	Severely affected neonates can have apnea, cyanosis, respiratory compromise; varying degrees of fatigueable ocular, bulbar and limb weakness. Respiratory distress can be triggered by infection, fever, or excitement.	Myriad of genes cause them; autosomal recessive inheritance, occasionally autosomal dominant.	Cholinesterase inhibitors are used to treat patients with presynaptic CMS. Postsynaptic fast-channel CMS is treated with cholinesterase inhibitors and 3,4-diaminopyridine; postsynaptic slow-channel CMS is treated with quinidine or fluoxetine. Synaptic CMS has no effective drug treatment.
X-linked myotubular myopathy	Hypotonia and respiratory distress in newborn.	X-linked recessive; 80%–85% have MTM1 gene defect.	Treatment is symptomatic. Death in infancy is common.
Multiminicore disease	Hypotonia, delayed motor development, axial muscle weakness, later scoliosis, and respiratory compromise.	Minicores on muscle biopsy using oxidative stains; mutations in SEPN1 and RYR1 genes.	Multidisciplinary supportive care with aggressive management of complications.
MECP2 encephalopathy	Neonatal male presents with generalized hypotonia, irregular breathing, and hypoxia caused by hypoventilation.	MECP2 null mutations.	Progressive encephalopathy; treatment is mainly supportive. Associated seizures can be managed with medication.
Mobius syndrome	Poor suck, facial paralysis, strabismus, and difficulty blinking due to underdevelopment of CN VI and VII	Child with mask-like facies and inability to move eyes laterally; may also be associated with limb and chest wall abnormalities.	Supportive care, which may include speech therapy, feeding tube, and lubrication of eyes.

asleep was 21-fold greater in children with dyskinetic CP, 13-times higher in those with either severe visual impairment or spastic quadriplegia.

PSG is often helpful in clarifying the nature of the sleep problems including SDB, PLMS, sleep-related seizures, and identifying comorbid sleep disruptors.[177] PSG studies have shown that children with CP compared to TD controls are more likely to have: less gross body movements; fewer body shifts; more respiratory disturbances; increased arousals; delayed REM sleep latency; and shorter duration of REM sleep.[178,179]

Sleep in infants with CP can be fragmented or disrupted by SDB reflux, seizures, involuntary motor movements but especially pain. Pain disrupting sleep in CP can be due to: reflux, constipation, muscle spasms, involuntary motor postures, reduced ability to shift body positions, and/or hip displacement. A third of parents of children with CP (especially those severely affected) complained of feeling sleep deprived often or always by their child's trouble sleeping.[180]

Obstructive Sleep Disordered Breathing Common in Children With Cerebral Palsy

SDB in children with severe CP often consists of varying combinations of obstructive and central events, central and obstructive hypoventilation, and hypoxemia during REM sleep. Recurrent aspiration, airway colonization with pathogenic bacteria, bronchiectasis, and SDB are major contributors to mortality and morbidity in individuals with CP. SDB was found in 18% of 94 children with CP.[181] The prevalence of SDB was 67% in children with CP who had epilepsy and severe motor disabilities in another cross-sectional study.[182]

Clinical features which predispose children with CP to SDB include: pharyngeal hypotonia, adenotonsillar hypertrophy, glossoptosis, disproportionate midface anatomy, restricted lung volumes, recurrent aspiration, GERD, hypersalivation, excessive oral secretions, and scoliosis. Symptoms of SDB were present in 80% of children with CP who had intrathecal baclofen pumps placed to treat spasticity.[183]

Adenotonsillectomy is usually the first treatment option for OSA in children with CP even though OSA is less likely to remit with adenotonsillectomy in CP.[184,185] Children with CP are at higher risk for postoperative complications following adenotonsillectomy (especially pneumonia and additional airway management problems) and should be hospitalized overnight after surgery.[186] Since residual postoperative OSA is likely to remain, a PSG should be performed 2 to 3 months following surgery.[187]

If significant SDB persists following adenotonsillectomy in children with CP, consider: (1) a repeat sleep study titrating CPAP for OSA, or BPAP if needed for tolerance or concomitant hypoventilation, or high flow nasal cannula (HFNC) if neither tolerated, best preceded by a PAP desensitization trial; (2) drug-induced sleep endoscopy (DISE) is useful to identify remaining sites of obstruction in the upper airway, helping guiding further upper airway surgeries such as mandibular distraction, tongue base reduction/suspension, and/or skeletal advancement or expansion; and (3) aggressive treatment of comorbidities including excessive oral secretions, swallowing problems, epilepsy, and reflux to possibly improve overall sleep quality.[185,188,189] Other treatment strategies for SDB in children with CP, with or without ID or spastic quadriparesis are: (1) nocturnal postural devices as long as they do not worsen the SDB[190]; (2) oral appliances[191]; and (3) botulinum toxin injections of submandibular salivary glands to reduce hypersalivation.[192]

Sleep Breathing Disorders Associated With Skull Base and Hindbrain Malformations

SDB is common in people with skull base and hind brain malformations such as CM, spina bifida, achondroplasia, and Joubert syndrome. SDB in hind brain malformations can be predominantly OSA, predominantly CSA, or a combination of OSA and CSA. Compression of the brainstem and respiratory centers is thought to be mechanism producing CSA whereas compression of lower cranial nerves decreased upper airway patency and obstruction.

Finding predominantly CSA on PSG in infants and children prompts consideration of posterior fossa lesions and/or hydrocephalus but neuroimaging is more often negative. Worse yet, CSA in patients with hindbrain malformations often does not correlate with the severity of brainstem compression/herniation evident on neuroimaging.

A 2021 retrospective analysis of 65 children (median age 6 years, range 1–18 years) diagnosed with CSA by PSG found normal brain MRI in 70%.[193] Twenty percent had abnormalities on MRI unrelated to CSA. Only 11% had brainstem pathology on MRI which could be attributed to hindbrain abnormalities. They further found a central apnea-hypopnea (CAHI) $\geq$9.5 events/hour, $\geq$6.4% of TST with an end-tidal CO_2 $\geq$50 mmHg best predicted brainstem pathology would be found on MRI.

Another 2021 retrospective study of CSA found on PSG in 3% (95) of 2981 children (>1 month old, 41% 1–6 years old, 19% $\geq$6 years) with mean CAI of 20 $\pm$ 30/hour.[194] SDB was exclusively central in type in 61%; periodic breathing in 81% with mean percentage of time with periodic breathing of 9 $\pm$ 16%. Among periodic breathing episodes, 40% appeared after a sigh, 8% after an obstructive event, 6% after breathing instability, and 2% after bradypnea. Watchful waiting over 6 months was performed in 22 (23%) patients with spontaneous improvement in 20. The most common brain pathology among them were CM. CSA was most severe in those with encephalopathy and/or epilepsy.

EPILEPSY

Sleep and epilepsy are too often poor bedfellows. Complex bidirectional relationships are observed between sleep and epilepsy.[195] Epilepsy (and perhaps some treatments for it) disrupts sleep, and seizures can fragment sleep and/or alter sleep architecture and circadian rhythms. Sleep problems and SWDs are far more likely to be found in children with epilepsy (CWE) than the general pediatric population.

A 2021 metaanalysis (19 studies, 901 CWE compared with 1470 healthy children) found CWE had an average of 34 minutes less nighttime sleep, and more nighttime awakenings, parasomnias, and sleep-disordered breathing than healthy controls.[196] The presence of SWDs in CWE has been associated with behavior problems and impaired academic performance.[197-199] Comorbidities such as NDDs, ID, ASD, and ADHD increase the likelihood of problematic sleep and SWDs in CWE.[200] Even in the absence of nighttime seizures, sleep problems were reported by parents as 12 times more common in 4- to 10-year-old children with focal-onset epilepsy (CWE) than children without epilepsy and associated with lower health-related QoL.[201]

Using different pediatric sleep questionnaires, a 2012 study of 105 households with a child with epilepsy and 79 controls found CWE compared to healthy controls had increased rates of parent-child roomsharing and cosleeping and more sleep disturbances especially parasomnias, nocturnal awakenings, sleep duration, daytime sleepiness, sleep onset delay, and bedtime resistance.[202] Further findings are worthy of mention: (1) severity of a child's epilepsy correlated with the severity of child and parent sleep dysfunction and parental fatigue; (2) antiseizure medication (ASM) polypharmacy predicted greater childhood sleep disturbances would be reported; (3) sleep problems in CWE were associated with roomsharing and cosleeping; (4) 62% of parents described decreased quantity and/or quality of sleep when cosleeping; and (5) 42% of parents reported never/rarely feeling rested because they were concerned about their children having seizures during sleep.[202]

Sleep Problems in Infants and Toddlers With Epilepsy

Very few studies have evaluated the relationship between sleep and epilepsy in children <2 years of age. One case-control study evaluated sleep duration and fragmentation in 32 infants with early onset epilepsy (ages 1–11 months) comparing them to 160 TD babies (ages 3.5–11 months) (Pisch et al., 2015). They found that the infants with epilepsy had shorter nocturnal sleep duration and greater night waking frequency than TD infants. The earlier the age of epilepsy onset, the shorter the night sleep duration. The number of night waking was reduced when seizures were controlled.

Epileptic Seizures Often Quite Different Looking in Children Less Than Age 2 Years

Epileptic seizures in children <2 years of age often have limited clinical expression and are different from seizures observed in older children and adults (even though they emanate from the same brain areas). Infant seizure types are easier to recognize as seizures are: sustained tonic eye (and head) deviation; unilateral clonic twitching of face and/or limbs; symmetric or asymmetric tonic postures; and infant spasms. Seizure types more difficult to identify as seizures are: stares; subtle changes in behavior; pallor or perioral cyanosis; and/or rhythmic eye blinking.

Clinical features which warrant concern for sleep-related epileptic seizures are: (1) events occur any time in the night, just after falling asleep, or shortly before awakening in the morning; (2) multiple events a night; (3) occasional occurrence of these events awake or during a brief nap. If you suspect the parasomnia may be sleep-related seizures and the child has not had an EEG with sleep, request one first. Repetitive sleep starts (hypnic jerks) can be observed in neurologically compromised infants in transitions to NREM 1 sleep and in the absence of ictal EEG activity should not be misdiagnosed as infantile spasms.[203-205]

The first best test to confirm sleep-related seizures in an infant is a routine EEG with sleep. A prospective study of EEG done on 534 children referred for possible epilepsy reported epileptiform activity was found in 37% of the children with definite epilepsy and 13% of clinically suspected cases.[206] However, the initial EEG will be normal in approximately one-half of children with clinically diagnosed epilepsy.[207,208] If a child is having spells daily, 4 to 8 hours of outpatient video-EEG often captures and confirms the nature of the events. Fig. 10.5 shows an example of an electrographic seizure recorded during sleep in an infant.

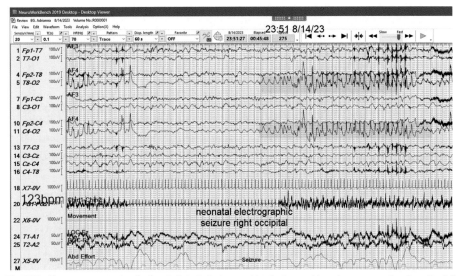

Fig. 10.5 Shows an example of a focal clinical-electrographic electrographic seizure emanating from the left posterior during sleep in a 6-months-old infant.

Sleep-Related Movements and Sleep-Related Movement Disorders in Infants and Toddlers

ONTOGENY OF MOVEMENT IN FETUS AND INFANTS

By 16 weeks gestational age (wGA), almost the entire repertoire of movements observed in infants at term are present: general body movements, startle and twitch movements, isolated limb movements, breathing movements, hiccups, isolated head and neck movements, sucking the thumb and swallowing, jaw movements (including yawning), hand-face contact, stretch, and rotation.[209] Purposeful movements are observed by 18 wGA, gradually replacing reflex movements, and purposeful voluntary movements develop further after birth. Fig. 10.6 shows the ontogeny of body and limb movements in utero.

A circadian rhythm of rest-activity can be detected by fetal ultrasound and EKG by 14 to 18 wGA. By week 21, the fetus exhibits a regular schedule of movement. Cycles of rest-activity of motor movements are observed in fetuses as young as 20 to 28 wGA, and last 40 to 60 minutes at 24 wGA.[210,211] The median percentage of time spent in fetal body movements decreases from 17% at 24 wGA to 7% near term. Of note, rest-activity cycles in fetus are not synced with the mother; fetuses are most active from 9 a.m. to 2 p.m. and again from 7 p.m. to 4 a.m. Most of the kicking or jabbing movements after 32 to 34 wGA occur when the fetus is sleeping.

As fetuses approach term, they appear cramped; movements become smaller, and major joint movements limited to rotations and attempts to extend the spine are present.[209] Whereas, numbers of facial movements including chewing, swallowing, jaw opening and closure increase. Fetal behavior patterns change as the nervous system matures and an index of fetal health.[212,213]

A longitudinal study of sleep-related movement between ages 30 wGA and 18 months found these decrease with increasing age.[214] Phasic muscle activity decreases first, then localized body movements next. The frequency of gross body motor movements during sleep remained unchanged until a basal level of 9 to 13 months term. The number of PSG epochs without body movements increased steadily until about 8 months term.

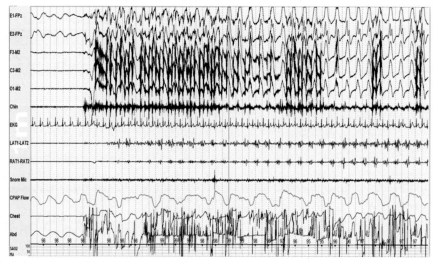

Fig. 10.6   A 60-second epoch of repetitive head banging and humming in an 18-months-old child consistent with sleep-related rhythmic movement disorder.

NIGHTTIME NONNUTRITIVE SUCKING

Nighttime nonnutritive sucking common infants especially half hour before and after feeds. Nonnutritive sucking: state regulation (i.e., self-soothing behavior), cope with stressors, central pattern generator, and foster maturation of swallow reflex.

RECOGNIZING NORMAL REM SLEEP BEHAVIORS IN INFANTS

During REM sleep, rapid eye movements (at times dysconjugate) are observed with closed eyes; slight opening and closing of eyes can be seen. The chin EMG is atonic but bursts of sucking, brief runs of clonic jaw jerks, twitching, and small phasic muscle activity are common. Smiles, facial grimaces, sighs, and sobs are observed. Isolated limb jerks, body and limb tremors; intermittent stretching; writhing body; and large athetoid limb movements are common.[215]

It is important to recognize the behavioral and movement correlates of Active Wake, Quiet Wake, Quiet/NREM, Active/REM, and behaviors heralding sleep/wake transitions in term infants (Fig. 10.7).

Sleep-Related Movement Disorders in Infants

BENIGN SLEEP-RELATED MYOCLONUS

Benign neonatal sleep myoclonus (BNSM) is a parasomnia characterized by myoclonic jerks that occur during sleep which abruptly stop when the infant is aroused.[216-218] One case series of 38 infants with BNSM found it was observed at a median age of 3 days (range 1–16 days) and spontaneously remitted at a median age of 2 months (range 2 weeks to 10 months).[218] Video-PSG studies show BNSM: (1) can occur in any stage of sleep; (2) the limb movements are more often bilateral, symmetrical, and involve the arms and/or legs; (3) usually occur in clusters lasting a few seconds but occasionally 5 minutes; (4) most often begin at sleep onset; and (5) but sometimes appear after the infant has been sleeping for more than 20 minutes or, more rarely, before awakening.

BNSM can initially be misdiagnosed as multifocal myoclonic seizures.[219-221] The nonepileptic nature of BNSM confirmed by: (1) absence of epileptiform/ictal EEG activity accompanying jerks; (2) occurrence during sleep, disappearing with awakening or arousal. A recent small case-control study recorded video-PSG with expanded EEG in four term infants with BNSM and two controls.[222] EEG averaging time-locked to myoclonic jerks and the somatosensory stimuli provoked by tapping on palms and feet showed: (1) theta activity central and midline central electrodes time-locked to the myoclonic jerks; and a series of (2) late somatosensory evoked potential responses which back-averaging showed followed the jerk, and maximal at the midline central (vertex, Cz) electrode. They emphasized it is important not to mistake these waveforms in theta band as ictal activity.

SLEEP-RELATED RHYTHMIC MOVEMENT DISORDER

Sleep-related rhythmic movement disorder (SRMD) is another parasomnia which is most common in infants and young children.[223] SRMD is characterized by: (1) repetitive episodes of movements involving large muscle groups (most often head and neck) which are associated with rhythmic head banging, head rolling, body rocking, or body rolling; (2) usually occurs just before sleep onset, but may persist into NREM 1 or 2 sleep, and rarely recurs in REM sleep; (3) often accompanied by humming or rhythmic vocalization; and (4) more common in infants and young children.[223-225] RMD usually occurs just before sleep onset, but may persist into NREM 1 or 2 sleep, and rarely recur in REM sleep. May represent vestibular stimulation for motor system and/or central pattern generator.

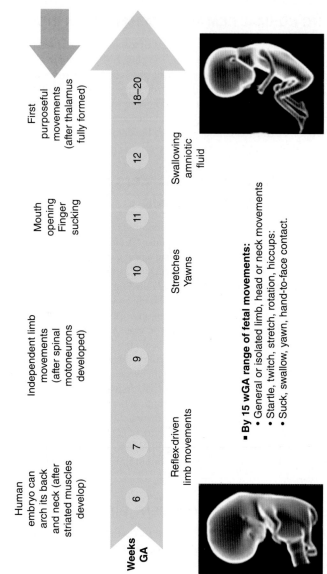

Ontogeny of Body and Limb Movements in Utero

Weeks GA

6 — Human embryo can arch its back and neck (after striated muscles develop)

7 — Reflex-driven limb movements

9 — Independent limb movements (after spinal motoneurons developed)

10 — Stretches Yawns

11 — Mouth opening Finger sucking

12 — Swallowing amniotic fluid

18–20 — First purposeful movements (after thalamus fully formed)

- **By 15 wGA range of fetal movements:**
  - General or isolated limb, head or neck movements
  - Startle, twitch, stretch, rotation, hiccups:
  - Suck, swallow, yawn, hand-to-face contact.

Fig. 10.7   Ontogeny of body and limb movements *in utero*.

Nearly 66% of 9-month-old infants (both neurodevelopmental normal and abnormal) exhibit SRMD but the prevalence falls to 8% age 4, 5% age 5, and most cases remit by age 10.[225] SRMD which persists in later childhood is more likely to occur in children with neurodevelopmental, psychiatric and/or ASDs. SRMD relatively rarely persists in adults.[223,224,226]

Polysomnographic features of RMD: 0.5 to 2 Hz rhythmic repetitive stereotyped movements involve large muscle groups (Fig. 10.8). Most often: presleep W, sleep/wake transitions, N1, N2 (especially with K-complexes). During NREM, RMD most often begins after start of cyclic alternating pattern (CAP) phase A.

Treatment strategies: (1) reassurance, usually resolves with age; (2) protective measures (e.g., headbanging padding and helmet if needed); (3) metronome near bed; (4) allow infant to rock before bed on chair or rocking horse; (5) if severe, low dose clonazepam (e.g., 0.25 mg).

SLEEP STARTS (HYPNIC JERKS)

Sleep starts (also known as hypnic jerks) are normal physiological events which most often occur in the transition from wakefulness to sleep. They are characterized by one or two abrupt myoclonic flexion jerks which in older children and adults are often accompanied by a feeling of falling, a sensory flash, and/or dream-like imagery.[227] Sleep starts: (1) can be spontaneous or induced by stimuli; (2) are usually associated with tachycardia and/or irregular breathing; and (3) occasionally a noisy gasp accompanies a jerk.

SLEEP-RELATED RHYTHMIC TONGUE MOVEMENTS IN INFANTS WITH COSTELLO SYNDROME

Long-lasting episodes of repetitive tongue protrusions during NREM sleep are observed in infants and young children with Costello syndrome.[228,229] Costello syndrome is characterized by delayed development, FTT in infancy due to poor suck/feed, oromotor apraxia, and macrosomnia.[230] Movements of the tongue (and sometimes the lips) resemble repetitive licking and/or sucking and produce a peculiar noise; these disappear or are markedly reduced/absent during REM sleep and associated with the *HRAS* gene.

BENIGN NOCTURNAL ALTERNATING HEMIPLEGIA OF CHILDHOOD STARTS FIRST FEW MONTHS OF AGE

Benign nocturnal alternating hemiplegia of childhood (BNAHC) is characterized by episodes of unilateral (less often bilateral) weakness which occur upon awakening from sleep.[231] Episodes of hemiplegia usually last 15 to 20 minutes but can last up to 5 hours; often recur once a month. Episodes are heralded by inconsolable crying or screaming; then head deviation toward one side which progresses to hemiplegia (often worse in arm than leg) and be accompanied by difficulty with swallowing and breathing. The child typically awakens the next morning without deficits. Twelve cases have been reported in the literature as of 2018; these show a male predominance; stress and sleep deprivation triggers for some; and gradual decrease in attack frequency and usually complete remission. EEG performed during an attack often shows slowing of background on the side contralateral to the hemiplegia. A family history of hemiplegic migraine or intermittent headache reported in many of the children.[231]

BNAHC is quite different from ATP1A3-related alternating hemiplegia of childhood (AHC) in which attacks begin during wakefulness and are relieved by sleep.[232,233] BNAHC also needs to be distinguished from paroxysmal hypnogenic dyskinesia (PHD) characterized by brief attacks of dystonic, choreiform or ballistic movements during NREM sleep.[234-236] PHD attacks

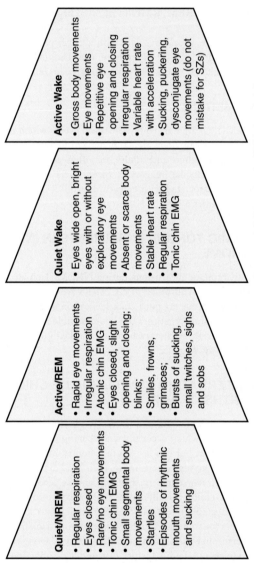

Behavioral Correlates of Sleep/Wake States

Quiet/NREM
- Regular respiration
- Eyes closed
- Rare/no eye movements
- Tonic chin EMG
- Small segmental body movements
- Startles
- Episodes of rhythmic mouth movements and sucking

Active/REM
- Rapid eye movements
- Irregular respiration
- Atonic chin EMG
- Eyes closed, slight opening and closing; blinks;
- Smiles, frowns, grimaces;
- Bursts of sucking, small twitches, sighs and sobs

Quiet Wake
- Eyes wide open, bright eyes with or without exploratory eye movements
- Absent or scarce body movements
- Stable heart rate
- Regular respiration
- Tonic chin EMG

Active Wake
- Gross body movements
- Eye movements
- Repetitive eye opening and closing
- Irregular respiration
- Variable heart rate with acceleration
- Sucking, puckering, dysconjugate eye movements (do not mistake for SZs)

Fig. 10.8 Behavioral correlates of active wake, quiet wake, quiet/NREM and active/REM sleep in infants.

respond to treatment with sodium channel blockers (oxcarbamazepine, phenytoin). A mutation of the PRRT2 gene has been found in a few patients with PND.

HEREDITARY GENIOSPASM AND RECURRENT NOCTURNAL TONGUE-BITING OF INFANCY

Paroxysmal movement disorder of mentalis (chin) muscle is another rare movement disorder which begins in infancy or childhood and characterized by involuntary trembling or quivering of the chin and lower lip due to involuntary repetitive contractions of the bilateral mentalis muscles.[237] Episodes last minutes/hours primarily during drowsiness or immediately upon awakening; and often triggered by stress or strong emotions, but can occur spontaneously.

Hereditary or sporadic geniospasm occurring during sleep has been reported to cause or be associated recurrent nocturnal tongue-biting (RNTB).[238,239] A 13-month-old boy had recurrent tongue-biting during sleep and found to be due to episodes of geniospasm occurring during NREM sleep.[239] Other cases have been reported. Patients awake from sleep with painful lacerations typically at the tip or sides of the tongue (compounded by repeated injuries to the same areas). RNTB tends to begin between ages 10 and 18 months; may decrease or abate during early childhood. RNTB can occur more than half the nights of the week and recur more than once a night.

In closing, sleep disturbances and disorders are highly prevalent in infants with particular neurogenetic syndromes, neurological and neurodevelopmental disorders. Cognizant of a particularly common sleep problems and disturbances seen in particular neurological conditions can be helpful when evaluating their sleep.

References

1. Uchitel J, Vanhatalo S, Austin T. Early development of sleep and brain functional connectivity in term-born and preterm infants. *Pediatr Res.* 2022;91(4):771-786.
2. Basile C, Gigliotti F, Cesario S, Bruni O. The relation between sleep and neurocognitive development in infancy and early childhood: a neuroscience perspective. *Adv Child Dev Behav.* 2021;60:9-27.
3. Henderson JMT, Blampied NM, France KG. Longitudinal study of infant sleep development: early predictors of sleep regulation across the first year. *Nat Sci Sleep.* 2020;12:949-957.
4. Pisch M, Wiesemann F, Karmiloff-Smith A. Infant wake after sleep onset serves as a marker for different trajectories in cognitive development. *J Child Psychol Psychiatry.* 2019;60(2):189-198. doi:10.1111/jcpp.12948.
5. Shaw KA, Maenner MJ, Bakian AV, et al. Early identification of autism spectrum disorder among children aged 4 years—autism and developmental disabilities monitoring network, 11 sites, United States, 2018. *MMWR Surveill Summ.* 2021;70:1-14.
6. Bourel-Ponchel E, Hasaerts D, Challamel MJ, Lamblin MD. Behavioral-state development and sleep-state differentiation during early ontogenesis. *Neurophysiol Clin.* 2021;51:89-98.
7. Hvolby A, Christensen J, Gasse C, Dalsgaard S, Dreier JW. Cumulative incidence and relative risk of sleep problems among children and adolescents with newly diagnosed neurodevelopmental disorders: A nationwide register-based study. *J Sleep Res.* 2021;30:e13122.
8. D'Souza D, D'Souza H, Horváth K, Plunkett K, Karmiloff-Smith A. Sleep is atypical across neurodevelopmental disorders in infants and toddlers: a cross-syndrome study. *Res Dev Disabil.* 2020;97:103549.
9. Abel EA, Tonnsen BL. Sleep phenotypes in infants and toddlers with neurogenetic syndromes. *Sleep Med.* 2017;38:130-134.
10. Kamara D, Beauchaine TP. A review of sleep disturbances among infants and children with neurodevelopmental disorders. *Rev J Autism Dev Disord.* 2020;7:278-294.
11. Robinson-Shelton A, Malow BA. Sleep disturbances in neurodevelopmental disorders. *Curr Psychiatry Rep.* 2016;18:6.
12. Angriman M, Caravale B, Novelli L, Ferri R, Bruni O. Sleep in children with neurodevelopmental disabilities. *Neuropediatrics.* 2015;46:199-210.

13. Paruthi S, Brooks LJ, D'Ambrosio C, et al. Recommended amount of sleep for pediatric populations: a consensus statement of the American Academy of Sleep Medicine. *J Clin Sleep Med.* 2016;12:785-786.

14. Scott N, Blair PS, Emond AM, et al. Sleep patterns in children with ADHD: a population-based cohort study from birth to 11 years. *J Sleep Res.* 2013;22:121-128.

15. Magee CA, Gordon R, Caputi P. Distinct developmental trends in sleep duration during early childhood. *Pediatrics.* 2014;133:e1561-e1567.

16. Wheaton AG, Claussen AH. Short sleep duration among infants, children, and adolescents aged 4 months-17 years—United States, 2016-2018. *MMWR Morb Mortal Wkly Rep.* 2021;70:1315-1321.

17. Valent F, Brusaferro S, Barbone F. A case-crossover study of sleep and childhood injury. *Pediatrics.* 2001; 107:E23.

18. Allotey J, Zamora J, Cheong-See F, et al. Cognitive, motor, behavioural and academic performances of children born preterm: a meta-analysis and systematic review involving 64 061 children. *BJOG.* 2018; 125:16-25.

19. Eyre M, Fitzgibbon SP, Ciarrusta J, et al. The Developing Human Connectome Project: typical and disrupted perinatal functional connectivity. *Brain.* 2021;144:2199-2213.

20. Grothe MJ, Scheef L, Bäuml J, et al. Reduced cholinergic basal forebrain integrity links neonatal complications and adult cognitive deficits after premature birth. *Biol Psychiatry.* 2017;82:119-126.

21. Meng C, Bäuml JG, Daamen M, et al. Extensive and interrelated subcortical white and gray matter alterations in preterm-born adults. *Brain Struct Funct.* 2016;221:2109-2121.

22. Weisman O, Magori-Cohen R, Louzoun Y, Eidelman AI, Feldman R. Sleep-wake transitions in premature neonates predict early development. *Pediatrics.* 2011;128:706-714.

23. Arditi-Babchuk H, Feldman R, Eidelman AI. Rapid eye movement (REM) in premature neonates and developmental outcome at 6 months. *Infant Behav Dev.* 2009;32:27-32.

24. Geva R, Yaron H, Kuint J. Neonatal sleep predicts attention orienting and distractibility. *J Atten Disord.* 2016;20:138-150.

25. Jaleel Z, Schaeffer T, Trinh C, Cohen MB, Levi JR. Prematurity: a prognostic factor for increased severity of pediatric obstructive sleep apnea. *Laryngoscope.* 2021;131:1909-1914.

26. Sadras I, Reiter J, Fuchs N, Erlichman I, Gozal D, Gileles-Hillel A. Prematurity as a risk factor of sleep-disordered breathing in children younger than two years: a retrospective case-control study. *J Clin Sleep Med.* 2019;15:1731-1736.

27. Crump C, Friberg D, Li X, Sundquist J, Sundquist K. Preterm birth and risk of sleep-disordered breathing from childhood into mid-adulthood. *Int J Epidemiol.* 2019;48:2039-2049.

28. Resta RG. Changing demographics of advanced maternal age (AMA) and the impact on the predicted incidence of Down syndrome in the United States: Implications for prenatal screening and genetic counseling. *Am J Med Genet A.* 2005;133A:31-36.

29. Cocchi G, Gualdi S, Bower C, et al. International trends of Down syndrome 1993–2004: Births in relation to maternal age and terminations of pregnancies. *Birth Defects Res A Clin Mol Teratol.* 2010;88:474-479.

30. Grieco J, Pulsifer M, Seligsohn K, Skotko B, Schwartz A. Down syndrome: Cognitive and behavioral functioning across the lifespan. *Am J Med Genet C Semin Med Genet.* 2015;169:135-149.

31. Lott IT, Dierssen M. Cognitive deficits and associated neurological complications in individuals with Down's syndrome. *Lancet Neurol.* 2010;9:623-633.

32. Lee CF, Lee CH, Hsueh WY, Lin MT, Kang KT. Prevalence of obstructive sleep apnea in children with down syndrome: a meta-analysis. *J Clin Sleep Med.* 2018;14:867-875.

33. Waters KA, Castro C, Chawla J. The spectrum of obstructive sleep apnea in infants and children with Down Syndrome. *Int J Pediatr Otorhinolaryngol.* 2020;129:109763.

34. Goffinski A, Stanley MA, Shepherd N, et al. Obstructive sleep apnea in young infants with Down syndrome evaluated in a Down syndrome specialty clinic. *Am J Med Genet A.* 2015;167A:324-330.

35. Guimaraes CV, Donnelly LF, Shott SR, Amin RS, Kalra M. Relative rather than absolute macroglossia in patients with Down syndrome: implications for treatment of obstructive sleep apnea. *Pediatr Radiol.* 2008;38:1062-1067.

36. Lagan N, Huggard D, Mc Grane F, et al. Multiorgan involvement and management in children with Down syndrome. *Acta Paediatr.* 2020;109:1096-1111.

37. Bertapelli F, Pitetti K, Agiovlasitis S, Guerra-Junior G. Overweight and obesity in children and adolescents with Down syndrome-prevalence, determinants, consequences, and interventions: a literature review. *Res Dev Disabil.* 2016;57:181-192.

38. Ferrari M, Stagi S. Autoimmunity and genetic syndromes: a focus on down syndrome. *Genes (Basel)*. 2021;12:268.
39. Huggard D, Kelly L, Worrall A, et al. Melatonin as an immunomodulator in children with Down syndrome. *Pediatr Res*. 2022;91(7):1812-1820.
40. Bull MJ. Health supervision for children with Down syndrome. *Pediatrics*. 2011;128:393-406.
41. Naime S, Weiss M, Lew J, et al. Central breathing abnormalities in children with trisomy 21: effect of age, sex, and concomitant OSA. *Pediatr Pulmonol*. 2021;56:472-478.
42. Trucco F, Chatwin M, Semple T, Rosenthal M, Bush A, Tan HL. Sleep disordered breathing and ventilatory support in children with Down syndrome. *Pediatr Pulmonol*. 2018;53:1414-1421.
43. Yau S, Pickering RM, Gringras P, et al. Sleep in infants and toddlers with Down syndrome compared to typically developing peers: looking beyond snoring. *Sleep Med*. 2019;63:88-97.
44. Fernandez F, Nyhuis CC, Anand P, et al. Young children with Down syndrome show normal development of circadian rhythms, but poor sleep efficiency: a cross-sectional study across the first 60 months of life. *Sleep Med*. 2017;33:134-144.
45. McKay SM, Angulo-Barroso RM. Longitudinal assessment of leg motor activity and sleep patterns in infants with and without Down syndrome. *Infant Behav Dev*. 2006;29:153-168.
46. Lukowski AF, Slonecker EM, Milojevich HM. Sleep problems and recall memory in children with Down syndrome and typically developing controls. *Res Dev Disabil*. 2020;96:103512.
47. Anand V, Shukla G, Gupta N, et al. Association of sleep apnea with development and behavior in Down syndrome: a prospective clinical and polysomnographic study. *Pediatr Neurol*. 2021;116:7-13.
48. Sibarani CR, Walter LM, Davey MJ, Nixon GM, Horne RSC. Sleep-disordered breathing and sleep macro- and micro-architecture in children with Down syndrome. *Pediatr Res*. 2022;91(5):1248-1256.
49. Deliens G, Peigneux P. Sleep-behaviour relationship in children with autism spectrum disorder: methodological pitfalls and insights from cognition and sensory processing. *Dev Med Child Neurol*. 2019;61:1368-1376.
50. National Institute for Health and Care Excellence. *Clinical Guidelines*. Autism Spectrum Disorder in Under 19s: Support and Management. London: National Institute for Health and Care Excellence (NICE); 2021.
51. Havdahl A, Niarchou M, Starnawska A, Uddin M, van der Merwe C, Warrier V. Genetic contributions to autism spectrum disorder. *Psychol Med*. 2021;51:2260-2273.
52. Hyman SL, Levy SE, Myers SM. Identification, evaluation, and management of children with autism spectrum disorder. *Pediatrics*. 2020;145:e20193447.
53. Hodge D, Carollo TM, Lewin M, Hoffman CD, Sweeney DP. Sleep patterns in children with and without autism spectrum disorders: developmental comparisons. *Res Dev Disabil*. 2014;35:1631-1638.
54. Verhoeff ME, Blanken LME, Kocevska D, et al. The bidirectional association between sleep problems and autism spectrum disorder: a population-based cohort study. *Mol Autism*. 2018;9:8.
55. Humphreys JS, Gringras P, Blair PS, et al. Sleep patterns in children with autistic spectrum disorders: a prospective cohort study. *Arch Dis Child*. 2014;99:114-118.
56. Goldman SE, Richdale AL, Clemons T, Malow BA. Parental sleep concerns in autism spectrum disorders: variations from childhood to adolescence. *J Autism Dev Disord*. 2012;42:531-538.
57. Malow BA, Crowe C, Henderson L, et al. A sleep habits questionnaire for children with autism spectrum disorders. *J Child Neurol*. 2009;24:19-24.
58. Cortesi F, Giannotti F, Ivanenko A, Johnson K. Sleep in children with autistic spectrum disorder. *Sleep Med*. 2010;11:659-664.
59. Kotagal S, Broomall E. Sleep in children with autism spectrum disorder. *Pediatr Neurol*. 2012;47:242-251.
60. MacDuffie KE, Munson J, Greenson J, et al. Sleep problems and trajectories of restricted and repetitive behaviors in children with neurodevelopmental disabilities. *J Autism Dev Disord*. 2020;50:3844-3856.
61. Lamônica DAC, Giacheti CM, Dias Hayssi Haduo M, Dias Dos Santos MJ, da Silva NC, Pinato L. Sleep quality, functional skills, and communication in preschool-aged children with autism spectrum disorder. *Res Dev Disabil*. 2021;116:104024.
62. Taylor MA, Schreck KA, Mulick JA. Sleep disruption as a correlate to cognitive and adaptive behavior problems in autism spectrum disorders. *Res Dev Disabil*. 2012;33:1408-1417.
63. Sikora DM, Johnson K, Clemons T, Katz T. The relationship between sleep problems and daytime behavior in children of different ages with autism spectrum disorders. *Pediatrics*. 2012;130 suppl 2:S83-S90.
64. Taylor BJ, Reynolds CF III, Siegel M. Insomnia subtypes and clinical impairment in hospitalized children with autism spectrum disorder. *Autism*. 2021;25:656-666.

65. Grigg-Damberger M, Ralls F. Treatment strategies for complex behavioral insomnia in children with neurodevelopmental disorders. *Curr Opin Pulm Med*. 2013;19:616-625.
66. Woodford EC, McLay L, France KG, et al. Endogenous melatonin and sleep in individuals with Rare Genetic Neurodevelopmental Disorders (RGND): a systematic review. *Sleep Med Rev*. 2021;57:101433.
67. Girault JB, Piven J. The neurodevelopment of autism from infancy through toddlerhood. *Neuroimaging Clin N Am*. 2020;30:97-114.
68. Barnevik Olsson M, Carlsson LH, Westerlund J, Gillberg C, Fernell E. Autism before diagnosis: crying, feeding and sleeping problems in the first two years of life. *Acta Paediatr*. 2013;102:635-639.
69. Horiuchi F, Kawabe K, Oka Y, Nakachi K, Hosokawa R, Ueno SI. The Association between Autistic Traits and Sleep Habits/Problems in Toddlers. *Dev Neuropsychol*. 2020;45:485-495.
70. MacDuffie KE, Shen MD, Dager SR, et al. Sleep onset problems and subcortical development in infants later diagnosed with autism spectrum disorder. *Am J Psychiatry*. 2020;177:518-525.
71. Seo WS. An update on the cause and treatment of sleep disturbance in children and adolescents with autism spectrum disorder. *Yeungnam Univ J Med*. 2021;38:275-281.
72. Rana M, Kothare S, DeBassio W. The assessment and treatment of sleep abnormalities in children and adolescents with autism spectrum disorder: a review. *J Can Acad Child Adolesc Psychiatry*. 2021;30:25-35.
73. Persico AM, Ricciardello A, Lamberti M, et al. The pediatric psychopharmacology of autism spectrum disorder: A systematic review—part I: the past and the present. *Prog Neuropsychopharmacol Biol Psychiatry*. 2021;110:110326.
74. Elkhatib Smidt SD, Gooneratne N, Brodkin ES, Bucan M, Mitchell JA. ss. *Autism*. 2022;26(4):814-826.
75. Schroder CM, Banaschewski T, Fuentes J, et al. Pediatric prolonged-release melatonin for insomnia in children and adolescents with autism spectrum disorders. *Expert Opin Pharmacother*. 2021;22: 2445-2454.
76. Malow BA, Findling RL, Schroder CM, et al. Sleep, growth, and puberty after 2 years of prolonged-release melatonin in children with autism spectrum disorder. *J Am Acad Child Adolesc Psychiatry*. 2021;60:252-261.e3.
77. Cassidy SB SS, I Seattle (WA): University of Washington S-, 03]. OuS. Prader-Willi Syndrome. In: Pagon RA, BT, Dolan CR, Stephens K, eds. Gene Reviews [Internet]. 1993-1998 Oct 06 [updated 2009 Sep 03]. ed: University of Washington, Seattle; 2009.
78. Yang L, Zhou Q, Ma B, et al. Perinatal features of Prader-Willi syndrome: a Chinese cohort of 134 patients. *Orphanet J Rare Dis*. 2020;15:24.
79. Gillett ES, Perez IA. Disorders of sleep and ventilatory control in Prader-Willi syndrome. *Diseases*. 2016;4(3):23.
80. Fermin Gutierrez MA, Mendez MD. Prader-Willi syndrome. In: *StatPearls*. Treasure Island, FL: StatPearls Publishing LLC.; 2021.
81. Feighan SM, Hughes M, Maunder K, Roche E, Gallagher L. A profile of mental health and behaviour in Prader-Willi syndrome. *J Intellect Disabil Res*. 2020;64:158-169.
82. Neo WS, Tonnsen BL. Brief report: challenging behaviors in toddlers and preschoolers with angelman, Prader-Willi, and Williams syndromes. *J Autism Dev Disord*. 2019;49:1717-1726.
83. Butler MG, Miller JL, Forster JL. Prader-Willi syndrome—clinical genetics, diagnosis and treatment approaches: an update. *Curr Pediatr Rev*. 2019;15:207-244.
84. Gillett ES, Perez IA. Disorders of sleep and ventilatory control in Prader-Willi syndrome. *Diseases*. 2016;4:23.
85. Urquhart DS, Gulliver T, Williams G, Harris MA, Nyunt O, Suresh S. Central sleep-disordered breathing and the effects of oxygen therapy in infants with Prader-Willi syndrome. *Arch Dis Child*. 2013;98: 592-595.
86. Cohen M, Hamilton J, Narang I. Clinically important age-related differences in sleep related disordered breathing in infants and children with Prader-Willi syndrome. *PLoS One*. 2014;9:e101012.
87. Khayat A, Narang I, Bin-Hasan S, Amin R, Al-Saleh S. Longitudinal evaluation of sleep disordered breathing in infants with Prader-Willi syndrome. *Arch Dis Child*. 2017;102:634-638.
88. Lu A, Luo F, Sun C, Zhang X, Wang L, Lu W. Sleep-disordered breathing and genetic findings in children with Prader-Willi syndrome in China. *Ann Transl Med*. 2020;8:989.
89. Carrel AL, Myers SE, Whitman BY, Eickhoff J, Allen DB. Long-term growth hormone therapy changes the natural history of body composition and motor function in children with Prader-Willi syndrome. *J Clin Endocrinol Metab*. 2010;95:1131-1136.

90. Corripio R, Tubau C, Calvo L, et al. Safety and effectiveness of growth hormone therapy in infants with Prader-Willi syndrome younger than 2 years: a prospective study. *J Pediatr Endocrinol Metab*. 2019;32: 879-884.

91. Donze SH, Damen L, Mahabier EF, Hokken-Koelega ACS. Cognitive functioning in children with Prader-Willi syndrome during 8 years of growth hormone treatment. *Eur J Endocrinol*. 2020;182:405-411.

92. Zimmermann M, Laemmer C, Woelfle J, Fimmers R, Gohlke B. Sleep-disordered breathing in children with prader-willi syndrome in relation to growth hormone therapy onset. *Horm Res Paediatr*. 2020; 93:85-93.

93. Caudri D, Nixon GM, Nielsen A, et al. Sleep-disordered breathing in Australian children with Prader-Willi syndrome following initiation of growth hormone therapy. *J Paediatr Child Health*. 2022;58:248-255.

94. McCandless SE. Clinical report—health supervision for children with Prader-Willi syndrome. *Pediatrics*. 2011;127:195-204.

95. Nagai T, Obata K, Tonoki H, et al. Cause of sudden, unexpected death of Prader-Willi syndrome patients with or without growth hormone treatment. *Am J Med Genet A*. 2005;136:45-48.

96. Festen DA, de Weerd AW, van den Bossche RA, Joosten K, Hoeve H, Hokken-Koelega AC. Sleep-related breathing disorders in prepubertal children with Prader-Willi syndrome and effects of growth hormone treatment. *J Clin Endocrinol Metab*. 2006;91:4911-4915.

97. Tauber M, Diene G, Molinas C, Hebert M. Review of 64 cases of death in children with Prader-Willi syndrome (PWS). *Am J Med Genet A*. 2008;146:881-887.

98. Miller JL, Shuster J, Theriaque D, Driscoll DJ, Wagner M. Sleep disordered breathing in infants with Prader-Willi syndrome during the first 6 weeks of growth hormone therapy: a pilot study. *J Clin Sleep Med*. 2009;5:448-453.

99. Wolfgram PM, Carrel AL, Allen DB. Long-term effects of recombinant human growth hormone therapy in children with Prader-Willi syndrome. *Curr Opin Pediatr*. 2013;25:509-514.

100. Maas AP, Didden R, Bouts L, Smits MG, Curfs LM. Scatter plot analysis of excessive daytime sleepiness and severe disruptive behavior in adults with Prader-Willi syndrome: a pilot study. *Res Dev Disabil*. 2009;30:529-537.

101. Richdale AL, Cotton S, Hibbit K. Sleep and behaviour disturbance in Prader-Willi syndrome: a questionnaire study. *J Intellect Disabil Res*. 1999;43(Pt 5):380-392.

102. Smith ACM, Boyd KE, Brennan C, et al. Smith-Magenis syndrome. In: Adam MP, Ardinger HH, Pagon RA, et al., eds. *GeneReviews(®)*. Seattle, WA: University of Washington, Seattle; 1993. Copyright © 1993-2022, University of Washington, Seattle. GeneReviews is a registered trademark of the University of Washington, Seattle. All rights reserved.

103. Gropman AL, Duncan WC, Smith AC. Neurologic and developmental features of the Smith-Magenis syndrome (del 17p11.2). *Pediatr Neurol*. 2006;34:337-350.

104. Trickett J, Oliver C, Heald M, et al. Sleep in children with Smith-Magenis syndrome: a case-control actigraphy study. *Sleep*. 2020;43:zsz260.

105. Kaplan KA, Elsea SH, Potocki L. Management of sleep disturbances associated with Smith-Magenis syndrome. *CNS Drugs*. 2020;34:723-730.

106. De Leersnyder H. Smith-Magenis syndrome. *Handb Clin Neurol*. 2013;111:295-296.

107. De Leersnyder H, De Blois MC, Claustrat B, et al. Inversion of the circadian rhythm of melatonin in the Smith-Magenis syndrome. *J Pediatr*. 2001;139:111-116.

108. De Leersnyder H, Bresson JL, de Blois MC, et al. Beta 1-adrenergic antagonists and melatonin reset the clock and restore sleep in a circadian disorder, Smith-Magenis syndrome. *J Med Genet*. 2003;40:74-78.

109. Smith ACM, Morse RS, Introne W, Duncan Jr WC. Twenty-four-hour motor activity and body temperature patterns suggest altered central circadian timekeeping in Smith-Magenis syndrome, a neurodevelopmental disorder. *Am J Med Genet A*. 2019;179:224-236.

110. Polymeropoulos CM, Brooks J, Czeisler EL, et al. Tasimelteon safely and effectively improves sleep in Smith-Magenis syndrome: a double-blind randomized trial followed by an open-label extension. *Genet Med*. 2021;23:2426-2432.

111. Morris CA. Williams syndrome. In: Adam MP, Ardinger HH, Pagon RA, et al., eds. *GeneReviews(®)*. Seattle, WA: University of Washington, Seattle; 1993. Copyright © 1993-2022, University of Washington, Seattle. GeneReviews is a registered trademark of the University of Washington, Seattle. All rights reserved.

112. Wilson M, Carter IB. Williams syndrome. In: *StatPearls*. Treasure Island, FL: StatPearls Publishing LLC.; 2021.

113. Kirchner RM, Martens MA, Andridge RR. Adaptive behavior and development of infants and toddlers with Williams syndrome. *Front Psychol.* 2016;7:598.

114. Annaz D, Hill CM, Ashworth A, Holley S, Karmiloff-Smith A. Characterisation of sleep problems in children with Williams syndrome. *Res Dev Disabil.* 2011;32:164-169.

115. Mason TB, Arens R, Sharman J, et al. Sleep in children with Williams syndrome. *Sleep Med.* 2011; 12:892-897.

116. Ashworth A, Hill CM, Karmiloff-Smith A, Dimitriou D. Cross syndrome comparison of sleep problems in children with Down syndrome and Williams syndrome. *Res Dev Disabil.* 2013;34:1572-1580.

117. Gwilliam K, Joyce A, Dimitriou D. Early manifestation of sleep problems in toddlers with Williams Syndrome using a mixed method longitudinal approach. *Res Dev Disabil.* 2020;104:103658.

118. Greiner de Magalhães C, O'Brien LM, Mervis CB. Sleep characteristics and problems of 2-year-olds with Williams syndrome: relations with language and behavior. *J Neurodev Disord.* 2020;12:32.

119. Axelsson EL, Hill CM, Sadeh A, Dimitriou D. Sleep problems and language development in toddlers with Williams syndrome. *Res Dev Disabil.* 2013;34:3988-3996.

120. Martens MA, Seyfer DL, Andridge RR, Coury DL. Use and effectiveness of sleep medications by parent report in individuals with Williams syndrome. *J Dev Behav Pediatr.* 2017;38:765-771.

121. Sniecinska-Cooper AM, Iles RK, Butler SA, Jones H, Bayford R, Dimitriou D. Abnormal secretion of melatonin and cortisol in relation to sleep disturbances in children with Williams syndrome. *Sleep Med.* 2015;16:94-100.

122. Yang L, Shu X, Mao S, Wang Y, Du X, Zou C. Genotype-phenotype correlations in Angelman syndrome. *Genes (Basel).* 2021;12:987.

123. Madaan M, Mendez MD. Angelman syndrome. In: *StatPearls.* Treasure Island, FL: StatPearls Publishing LLC.; 2021.

124. Trickett J, Heald M, Oliver C. Sleep in children with Angelman syndrome: parental concerns and priorities. *Res Dev Disabil.* 2017;69:105-115.

125. Wink LK, Fitzpatrick S, Shaffer R, et al. The neurobehavioral and molecular phenotype of Angelman Syndrome. *Am J Med Genet A.* 2015;167a:2623-2628.

126. Spruyt K, Braam W, Curfs LM. Sleep in Angelman syndrome: a review of evidence. *Sleep Med Rev.* 2018;37:69-84.

127. Ryan CS, Edlund W, Mandrekar J, Wong-Kisiel LC, Gavrilova RH, Kotagal S. Iron deficiency and its role in sleep disruption in patients with Angelman syndrome. *J Child Neurol.* 2020;35:963-969.

128. Wheeler AC, Okoniewski KC, Wylie A, et al. Anxiety-associated and separation distress-associated behaviours in Angelman syndrome. *J Intellect Disabil Res.* 2019;63:1234-1247.

129. Puckett Y, Mallorga-Hernández A, Montaño AM. Epidemiology of mucopolysaccharidoses (MPS) in United States: challenges and opportunities. *Orphanet J Rare Dis.* 2021;16:241.

130. Ademhan Tural D, Emiralioglu N, Dogru D, et al. Evaluation of sleep-disordered breathing and its relationship with respiratory parameters in children with mucopolysaccharidosis Type IVA and VI. *Am J Med Genet A.* 2021;185:2306-2314.

131. Leighton SE, Papsin B, Vellodi A, Dinwiddie R, Lane R. Disordered breathing during sleep in patients with mucopolysaccharidoses. *Int J Pediatr Otorhinolaryngol.* 2001;58:127-138.

132. Kasapkara ÇS, Tümer L, Aslan AT, et al. Home sleep study characteristics in patients with mucopolysaccharidosis. *Sleep Breath.* 2014;18:143-149.

133. Akyol MU, Alden TD, Amartino H, et al. Recommendations for the management of MPS VI: systematic evidence- and consensus-based guidance. *Orphanet J Rare Dis.* 2019;14:118.

134. Lin HY, Chen MR, Lin CC, et al. Polysomnographic characteristics in patients with mucopolysaccharidoses. *Pediatr Pulmonol.* 2010;45:1205-1212.

135. Lee CL, Lee KS, Chuang CK, et al. Otorhinolaryngological management in Taiwanese patients with mucopolysaccharidoses. *Int J Med Sci.* 2021;18:3373-3379.

136. Moreau J, Brassier A, Amaddeo A, et al. Obstructive sleep apnea syndrome after hematopoietic stem cell transplantation in children with mucopolysaccharidosis type I. *Mol Genet Metab.* 2015;116:275-280.

137. Pal AR, Langereis EJ, Saif MA, et al. Sleep disordered breathing in mucopolysaccharidosis I: a multivariate analysis of patient, therapeutic and metabolic correlators modifying long term clinical outcome. *Orphanet J Rare Dis.* 2015;10:42.

138. Wraith JE, Beck M, Lane R, et al. Enzyme replacement therapy in patients who have mucopolysaccharidosis I and are younger than 5 years: results of a multinational study of recombinant human alpha-L-iduronidase (laronidase). *Pediatrics.* 2007;120:e37-e46.

139. Sader N, Hader W, Hockley A, Kirk V, Adeleye A, Riva-Cambrin J. The relationship between Chiari 1.5 malformation and sleep-related breathing disorders on polysomnography. *J Neurosurg Pediatr*. 2021;27:452-458.
140. Ortiz JF, Ruxmohan S, Alli A, Halan T, Alzamora IM. Chiari malformation type III: a case report and review of literature. *Cureus*. 2021;13:e14131.
141. Azahraa Haddad F, Qaisi I, Joudeh N, et al. The newer classifications of the chiari malformations with clarifications: an anatomical review. *Clin Anat*. 2018;31:314-322.
142. Ciaramitaro P, Ferraris M, Massaro F, Garbossa D. Clinical diagnosis-part I: what is really caused by Chiari I. *Childs Nerv Syst*. 2019;35:1673-1679.
143. Moore M, Fuell W, Jambhekar S, Ocal E, Albert GW. Management of sleep apnea in children with chiari I malformation: a retrospective study. *Pediatr Neurosurg*. 2022;57(3):175-183.
144. Voutsas G, St-Laurent A, Hutchinson C, Amin R, Drake J, Narang I. The efficacy of neurosurgical intervention on sleep-disordered breathing in pediatric patients with Chiari malformation type I. *J Neurosurg Pediatr*. 2021;27:611-619.
145. Leu RM. Sleep-related breathing disorders and the Chiari 1 malformation. *Chest*. 2015;148:1346-1352.
146. Ferre Maso A, Poca MA, de la Calzada MD, Solana E, Romero Tomas O, Sahuquillo J. Sleep disturbance: a forgotten syndrome in patients with Chiari I malformation. *Neurologia*. 2014;29:294-304.
147. Losurdo A, Dittoni S, Testani E, et al. Sleep disordered breathing in children and adolescents with Chiari malformation type I. *J Clin Sleep Med*. 2013;9:371-377.
148. Alsaadi MM, Iqbal SM, Elgamal EA, Gozal D. Sleep-disordered breathing in children with Chiari malformation type II and myelomeningocele. *Pediatr Int*. 2012;54:623-626.
149. Grahovac G, Pundy T, Tomita T. Chiari type I malformation of infants and toddlers. *Childs Nerv Syst*. 2018;34:1169-1176.
150. McDowell MM, Blatt JE, Deibert CP, Zwagerman NT, Tempel ZJ, Greene S. Predictors of mortality in children with myelomeningocele and symptomatic Chiari type II malformation. *J Neurosurg Pediatr*. 2018;21:587-596.
151. Jha DK, Gosal JS, Kumar R, Khera P. Delayed post-operative aggravation of sleep related disturbances in patients of basilar invagination with Chiari malformation: case report and review of the literature. *Br J Neurosurg*. 2021:1-5.
152. Legare JM. Achondroplasia. In: Adam MP, Ardinger HH, Pagon RA, et al., eds. *GeneReviews(®)*. Seattle, WA: University of Washington, Seattle; 1993. Copyright © 1993-2022, University of Washington, Seattle. GeneReviews is a registered trademark of the University of Washington, Seattle. All rights reserved.
153. Hoover-Fong JE, Alade AY, Hashmi SS, et al. Achondroplasia Natural History Study (CLARITY): a multicenter retrospective cohort study of achondroplasia in the United States. *Genet Med*. 2021;23:1498-1505.
154. Hoover-Fong J, Scott CI, Jones MC. Health supervision for people with achondroplasia. *Pediatrics*. 2020;145(6):e20201010.
155. Boulet S, Althuser M, Nugues F, Schaal JP, Jouk PS. Prenatal diagnosis of achondroplasia: new specific signs. *Prenat Diagn*. 2009;29:697-702.
156. Orhant L, Anselem O, Fradin M, et al. Droplet digital PCR combined with minisequencing, a new approach to analyze fetal DNA from maternal blood: application to the non-invasive prenatal diagnosis of achondroplasia. *Prenat Diagn*. 2016;36:397-406.
157. Kumble S, Savarirayan R. Emerging therapies for Achondroplasia: changing the rules of the game. *Expert Opin Emerg Drugs*. 2021;26:425-431.
158. Afsharpaiman S, Sillence DO, Sheikhvatan M, Ault JE, Waters K. Respiratory events and obstructive sleep apnea in children with achondroplasia: investigation and treatment outcomes. *Sleep Breath*. 2011;15:755-761.
159. Booth KL, Levy DA, White DR, Meier JD, Pecha PP. Management of obstructive sleep apnea in children with achondroplasia: outcomes of surgical interventions. *Int J Pediatr Otorhinolaryngol*. 2020;138:110332.
160. Tenconi R, Khirani S, Amaddeo A, et al. Sleep-disordered breathing and its management in children with achondroplasia. *Am J Med Genet A*. 2017;173:868-878.
161. Sano M, Takahashi N, Nagasaki K, Oishi M, Yoshimura J, Fujii Y. Polysomnography as an indicator for cervicomedullary decompression to treat foramen magnum stenosis in achondroplasia. *Childs Nerv Syst*. 2018;34:2275-2281.
162. Hashmi SS, Gamble C, Hoover-Fong J, et al. Multicenter study of mortality in achondroplasia. *Am J Med Genet A*. 2018;176:2359-2364.

163. Okenfuss E, Moghaddam B, Avins AL. Natural history of achondroplasia: a retrospective review of longitudinal clinical data. *Am J Med Genet A*. 2020;182:2540-2551.
164. Pauli RM, Horton VK, Glinski LP, Reiser CA. Prospective assessment of risks for cervicomedullary-junction compression in infants with achondroplasia. *Am J Hum Genet*. 1995;56:732-744.
165. Shimony N, Ben-Sira L, Sivan Y, Constantini S, Roth J. Surgical treatment for cervicomedullary compression among infants with achondroplasia. *Childs Nerv Syst*. 2015;31:743-750.
166. Cheung MS, Irving M, Cocca A, et al. Achondroplasia Foramen Magnum Score: screening infants for stenosis. *Arch Dis Child*. 2021;106:180-184.
167. Weese-Mayer DE, Rand CM, Khaytin I, et al. Congenital Central Hypoventilation Syndrome. In: Adam MP, Ardinger HH, Pagon RA, et al., eds. *GeneReviews(®)*. Seattle, WA: University of Washington; 1993. Seattle Copyright © 1993-2022, University of Washington, Seattle. GeneReviews is a registered trademark of the University of Washington, Seattle. All rights reserved., 1993.
168. Porcaro F, Paglietti MG, Cherchi C, Schiavino A, Chiarini Testa MB, Cutrera R. How the management of children with congenital central hypoventilation syndrome has changed over time: two decades of experience from an Italian Center. *Front Pediatr*. 2021;9:648927.
169. Weese-Mayer DE, Shannon DC, Keens TG, Silvestri JM. Idiopathic congenital central hypoventilation syndrome: diagnosis and management. American Thoracic Society. *Am J Respir Crit Care Med*. 1999;160:368-373.
170. Marcus CL, Bautista DB, Amihiya A, Ward SL, Keens TG. Hypercapneic arousal responses in children with congenital central hypoventilation syndrome. *Pediatrics*. 1991;88:993-998.
171. Gozal D. Congenital central hypoventilation syndrome: an update. *Pediatr Pulmonol*. 1998;26:273-282.
172. Morgan C, Fahey M, Roy B, Novak I. Diagnosing cerebral palsy in full-term infants. *J Paediatr Child Health*. 2018;54:1159-1164.
173. Lang CP, Boucaut A, Guppy M, Johnston LM. Children with cerebral palsy: a cross-sectional study of their sleep and their caregiver's sleep quality, psychological health and well-being. *Child Care Health Dev*. 2021;47:859-868.
174. Novak I, Morgan C, Adde L, et al. Early, accurate diagnosis and early intervention in cerebral palsy: advances in diagnosis and treatment. *JAMA Pediatr*. 2017;171:897-907.
175. Newman CJ, O'Regan M, Hensey O. Sleep disorders in children with cerebral palsy. *Dev Med Child Neurol*. 2006;48:564-568.
176. Obrecht A, Fischer de Almeida M, Maltauro L, Leite da Silva WD, Bueno Zonta M, de Souza Crippa AC. The relationship between gross motor function impairment in cerebral palsy and sleeping issues of children and caregivers. *Sleep Med*. 2021;81:261-267.
177. Tanner K, Noritz G, Ayala L, et al. Assessments and interventions for sleep disorders in infants with or at high risk for cerebral palsy: a systematic review. *Pediatr Neurol*. 2021;118:57-71.
178. Hayashi M, Inoue Y, Iwakawa Y, Sasaki H. REM sleep abnormalities in severe athetoid cerebral palsy. *Brain Dev*. 1990;12:494-497.
179. Kotagal S, Gibbons VP, Stith JA. Sleep abnormalities in patients with severe cerebral palsy. *Dev Med Child Neurol*. 1994;36:304-311.
180. Hulst RY, Gorter JW, Voorman JM, et al. Sleep problems in children with cerebral palsy and their parents. *Dev Med Child Neurol*. 2021;63:1344-1350.
181. Koyuncu E, Türkkani MH, Sarikaya FG, Özgirgin N. Sleep disordered breathing in children with cerebral palsy. *Sleep Med*. 2017;30:146-150.
182. Garcia J, Wical B, Wical W, et al. Obstructive sleep apnea in children with cerebral palsy and epilepsy. *Dev Med Child Neurol*. 2016;58:1057-1062.
183. Mohon RT, Sawyer K, Pickett K, et al. Sleep-related breathing disorders associated with intrathecal baclofen therapy to treat patients with cerebral palsy: a cohort study and discussion. *NeuroRehabilitation*. 2021;48:481-491.
184. Magardino TM, Tom LW. Surgical management of obstructive sleep apnea in children with cerebral palsy. *Laryngoscope*. 1999;109:1611-1615.
185. Ali NE, Alyono JC, Kumar AR, Cheng H, Koltai PJ. Sleep surgery in syndromic and neurologically impaired children. *Am J Otolaryngol*. 2020;41:102566.
186. End C, Propst EJ, Cushing SL, et al. Risks and benefits of adenotonsillectomy in children with cerebral palsy with obstructive sleep apnea: a systematic review. *Laryngoscope*. 2022;132(3):687-694.
187. Wiet GJ, Bower C, Seibert R, Griebel M. Surgical correction of obstructive sleep apnea in the complicated pediatric patient documented by polysomnography. *Int J Pediatr Otorhinolaryngol*. 1997;41:133-143.

188. Hartzell LD, Guillory RM, Munson PD, Dunham AK, Bower CM, Richter GT. Tongue base suspension in children with cerebral palsy and obstructive sleep apnea. *Int J Pediatr Otorhinolaryngol.* 2013;77:534-537.
189. Cohen SR, Lefaivre JF, Burstein FD, et al. Surgical treatment of obstructive sleep apnea in neurologically compromised patients. *Plast Reconstr Surg.* 1997;99:638-646.
190. Hill CM, Parker RC, Allen P, Paul A, Padoa KA. Sleep quality and respiratory function in children with severe cerebral palsy using night-time postural equipment: a pilot study. *Acta Paediatr.* 2009;98:1809-1814.
191. Yoshida K. Elastic retracted oral appliance to treat sleep apnea in mentally impaired patients and patients with neuromuscular disabilities. *J Prosthet Dent.* 1999;81:196-201.
192. Sriskandan N, Moody A, Howlett DC. Ultrasound-guided submandibular gland injection of botulinum toxin for hypersalivation in cerebral palsy. *Br J Oral Maxillofac Surg.* 2010;48:58-60.
193. Stowe RC, Miranda-Schaeubinger M, Andronikou S, Tapia IE. Polysomnographic predictors of abnormal brainstem imaging in children. *J Clin Sleep Med.* 2021;17:1411-1421.
194. Ghirardo S, Amaddeo A, Griffon L, Khirani S, Fauroux B. Central apnea and periodic breathing in children with underlying conditions. *J Sleep Res.* 2021;30:e13388.
195. Grigg-Damberger M, Foldvary-Schaefer N. Bidirectional relationships of sleep and epilepsy in adults with epilepsy. *Epilepsy Behav.* 2021;116:107735.
196. Winsor AA, Richards C, Bissell S, Seri S, Liew A, Bagshaw AP. Sleep disruption in children and adolescents with epilepsy: a systematic review and meta-analysis. *Sleep Med Rev.* 2021;57:101416.
197. Chan S, Baldeweg T, Cross JH. A role for sleep disruption in cognitive impairment in children with epilepsy. *Epilepsy Behav.* 2011;20:435-440.
198. Parisi P, Bruni O, Pia Villa M, et al. The relationship between sleep and epilepsy: the effect on cognitive functioning in children. *Dev Med Child Neurol.* 2010;52:805-810.
199. Manni R, Terzaghi M. Comorbidity between epilepsy and sleep disorders. *Epilepsy Res.* 2010;90:171-177.
200. Hvolby A, Christensen J, Gasse C, Dalsgaard S, Dreier JW. Cumulative incidence and relative risk of sleep problems among children and adolescents with newly diagnosed neurodevelopmental disorders: a nationwide register-based study. *J Sleep Res.* 2021;30(3):e13122.
201. Gutter T, Brouwer OF, de Weerd AW. Subjective sleep disturbances in children with partial epilepsy and their effects on quality of life. *Epilepsy Behav.* 2013;28:481-488.
202. Larson AM, Ryther RC, Jennesson M, et al. Impact of pediatric epilepsy on sleep patterns and behaviors in children and parents. *Epilepsia.* 2012;53:1162-1169.
203. Fusco L, Pachatz C, Cusmai R, Vigevano F. Repetitive sleep starts in neurologically impaired children: an unusual non-epileptic manifestation in otherwise epileptic subjects. *Epileptic Disord.* 1999;1:63-67.
204. Maki Y, Kidokoro H, Okumura A, et al. Repetitive sleep starts: an important differential diagnosis of infantile spasms. *Epilepsy Behav.* 2021;121:108075.
205. Serino D, Fusco L. Epileptic hypnagogic jerks mimicking repetitive sleep starts. *Sleep Med.* 2015;16:1014-1016.
206. Aydin K, Okuyaz C, Serdaroglu A, Gucuyener K. Utility of electroencephalography in the evaluation of common neurologic conditions in children. *J Child Neurol.* 2003;18:394-396.
207. Camfield P, Gordon K, Camfield C, Tibbles J, Dooley J, Smith B. EEG results are rarely the same if repeated within six months in childhood epilepsy. *Can J Neurol Sci.* 1995;22:297-300.
208. Gilbert DL, Gartside PS. Factors affecting the yield of pediatric EEGs in clinical practice. *Clin Pediatr (Phila).* 2002;41:25-32.
209. Borsani E, Della Vedova AM, Rezzani R, Rodella LF, Cristini C. Correlation between human nervous system development and acquisition of fetal skills: an overview. *Brain Dev.* 2019;41:225-233.
210. Bourel-Ponchel E, Hasaerts D, Challamel MJ, Lamblin MD. Behavioral-state development and sleep-state differentiation during early ontogenesis. *Neurophysiol Clin.* 2021;51(1):89-98.
211. Nijhuis JG, Prechtl HF, Martin Jr CB, Bots RS. Are there behavioural states in the human fetus? *Early Hum Dev.* 1982;6:177-195.
212. Lai J, Nowlan NC, Vaidyanathan R, Shaw CJ, Lees CC. Fetal movements as a predictor of health. *Acta Obstet Gynecol Scand.* 2016;95:968-975.
213. Kurjak A, Stanojević M, Predojević M, Laušin I, Salihagić-Kadić A. Neurobehavior in fetal life. *Semin Fetal Neonatal Med.* 2012;17:319-323.
214. Fukumoto M, Mochizuki N, Takeishi M, Nomura Y, Segawa M. Studies of body movements during night sleep in infancy. *Brain Dev.* 1981;3:37-43.
215. Grigg-Damberger MM. The visual scoring of sleep in infants 0 to 2 months of age. *J Clin Sleep Med.* 2016;12:429-445.

216. Suzuki Y, Toshikawa H, Kimizu T, et al. Benign neonatal sleep myoclonus: our experience of 15 Japanese cases. *Brain Dev.* 2015;37:71-75.
217. Maurer VO, Rizzi M, Bianchetti MG, Ramelli GP. Benign neonatal sleep myoclonus: a review of the literature. *Pediatrics.* 2010;125:e919-e924.
218. Paro-Panjan D, Neubauer D. Benign neonatal sleep myoclonus: experience from the study of 38 infants. *Eur J Paediatr Neurol.* 2008;12:14-18.
219. Goraya JS, Singla G, Mahey H. Benign neonatal sleep myoclonus: frequently misdiagnosed as neonatal seizures. *Indian Pediatr.* 2015;52:713-714.
220. Kakisaka Y, Ohara T, Hino-Fukuyo N, Uematsu M, Kure S. Neonatal "seizure" while riding in a car: a peculiar but key episode for diagnosis of benign neonatal sleep myoclonus. *Clin Pediatr (Phila).* 2014; 53:605-606.
221. Ramelli GP, Sozzo AB, Vella S, Bianchetti MG. Benign neonatal sleep myoclonus: an under-recognized, non-epileptic condition. *Acta Paediatr.* 2005;94:962-963.
222. Losito E, Eisermann M, Vignolo P, Hovhannisyan S, Magny JF, Kaminska A. Benign neonatal sleep myoclonus evokes somatosensory responses. *J Clin Neurophysiol.* 2017;34:484-491.
223. DelRosso LM, Cano-Pumarega I, E SSA. Sleep-related rhythmic movement disorder. *Sleep Med Clin.* 2021;16:315-321.
224. Prihodova I, Skibova J, Nevsimalova S. Sleep-related rhythmic movements and rhythmic movement disorder beyond early childhood. *Sleep Med.* 2019;64:112-115.
225. Mayer G, Wilde-Frenz J, Kurella B. Sleep related rhythmic movement disorder revisited. *J Sleep Res.* 2007;16:110-116.
226. Stepanova I, Nevsimalova S, Hanusova J. Rhythmic movement disorder in sleep persisting into childhood and adulthood. *Sleep.* 2005;28:851-857.
227. Baldelli L, Provini F. Fragmentary hypnic myoclonus and other isolated motor phenomena of sleep. *Sleep Med Clin.* 2021;16:349-361.
228. Tuxhorn I, Hoppe M. Parasomnia with rhythmic movements manifesting as nocturnal tongue biting. *Neuropediatrics.* 1993;24:167-168.
229. Della Marca G, Rubino M, Vollono C, et al. Rhythmic tongue movements during sleep: a peculiar parasomnia in Costello syndrome. *Mov Disord.* 2006;21:473-478.
230. Gripp KW, Rauen KA. Costello syndrome. In: Adam MP, Ardinger HH, Pagon RA, et al., eds. *GeneReviews(®).* Seattle, WA: University of Washington, Seattle; 1993.
231. Maas R, Kamsteeg EJ, Mangano S, et al. Benign nocturnal alternating hemiplegia of childhood: A clinical and nomenclatural reappraisal. *Eur J Paediatr Neurol.* 2018;22:1110-1117.
232. Salles PA, Mata IF, Brünger T, Lal D, Fernandez HH. ATP1A3-related disorders: an ever-expanding clinical spectrum. *Front Neurol.* 2021;12:637890.
233. Capuano A, Garone G, Tiralongo G, Graziola F. Alternating hemiplegia of childhood: understanding the genotype-phenotype relationship of ATP1A3 variations. *Appl Clin Genet.* 2020;13:71-81.
234. Liu XR, Huang D, Wang J, et al. Paroxysmal hypnogenic dyskinesia is associated with mutations in the *PRRT2* gene. *Neurol Genet.* 2016;2:e66.
235. Almeida L, Dure LS. Paroxysmal hypnogenic dyskinesia. *Neurology.* 2014;82:1935.
236. Benbir G, Senturk A, Tan F, Karadeniz D. Polysomnographic recording of a child with paroxysmal hypnogenic dyskinesia and NREM parasomnia. *Sleep Med.* 2013;14:215-216.
237. Hull M, Parnes M. Effective treatment of geniospasm: case series and review of the literature. *Tremor Other Hyperkinet Mov (N Y).* 2020;10:31.
238. Mahmoudi M, Kothare SV. Tongue biting: a case of sporadic geniospasm during sleep. *J Clin Sleep Med.* 2014;10:1339-1340.
239. Goraya JS, Virdi V, Parmar V. Recurrent nocturnal tongue biting in a child with hereditary chin trembling. *J Child Neurol.* 2006;21:985-987.

Behavioral Sleep Disorders in Infancy

CHAPTER 11

Insomnia in Infancy: Phenomenology and Links With Parental Factors

Liat Tikotzky ▪ Michal Kahn

Introduction

The main purpose of this chapter is to highlight the various factors that contribute to the development of early childhood insomnia in the context of the transactional model of infant sleep, as described in Fig. 11.1.[1,2] This model reflects the idea that the development of insomnia in infants results from a dynamic, complex, and interactive process between the infant and various proximal and distal environmental factors, mediated mainly through sleep-related interactions between infants and their parents.[2-5] Understanding the role of these different factors is crucial for the assessment and treatment of sleep problems in infancy.

Specifically, the current chapter will review research **on the role of parental factors and the parent-infant relationship** in early childhood insomnia. The chapter will not cover other important parts of the model, such as physiological and constitutionally based factors (e.g., temperament, medical problems) or sociodemographic and cultural aspects that are related to infant sleep development. These domains are covered and discussed in other chapters of this book.

Throughout the chapter, we will refer to various sleep variables that reflect the behavioral aspects of sleep. These aspects include both sleep **quantity** variables, such as sleep duration and time in bed, and sleep **quality** variables. Sleep quality refers to both sleep initiation (sleep onset latency) and sleep consolidation (e.g., number and duration of night-awakenings, sleep percent, and longest period of uninterrupted sleep). Sleep regulation and self-soothing skills will also be covered, given their role in sleep initiation and maintenance.

Phenomenology of Insomnia in Infancy

The evolution of sleep consolidation and regulation is one of the main developmental processes during infancy. During the first months of life, infants wake frequently during the night, and these awakenings are usually accompanied by feeding and other types of external regulation (e.g., holding, rocking). However, the associations between feeding, external regulation, and falling asleep gradually weaken as the physiological sleep-wake system matures (i.e., circadian and homeostatic processes); the ability to retain calories increases; and adaptive sleep associations are learned. Throughout the second half of the first year of life, most infants develop consolidated and regulated sleep. Whereas sleep consolidation refers to the reduction in the length and number of night-wakings, sleep regulation refers to the capacity of the infant to independently resume sleep following natural nocturnal night-wakings.[6-9]

Although most infants attain the ability to "sleep through the night" during the first year of life, there is substantial variability between infants.[8,10] In fact, bedtime problems and difficulties

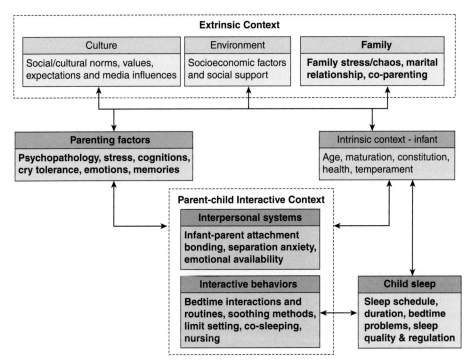

Fig. 11.1 A transactional model of child sleep. *(From Sadeh A, Anders TF. Infant sleep problems: origins, assessment, interventions.* Infant Ment Health J. *1993;14:17–34)*

in the process of nighttime sleep consolidation and regulation affect 15% to 30% of all young children between the ages of 6 months and 3 years.[11-14] These problems are among the most common concerns brought to the attention of pediatricians and other child-care professionals.[15,16] If not treated, they may persist in 20% to 50% of children[17,18] and may have negative consequences for children's socioemotional, behavioral, and cognitive development, as well as for parental sleep and mental health.[19-26]

Early childhood bedtime and night-waking problems are classified in the *International Classification of Sleep Disorders* (3rd ed., 2014) under the general diagnostic category of Chronic Insomnia Disorder, which refers to both adults and children. The main criteria (criteria A) specifies that the patient reports or **the patient's parents or caregiver observes** one or more of the following: (1) Difficulty initiating sleep; (2) Difficulty maintaining sleep; (3) Waking up earlier than desired; (4) Resistance going to bed on appropriate schedule; and (5) Difficulty sleeping without parent or caregiver intervention. In addition to criteria A, associated daytime dysfunction (e.g., fatigue, sleepiness, mood disturbance/irritability) is observed or reported (criteria B). Moreover, the sleep problems exist despite adequate sleep opportunities. Finally, disturbances occur at least 3 times per week, have been present for at least 3 months, and cannot be explained by another sleep disorder (e.g., obstructive sleep apnea). Similarly, the diagnostic criteria for an Insomnia Disorder according to the *Diagnostic and Statistical Manual of Mental Disorders* (DSM-5) specify that in children, sleep onset and night-waking problems may manifest as difficulies initiating sleep and returning to sleep **without caregiver intervention**. Thus, both the ICSD and the DSM emphasize that early childhood insomnia involves self-regualtion difficulties. These difficulties are manifested by infant signaling (e.g., by crying, fussing, refusing to lie down, etc.) at bedtime and upon waking at night, and by infant reliance on caregiver assitance to transition from wakefulness to sleep.

It is important to emphasize that the diagnosis of insomnia in infants depends largely on parents' experiences and perceptions. Parents may perceive their infant as having a sleep problem to the extent that the infant's night-wakings exceed the parents' expectations of "normal" awakenings with respect to the infant's age, the awakenings cause disruption to their own sleep, and/or cause considerable emotional distress.[1,6,13] However, not all parents of "signalers" are troubled by their infants' awakenings. For instance, they may not consider their infant to have a sleep problem when the night-wakings are short and require only short parental involvement, and the parents have no difficulty resuming their own sleep. A certain frequency of awakenings per night could thus be seen as problematic by some parents, and not by others. Likewise, a similar extent of sleep fragmentation or resistance could be perceived as a problem at age of 18 months, despite being perceived as normal by the same parents only a few months earlier. Thus, the subjective experience of the parent is a critical factor to consider as part of the assessment process.

One term which is frequently used to describe the dependency of infants on external help to fall asleep is "sleep-onset associations"—a certain set of conditions that the child learns to rely on at the time of sleep onset in order to fall asleep. Usually, this term refers to the caregiver's help and involvement, but it can also refer to other external objects that the infant associates with falling asleep, such as music or media screens. In the progress of their development, most infants acquire sleep-onset associations that allow for self-regulation and independent sleep initiation. These sleep-onset associations may include engaging with objects within their control (e.g., baby blanket, pacifier) or being in the same external conditions (e.g., dark, quiet room) at sleep onset and during the night. Infants who are capable of using these sleep-onset associations (i.e., "self-soothers") tend to experience brief natural arousals rather than prolonged night-wakings and resume sleep without signaling or requiring their parents' help. In contrast, "signalers" are usually unable to reastablish sleep on their own and typically present frequent and/or prolonged awakenings.[9,13,27]

A major question in the field of early childhood insomnia is how could these differences between infants be explained? Why do some infants become "self-soothers" while others become "signalers?" The following sections of this chapter will describe the role of parent and parent-infant relationship factors in the development of early childhood insomnia.

The various sections of this chapter are organized according to the different levels of influence, as suggested in the transactional model (Fig. 11.1).[1,2] First, the "parent-child interactive context" (interactive behaviors and interpersonal system) will be described, followed by "parenting factors" (parental mental health, cognitions, and cry tolerance), ending with the role of the broader "family" context (coparenting, chaos).

Parental Sleep-Related Behaviors and Infant Sleep

PARENTAL BEDTIME AND NIGHTTIME INVOLVEMENT

Based on the transactional model, the link between parental sleep-related behaviors and infant sleep is both direct and bidirectional. Infants for whom it is more difficult to self-soothe are more likely to elicit excessive parental nighttime help. At the same time, when parents actively settle their infant to sleep, infants learn to associate falling asleep with parental assistance and this may hinder the development of nocturnal self-soothing skills that are necessary for consolidated sleep.[1,2,5]

A few early studies examined the links between parental bedtime involvement and infant sleep.[6,28] In a seminal longitudinal study on this topic conducted by Anders, Halpern, and Hua,[6] 21 parents and their infants were assessed with videosomnography, so that both parental behaviors at bedtime and infant sleep were observed. The findings demonstrated significant concurrent associations between parent-infant interactions at bedtime and infant self-soothing behaviors at 3 and 8 months. Infants who were put into the crib awake and fell asleep on their own at bedtime were more likely to resume sleep on their own following awakenings later in the night, whereas infants who were settled to sleep by their parents at the beginning of the night were significantly more likely to receive similar help from their parents following night-wakings. However, no longitudinal links were found between parent-infant bedtime interactions at 3 months and infant sleep and self-soothing behaviors at 8 months, and hence the directionality of the links could not be established.

During the last decades, a vast body of empirical research around the world has consistently demonstrated that parental presence and active involvement in settling the infant to sleep (e.g., by feeding, holding, rocking) are strongly associated with frequent and/or prolonged infant night-wakings and with lower nighttime self-soothing. In contrast, infants who are placed into their cribs awake at the beginning of the night and/or use a sleep aid, show less nighttime wakefulness and are more likely to self-soothe during the night.[3,29-40] However, most of the research on this topic has been correlational, making it difficult to infer about the directionality of effects.

Overall, research on the effectiveness of clinical sleep interventions (see Chapter 14) and developmental-longitudinal studies conducted during the last two decades support the assumption that parental bedtime and nighttime involvement influence the development of infant sleep. For example, in a study of 80 infants, in which parent-infant nighttime interactions and infant sleep were studied through the use of videosomnography at five time points across the first year of life, one of the main factors that significantly predicted infant nighttime self-soothing at 12 months was longer parental response delays to infant awakenings at 3 months (the other two significant factors were time out of crib and percentage of quiet sleep).[29] A recent study similarly found that when parents introduced a short interval before feeding in the first weeks of life, infants had longer nighttime sleep periods at 3 months, based on both video and parent-report measures. However, no significant links were observed with infant sleep at 6 months.[41] In another recent longitudinal study, parental presence at sleep onset and the overall frequency of parent settling activities at 1 month of age predicted worse infant sleep at 6 and 12 months, based on sleep diaries.[42]

Most studies on parenting and infant sleep have focused on whether parents are present or not at bedtime, and on their level of involvement and response latency to infant awakenings. Recent research has examined whether beyond these factors, the **type or quality** of parental intervention might also be an important factor. For example, Voltaire and Teti examined whether the manner in which parents intervene with their infants during the first 3 months of life predicts infant night-wakings (as reported by the parents) across the first 9 months in a group of cosleeping and solitary sleeping infants.[43] Through direct observations these authors differentiated between non-distress-initiated interventions (i.e., interventions initiated by parents in response to a calm infant awakening or during infant sleep) and distress-initiated interventions (e.g., in response to infant crying). The authors found that only non-distress-initiated parent interventions predicted worse infant sleep outcomes, but this was only significant for infants who were sleeping in a separate room. Higher frequencies of distress-initiated interventions, on the other hand, predicted a sharper decrease in infant diary-based night-wakings in both cosleeping and solitary sleeping infants.

The links between parental quality and infant sleep were further studied by Philbrook and Teti who examined the role of maternal emotional availability at bedtime in predicting observed infant sleep at 1, 3, and 6 months of age.[35] Maternal emotional availability refers to the overall quality of emotional attunement with the infant, expressed through aspects such as sensitivity, structuring, and low hostility. The findings demonstrated significant within-subject effects. That is, when mothers were more emotionally available than usual, infants slept more and displayed less distress during the night. Moreover, an interaction between maternal bedtime practices and emotional availability was found in the prediction of infant sleep; infants whose mothers were more emotionally available at bedtime and used fewer arousing activities developed consolidated sleep faster. In addition, higher maternal emotional availability in combination with less close contact at bedtime was associated with more infant sleep across the night.

Altogether, these longitudinal studies suggest that parental difficulty in withholding their response to infant awakenings and low maternal emotional availability may hinder the acquisition of infant self-soothing abilities that promote better sleep consolidation (i.e., parent-driven effect). However, the question of whether infant sleep problems elicit more parental presence and intervention at bedtime and nighttime remains quite open, as this line of influence (i.e., infant-driven effect) has seldom been studied directly. In one study, both mother-driven and infant-driven mediational models were assessed, but only the mother-driven model showed significance.[44] However, this was a cross-sectional study and therefore directionality could not be accurately assessed. In a longitudinal study, neither infant night-wakings nor infant distress (e.g., crying) predicted later parenting practices (e.g., nursing, physical contact), although higher infant distress did predict lower maternal emotional availability at the following time point.[35] Thus, these findings provide partial support for infant-driven effects. As studies on infant-driven effects are extremely limited, additional longitudinal research is needed to examine the bidirectional paths of influence between parental behaviors and infant sleep-wake behaviors.

BREASTFEEDING AND COSLEEPING

Two specific and interrelated parental nighttime practices, which have been investigated in relation to infant sleep development, are breastfeeding and cosleeping.[45] Breastfeeding provides a myriad of benefits for the development of infants, making it a highly recommended practice. Nevertheless, in the context of sleep, breast milk is more easily digested and thus breastfed infants need to be fed more frequently. Around the age of 6 months, when nighttime feeding is usually no longer physiologically necessary to satisfy hunger, breastfed infants who are nursed to sleep at bedtime are more likely to become dependent on nursing to resume sleep during the night.[2,9] In fact, both breastfeeding and cosleeping allow the infant to spend prolonged periods of time in close contact to the mother and may therefore limit the infant's opportunity to practice nighttime self-soothing. Indeed, research demonstrates that both breastfeeding and cosleeping are associated with more night-wakings, shorter sleep duration, and less self-regulated sleep.[2,46-49]

With regards to cosleeping (roomsharing and/or bedsharing), new studies are consistent with previous findings[30,50] of mothers reporting more disturbed infant sleep (more night-wakings, shorter sleep duration) in cosleeping arrangements.[11,47,49,51,52] However, recent longitudinal studies comparing *objectively* measured infant sleep patterns (e.g., via actigraphy) of roomsharing versus solitary sleeping infants found no significant differences between groups.[25,52] Thus, it could be that mothers of roomsharing infants report more night-wakings as they are more aware of infant awakenings because of their physical proximity to the infant, and/or that infants who sleep in a separate room do not wake less than roomsharing infants but are more capable of self-soothing.

Notably, the research on cosleeping and infant sleep problems is mostly correlational and thus it is impossible to attribute causality to the findings. It could be that parents of cosleeping infants are more likely to intervene faster when the infant wakes up, and this may delay the acquisition of self-soothing skills (parent-driven effect). However, it is also possible that parents of infants with sleep problems are more likely to bring their infants to their room/bed as a way to cope with the infant's awakenings (i.e., reactive cosleeping; infant-driven effect).[25] Moreover, decisions regarding sleeping arrangements are heavily influenced by cultural and societal norms, and therefore findings concerning the links between infant sleep quality and cosleeping that are based on Western samples should be considered in the context of Western norms that overall encourage solitary sleeping arrangements.[53]

BEDTIME ROUTINES

Another aspect of parental bedtime behavior that is linked with children's bedtime behaviors and nighttime sleep patterns is parental consistency during bedtime routines. Bedtime routines are defined as the predictable and pleasant/calming activities that occur in the time preceding lights out, such as parent-child interactive activities (e.g., reading, singing) and hygiene-related activities (e.g., bathing).[54] Parental soothing behaviors that are aimed at helping the infant fall asleep, such as rocking or feeding to sleep, are not conceptualized as part of the bedtime routine, and as described above, these are associated with delayed self-soothing capacities and with more problematic sleep. Bedtime routines are thought to exert their positive influence on sleep by providing the infant with a sense of predictability, calmness, and security.[55] These aspects promote down-regulation, facilitating the infant's transition between wakefulness and sleep. Indeed, evidence from both cross-sectional[56-58] and longitudinal studies,[59,60] conducted on infants and preschool children, suggests that a consistent bedtime routine is associated with earlier bedtimes, shorter sleep latency, reduced night-awakenings, less bedtime resistance, longer nighttime sleep duration, and better caregiver-reported sleep quality.[54] For example, a large cohort study including more than 10,000 children (0–5 years old) from 14 different countries found that having a bedtime routine was associated with better sleep outcomes as reported by the parent. Moreover, within both predominantly Asian and predominantly Caucasian cultural regions, there was a dose-dependent relationship with better sleep outcomes associated with more frequent use of having a bedtime routine, underscoring the importance of bedtime routine consistency for both infants and preschoolers across countries and cultures.[61] In a longitudinal study, parents of 468 children completed a questionnaire asking about bedtime and bedtime routines, their child's sleep duration, nighttime waking, sleep latency, and sleep problems at 3, 12, 18, and 24 months of age. The findings demonstrated a few longitudinal associations between more bedtime routine consistency and better sleep outcomes at later assessment points. Specifically, consistency of bedtime routines at 12 months predicted fewer nighttime waking and sleep problems at 18 months, and an earlier bedtime at 18 months predicted consistency of bedtime routines at 24 months. Moreover, bedtime routine consistency was concurrently associated with longer sleep duration and earlier bedtimes.[55]

However, not all studies support an association between bedtime routine consistency and sleep quality in infants. Recently, Adams, Savage, Master, and Buxton examined the associations between bedtime routine consistency and actigraphic sleep in infants aged 6 to 24 weeks.[62] Significant associations between more consistent bedtime routines and longer true sleep time (excluding nighttime wakefulness) were found only at 6 weeks, but not at later ages, and no significant associations were found with sleep percent. These restricted findings, in comparison to other studies on bedtime routines, might be related to the young age of the infants and to the fact that sleep was measured using actigraphy, whereas most research in the field so far has been based on parental reports of both bedtime routines and child sleep.

Attachment and Infant Sleep

The attachment relationship refers to the enduring bond of the infant to the caregiver. A prominent factor in the development of a secure attachment relationship is the ability of the primary caregiver to provide physical proximity and emotional security to the child in threatening or stressful situations.[63,64] Going to sleep represents a separation from the ongoing interactions with the attachment figure and is therefore a potentially stressful situation for the infant.[27] Theoretically, a secure attachment relationship facilitates feelings of emotional safety in the child, which in turn is thought to enhance the infant's capacity to separate from the caregiver when going to sleep leading to better infant sleep regulation. On the other hand, an insecure attachment that is characterized by a high level of anxiety and worry, might manifest in difficulties separating from the caregiver at bedtime and in heightened vigilance, which is contrary to the physiological and psychological state of relaxation required for falling asleep.[27,65-67] In light of these assumptions, the links between attachment and infant sleep-wake regulation have been a topic of theoretical and empirical interest.[67-72] Studies on attachment and infant sleep have theoretically posited that insecure attachment styles, and in particular ambivalent attachment, would lead to more infant sleep problems. Consistent with the transactional model, another possibility is that sleep problems would compromise the attachment relationship, through their effect on parental sensitivity or emotion regulation. However, most research on the links between attachment and sleep has been cross-sectional, preventing the possibility to infer about directionality. Moreover, the empirical findings in this area are rather mixed, with some studies finding significant associations between insecure attachment and sleep problems, and others not.[2,70] For example, in a study of 94 nonrisk 12-month-olds,[66] the prevalence of infants who were defined by their mothers as "night-wakers" was high in the majority of cases and was only marginally different between the secure and insecure attachment groups (based on the Strange Situation Procedure). In a subgroup of 37 infants, actigraphic sleep measures were not related to attachment security, revealing similar levels of sleep efficiency and awakening in secure and insecure groups.[66] In a subsequent study with 57 low-risk 12-month-old infants, sleep was assessed using actigraphy and maternal reports, and the Attachment Q-Set procedure was used to assess the infant's level of attachment security and dependency. Findings showed that only mothers' reports of infant sleep problems (and not actigraphy) were associated with the child's dependency score, but not with the security score. The authors suggested that dependency might be a more relevant factor than security in explaining sleep regulation problems.[71] On the contrary, another study found that mothers of infants with an insecure-ambivalent/resistant attachment style reported more frequent and prolonged infant night-wakings than mothers of infants with an insecure-avoidant attachment style.[73] Morrell and Steele compared attachment (assessed with the Strange Situation Procedure) between 14- and 16-month-old infants with and without reported sleep problems.[74] There was a higher percentage of ambivalent attachment in the sleep problems group (12.5%) as compared to the good sleepers (1.7%). A follow-up assessment indicated that ambivalent attachment was predictive of persistent sleep problems a year later.[74]

More recent studies that examined the longitudinal associations between attachment security and infant sleep have also provided mixed results.[67,69,72,75-77] For example, Simard, Bernier, Bélanger, and Carrier investigated the relations between attachment assessed with the Strange Situation Procedure and infants' sleep quality, using both objective and subjective measures. Insecure-ambivalent attachment, assessed at 18 months, was not associated with actigraphy-assessed sleep, but was associated with longer nocturnal wake duration as reported by mothers at the age of two years.[67] In another study by the same group[75] attachment security at 15 months (assessed with the Attachment Q-set) was prospectively associated with more actigraphic minutes of sleep and with greater sleep efficiency at 2 years. In contrast, in a study assessing family predictors of reported infant sleep problems at the ages of 6, 15, 24, and 36 months, attachment security, measured with the Strange Situation Procedure, was not predictive of infant sleep trajectories.[78] In another longitudinal study, Pennestri et al. examined the relations between maternal report of infant sleep at four different time points (6, 12, 24, and 36 months) and attachment (assessed with Strange Situation Procedure at 36 months).[69] Children with a disorganized attachment style went to bed later and had shorter sleep duration and more night-wakings, compared to both insecure-ambivalent and secure children. However, no significant differences were found between the secure and ambivalent groups for any of the sleep parameters.

As can be noticed, most studies in the field examined whether attachment security predicts infant sleep. A recent longitudinal study examined the opposite direction of prediction by assessing whether infant sleep predicts later infant-father and infant-mother attachment security.[79] Opposite association patterns were found for mothers compared to fathers; longer infant nighttime awakenings at 3 months were predictive of lower infant-mother attachment security at 24 months, but a higher number and longer duration of infant nighttime awakenings at 3 months were unexpectedly associated with higher infant-father attachment security at 24 months.

The authors examined whether the surprising findings regarding fathers could be explained by paternal involvement in nighttime caregiving, but the data did not support this possibility. They recommended that future research would include a more comprehensive measure of paternal nighttime caregiving to further examine its role in the links between infant sleep and infant-father attachment.[79]

In summary, although there is a solid theoretical basis to assume that attachment security and sleep regulation will be strongly associated, the empirical findings in this area are overall inconclusive. The mixed findings based on the Strange Situation Procedure might be related to the small variance this procedure tends to yield in low-risk samples. However, inconclusive findings arose also from the few studies using the continuous, and thus more variable, scales of the Q-sort procedure. Additional research is needed that would examine the bidirectional links between sleep and attachment in more diverse samples. Moreover, as previous research has demonstrated significant links between maternal parenting quality (e.g., sensitivity, emotional availability) and infant attachment security, it would be interesting to explore how both domains interact to predict infant sleep development.

Parenting Factors and Infant Sleep

PARENTAL PSYCHOPATHOLOGY

Parental psychopathology plays a major role in the way parents perceive their children and interact with them. Research on maternal depression and child development has clearly demonstrated that depressed mothers are more likely to show poorer parenting practices and compromised mother-infant interactions, which may be responsible for long-term negative outcomes for the child.[80,81] According to the transactional model, parents who suffer from mental health problems may engage in less adaptive bedtime and nighttime behaviors, which may lead to the development of sleep disturbances.[1,2] On the other hand, persistent infant night-wakings that require intensive parental intervention may elicit parental stress and chronic sleep disturbances, that over time may lead to more parental emotional distress.[2,44,82]

Empirical research on the links between infant sleep and parental psychopathology has so far focused mainly on the role of maternal prenatal or postnatal depression/depressive symptoms. A few studies have demonstrated that newborns and young infants born to mothers with clinical prenatal depression were more likely to show less efficient and more fragmented sleep as assessed with actigraphy and with polysomnography, compared to infants born to nondepressed mothers.[83,84] Moreover, newborns of depressed mothers who were observed during sleep spent less time in deep sleep and more time in indeterminate (disorganized) sleep.[85] It has been suggested that because these changes in sleep-wake organization are observed so early in life, they might be influenced by biological factors. Specifically, genetic factors or fetal exposure to maternal hormonal abnormalities and changes in the maternal hypothalamic pituitary adrenal axis may put the infant at risk of developing regulatory problems, including sleep problems.[83,86] However, not all studies on sleep in infants of depressed pregnant women demonstrate significant changes. For instance, Galbally et al.[87] compared sleep of 6- and 12-month-old infants who were born to depressed and control women and found no significant differences in reported sleep problems between the groups.

Interestingly, there are only a few studies that have investigated the links between maternal postpartum clinical depression and infant sleep problems. This is surprising considering the high prevalence of postpartum depression, which is estimated to stand at 10% to 15%.[82,88] In one study that examined the relations between maternal depression in the postpartum and maternal reports of infant sleep problems, the rate of clinically significant depression scores (based on the clinical cutoff of the Center for Epidemiological Studies Depression Scale—CES-D) was about double in mothers of night-waking infants than in mothers whose infants did not usually wake up during the night at 6 months postpartum.[89] Furthermore, in a study of women with a history of clinical depression, disturbed infant sleep at 6 weeks, as reported by the mother, was associated with a higher depression score both concurrently at 6 weeks postpartum and longitudinally at 16 weeks postpartum.[90] A recent large longitudinal study, based on data from 2222 mothers and infants, examined the predictive links between maternal depression in the perinatal period (pregnancy and 3 months postpartum) and infant actigraphic and reported sleep at 12 months. Mothers who scored ≥13 points on the Edinburgh Postnatal Depression Scale (EPDS) during pregnancy and/or at 3 months postpartum were considered perinatally depressed. Whereas depressed mothers were more likely to consider their infant's sleep as problematic and to report >3 night-wakings per night than nondepressed mothers, no significant differences were found for the actigraphic sleep measures. Moreover, there were no differences in soothing techniques employed by depressed versus nondepressed mothers.[91]

The associations between maternal prenatal and postnatal *depressive symptoms* (distinct from clinical depression) and infant sleep have been studied quite extensively, and most show small to medium correlations.[44,89,92-103] Most of these studies are based on maternal reports of infant sleep. The few studies that assessed the links between maternal depressive symptoms and objective measures of infant sleep found only limited support for significant findings. In a study assessing infant sleep-wake patterns with videosomnography, mothers with higher depressive symptoms at 1-month postpartum were more likely to have infants who fell asleep independently at 12 months.[29] The authors suggested that these mothers might have waited longer before responding to their infants' awakenings, which may have led to the development of self-soothing skills. Another study found that greater postpartum maternal depressive symptoms were associated with more inconsistent total sleep duration, as assessed by actigraphy. However, sleep quality measures, such as infant awakenings, were not included in this study.[104]

Most research on parental depression and infant sleep has focused on mothers, but a few studies have also found significant concurrent associations between paternal depressive symptoms and infant sleep.[105-107] For instance, in one study, fathers of infants who perceived their infant's sleep as problematic at 4 months of age had increased depressive symptoms concurrently and also at 6 months of age.[105] Another study found significant associations between paternal emotional distress symptoms and 8- to 12-month-old infants' bedtime difficulties, as perceived by mothers.[107]

Clearly, most research on parental psychopathology and infant sleep has focused on maternal depression or depressive symptoms. Recent studies have contributed to this growing field by examining other aspects of parental emotional distress, such as maternal anxiety and stress.[96,108-113] Probably, the only study so far which examined mothers with a clinical prenatal and postpartum anxiety disorder did not find support for a significant association with infant sleep.[111] Similarly to studies on maternal depressive symptoms, studies on nonclinical samples found that prenatal anxiety symptoms[114] and postnatal anxiety, stress, and PTSD symptoms were moderately associated with more maternal reports of infant sleep problems.[90,92,96,109] Some of these studies found significant associations with fathers' stress symptoms as well.[23,115,116] A recent longitudinal study of 225 mothers and their infants examined the links between maternal depressive, anxiety, and stress symptoms and infant actigraphic and reported sleep. The findings demonstrated that mothers with higher emotional distress symptoms—and especially those with parenting-stress symptoms—were more likely to experience their infant's sleep as problematic. However, no significant correlations were found between maternal emotional distress symptoms and objective-actigraphic sleep measures. Moreover, trajectory analyses indicated no significant effects of changes in maternal emotional distress variables on changes in infant subjective or objective sleep.[117] These findings support growing evidence suggesting that mothers who suffer from emotional distress symptoms are more likely to experience the sleep of their infants as problematic, though there is little evidence to suggest that maternal emotional distress leads to the development of objective sleep difficulties.

Although the transactional model postulates that the links between maternal emotional distress and infant sleep problems are mediated through maternal bedtime and nighttime behaviors, underlying mechanisms of the links between maternal depression and infant sleep have hardly been investigated. Teti and Crosby examined such a mediation model in 45 infants (1–24 months old).[44] Mothers' depressive symptoms were associated with more maternal presence and close physical contact with infants during the night, though no significant associations were found between depressive symptoms and bedtime practices. Furthermore, the mediation analyses provided support for a mother-driven model in which maternal presence with infants during the night mediated the links between maternal depressive symptoms and infant night-waking. However, the authors emphasized that no causal relations from these results could be inferred, given the cross-sectional design of the study. One longitudinal study of 5568 mothers looked at infant temperament as a possible mediator and found that maternal antenatal depression, measured with the EPDS, predicted infant negative affectivity at 9 months which in turn predicted more reported infant night-wakings at 2 years of age.[118]

Overall, only a few studies examined whether infant sleep disturbances predict maternal emotional distress (i.e., infant-driven effects). In the study of Teti and Crosby described above, no statistical support was obtained for the infant-driven model, in which infant night waking predicted maternal depressive symptoms via maternal nighttime presence.[44] However, since the mediated paths in the infant-driven models approached significance, the authors concluded that it is possible that both mother- and infant-driven influences are relevant in explaining the links between maternal depressive symptoms and infant sleep.

Maternal sleep disturbances have been suggested to underlie the predictive links between infant sleep problems and maternal emotional distress.[82,95] Consistent with this asumption, links between poorer maternal sleep and increased severity of depressive symptoms have been reported,[119-121] and infant sleep has been shown to be strongly associated with maternal sleep.[61,122] However, to the best of our knowledge, there are no longitudinal studies that examined the role of maternal sleep as a mediator of the link between infant sleep and maternal emotional distress. Nevertheless, indirect support for this notion comes from infant sleep intervention studies which documented, in addition to improvements in infant sleep, alleviation in maternal sleep and mood.[123-125]

A few studies have tried to identify moderators of the links between maternal emotional distress and infant sleep.[77,92,98,126] These studies may shed light on the mixed findings regarding the direct links between these domains. For instance, in a study with two large longitudinal cohorts, infant reactivity and gender were examined as moderators of the association between maternal symptoms of antenatal depression and infant sleep. The findings demonstrated that reactive boys had a higher number of reported awakenings and shorter sleep duration when previously exposed to maternal symptoms of antenatal depression in comparison to girls and to infants with lower reactivity.[98] Another study examined family structure as a possible moderator of the link between maternal depressive and anxiety symptoms and infant sleep, by comparing the strengths of these links between two-parent families and solo-mother families (i.e., mothers who decided to parent alone). The findings demonstrated that only in solo-mother families higher maternal emotional distress was associated with more infant diary-based night-wakings.[126] The authors suggested that paternal involvement in two-parent families may mitigate the association between maternal poor sleep quality and emotional distress, explaining the stronger links found in solo-mother families.

To summarize, research based on clinical samples has demonstrated that mothers' prenatal clinical depression is a risk factor for the development of infant sleep problems in the beginning of the infant's life. Moreover, findings consistently show that mothers with elevated depressive symptoms are more likely to perceive their infants' sleep as problematic. However, the few studies that are based on objective sleep measures are scarce and do not support the notion that maternal emotional distress contributes to the development of poor objective infant sleep quality. Future studies are needed to further examine these links within longitudinal designs using objective and subjective measures of sleep. These studies might shed light on the directionality of the effects and may clarify whether these links are restricted to the subjective experience of the mother. Also, studies examining various mediators and moderators of these links are needed to elucidate possible underlying mechanisms.

PARENTAL COGNITIONS, CRY REACTIVITY, AND INFANT SLEEP

According to the transactional model, parental cognitions regarding infant sleep may impact their sleep-related behaviors and levels of nighttime involvement, which as described above, directly influence infant sleep. Parental cognitions refer to perceptions, attitudes, attributions, expectations, interpretations, and beliefs parents have regarding their children. Parental cognitions regarding child behavior have been significantly associated with the way parents respond to their children and have been associated with child development and parent-child interactions.[127] Increasing evidence suggests that parental cognitions are an important factor to consider in the development of infant sleep problems.[38,74,105,128-130] For instance, in one of the first studies on this topic, mothers of infants with sleep problems reported more cognitions related to difficulty with limit-setting, increased doubts about parenting competence, and increased anger at the infant's demands.[131] A follow-up study demonstrated that the most relevant factors for concurrent sleeping problems were maternal cognitions reflecting concerns about setting limits and fussy-difficult temperament.[74] Moreover, these variables explained the degree to which parents used active physical soothing to settle their infants to sleep, which in turn predicted the persistence of sleeping problems. In a study assessing the links between infant sleep and parental sleep-related cognitions in clinical and control samples, parents of sleep-disturbed infants reported more concerns and difficulties with limiting their nighttime involvement than did control parents. Furthermore, significant differences in sleep-related cognitions were found between fathers and mothers. Given hypothetical examples of infants with sleep problems, fathers were more likely than mothers to endorse an approach that encourages infant self-soothing ("limit-setting"). Moreover, the findings revealed that fathers' cognitions reflecting difficulties in limit setting were linked to more infant night-wakings, in addition and independently of maternal cognitions, implying that the likelihood of infant sleep problems increases when both parents have trouble in limiting their involvement.[130] In a longitudinal study (from pregnancy through the first year) aimed at assessing the prospective links between maternal sleep-related cognitions and infant sleep, significant predictive and concomitant links were demonstrated.[38] Specifically, maternal cognitions which emphasized the possibility that infants experience distress upon awakening and that parents should therefore help them, predicted and were associated with more disturbed infant sleep at 6 and 12 months of age. On the other hand, maternal cognitions emphasizing the importance of limiting parental nighttime involvement predicted and were associated with more consolidated sleep. In addition, parental soothing techniques mediated the links between maternal cognitions and infant sleep. Mothers who tended to interpret infant night-wakings at 6 months as a sign of distress that requires immediate attention were more actively involved in bedtime soothing at 12 months, and this, in turn, was related to more infant night-wakings. Consistent with transactional perspectives on this topic,[2] infant sleep also predicted a change in maternal cognitions, although this link seemed to be weaker than the direction of prediction from maternal cognitions to infant sleep.[38] Similarly, Teti and Crosby[44] also found support for a mediation model showing that mothers' nighttime presence with the infant mediated the relations between maternal worries about infant nighttime needs, and infant night waking. Relatedly, maternal separation anxiety (i.e., feelings of guilt, worry, and sadness that accompany short-term separations from the child) has been studied in relation to infant sleep. Higher levels of separation anxiety were found to be associated with greater maternal physical proximity at bedtime, more involvement during the night, and more actigraphic nighttime awakenings.[132,133]

Another related parenting factor that seems to be associated with parental cognitions and infant sleep and has been the focus of recent research is parental cry tolerance (PCT). In the first study on this topic, Sadeh and colleagues found that parents of infants with night-waking problems were less tolerant to infant crying compared to parents of infants without sleep problems and to childless controls.[134] PCT in this study was measured using parental responses to audio and video recording of infant crying. In the video procedure, participants were presented with a 2-minute video clip of a crying infant, with gradually increasing crying intensity. Prior to watching the video, a written cover story was presented to the participants with a rationale that delayed response is recommended because the infant they observed is very demanding and his parents are trying to encourage him to self-soothe. The delay to intervene was used as a measure of PCT. The findings of this study, showing lower cry tolerance in parents of sleep-disturbed infants, may suggest that PCT may be an important factor in the development of infant sleep. It could be that parents with lower PCT show faster responses and more active involvement in soothing their infants to sleep, which may lead to less consolidated infant sleep. However, consistent with the transactional model, it could also be that parents develop lower cry tolerance in reaction to their infant's sleep problems. To further clarify the direction of these links, a longitudinal study was conducted in which PCT was measured at pregnancy and 6 months, and infant sleep was assessed at 3 and 6 months.[135] Concurrent associations were found between lower maternal cry-tolerance and poorer actigraphic infant sleep at 6 months, as well as between lower PCT and more active nighttime soothing. Furthermore, lower cry-tolerance at pregnancy predicted better infant sleep at 3 months, whereas more disrupted sleep at 3 months predicted lower cry-tolerance at 6 months. The authors suggested that this shift in directionality may be explained by the evolving needs of the infant throughout the first months of life; lower PCT during late pregnancy may represent a parenting attitude more attuned to the infant needs and regulatory capacities. Later, parents may become more sensitive to infant crying when they need to continuously take care of a night-waking infant, as manifested in the reduction in cry tolerance at 6 months. In line with these notions, decreases in both PCT and cognitions attributing distress to nighttime awakening have been demonstrated following behavioral interventions for infant sleep problems.[136] These decreases were associated with parent-reported and actigraphic improvements in infant sleep following treatment, providing further evidence for the mutual evolution of these constructs.

Taken together, the findings of these studies highlight the role of parental sleep-related cognitions and cry-tolerance in infant sleep development and, consistent with the transactional model, demonstrate that these links are mediated through parental bedtime practices.

Family Factors and Infant Sleep: The Role of Fathers, Couple Relationship, and Family Chaos

At the distal level of influences on child sleep, the transactional model stipulates that family stressors, such as low-quality marital relationships, will influence infant sleep through their impact on parental sleep-related behaviors.[1,2] In practice, most studies on parenting and infant sleep problems have focused primarily on mothers, paying little attention to the role of other family variables such as the couple's relationship and coparenting.

A few studies have demonstrated the importance of the couple relationship as a factor that may contribute to infant sleep development.[24,52,137] For example, lower coparenting quality and lower marital adjustment as perceived by the mother have been found to predict continuing infant cosleeping arrangements through the first year of life.[52,138] Moreover, Bernier and colleagues reported that greater paternal marital satisfaction as well as mothers' perceived social support were predictive of better maternal reports of child sleep consolidation at 2 years.[108] These relations were stronger in families from lower SES backgrounds. Evidence for infant-driven effects on coparenting has also been found. Reported infant night-wakings predicted coparenting quality, with parent sleep quality mediating these links.[139] Another line of research has demonstrated better infant sleep quality and less bedtime resistance in families where both parents shared caregiving.[24,107] For example, in two studies, a relatively higher involvement of fathers in overall infant caregiving (as reported by mothers and fathers) when infants were 1 and 3 months old was predictive of more consolidated infant sleep, as assessed with actigraphy, at 6 months of age.[24,140] Whereas father involvement and the marital relationship seem to play a role in infant sleep development in two-parent families, a recent study suggests that the absence of a father does not seem to play a role when the mother has decided in advance to bring a child to the world on her own; in a study comparing infant sleep in families of solo-mothers (single women who have decided to parent alone) compared to two-parent families, there were no significant differences between the groups in mother or infant sleep quality, though solo-mothers were more likely to cosleep with their infants.[126]

Another family variable that seems to be associated with infant sleep problems is family chaos, although its impact has mainly been studied in families with preschool and older children.[141] One longitudinal study of 167 families, with 5 assessment points during the first year, examined the role of family chaos in infant sleep. Infants in homes characterized by higher chaos demonstrated delays in actigraphic sleep consolidation, manifested in greater sleep fragmentation and more variable sleep duration. However, chaos was also associated with longer sleep duration, maybe as a way to compensate for fragmented sleep.[142]

Overall, these studies suggest that exposure to family chaos, parent conflict, and low paternal involvement in two-parent families acts as a risk factor for the development of infant sleep problems. These couple and family variables may exert their influence through undermining the infant's sense of security.[143] It is also possible that they lead to less adaptive parental bedtime and nighttime behaviors which in turn negatively impact infant sleep.[1,2]

Conclusions and Research Limitations

The research reviewed in this chapter fits well into the conceptual framework of the transactional model describing bidirectional and dynamic links between various parenting and parent-infant relational factors and the development of early childhood insomnia. Recent findings, especially those that are based on longitudinal designs, have highlighted the important role of parenting factors, such as parental behaviors, emotional availability, cognitions, cry tolerance, mental health, and coparenting in the development of infant sleep.

Nevertheless, some significant research gaps still exist. Although the number of longitudinal studies has increased considerably during the last decade, most research is still based on cross-sectional designs, and thus it is difficult to ascribe causality or even directionality to the links. Moreover, most longitudinal studies have explored the role of parental factors in infant sleep development, but research regarding the influence of infant sleep problems on parental behavior and mental health has surprisingly been very limited. Thus, the relative influence of parent-driven effects versus infant-driven effects should be further explored. In addition, most studies are based on parental reports of infant sleep, and the restricted research that included objective methods, such as actigraphy and videosomnography, often shows less robust findings. It is unclear if this discrepancy is a result of inflated correlations due to shared method variance in studies using parent reports alone. More research that is based on objective methods is needed to clarify this question. Furthermore, although the transactional model assumes complex relations between the different levels of parental influences, most studies to date have examined the effect of parenting variables on infant sleep separately, and there has been very little research on the interaction between these variables, or between parenting factors and infant intrinsic variables (i.e., moderation analysis).

Likewise, only a few studies have so far examined the mediating role of parent-infant bedtime and nighttime interactive factors (e.g., bedtime soothing), in the links between distal parenting factors (e.g., mental health, coparenting) and infant sleep problems, within the context of longitudinal research. Lastly, although accumulating evidence has started to underscore the role of fathers and the broader family context (e.g., family chaos), this area of research is still in its infancy. In sum, future research should examine more complex models taking into account the bidirectional prospective links between parenting and different facets of infant sleep and the possible mediators (e.g., parent-infant relationship/interaction) and moderators (e.g., interaction between parental depression and infant temperament) relating to the different distal and proximal levels of the transactional model.

Clinical Implications

Early childhood insomnia is a major concern in infancy and a source for parental concern and distress that can significantly impact the well-being of the family. The findings reviewed in this chapter linking various parenting and parent-infant relationship factors to infant sleep problems imply that all these variables should be comprehensively evaluated during clinical assessment of early childhood insomnia, in addition to the assessment of potential medical and physiological sources for the sleep problem. Naturally, the role of these variables will vary from one family to the other. Whereas in some families, parental sleep-related cognitions may play a significant role in influencing parent-infant interactions around bedtime, in other families it might be low coparenting or mental health problems that may be more relevant in explaining the dynamics around sleep, and yet in other families the sleep problems might be more directly and specifically related to bedtime practices such as extensive feeding or inconsistent bedtime routines. Hence, it is important that health care professionals who conduct clinical assessments of infant sleep problems will be aware of the various factors that may contribute to the maintenance of the sleep problem and assess their possible influence in every single family. Accordingly, infant sleep interventions could be adjusted and tailored to the specific and unique characteristics of the infant and the family. The different parenting factors that were described in this chapter are all modifiable. Targeting the specific factors that contribute to the sleep problem in an individualized manner may increase the likelihood of successful intervention.

References

1. Sadeh A, Anders TF. Infant sleep problems: origins, assessment, interventions. *Infant Ment Health J.* 1993;14(1):17-34.
2. Sadeh A, Tikotzky L, Scher A. Parenting and infant sleep. *Sleep Med Rev.* 2010;14(2):89-96. Available at: https://doi.org/10.1016/j.smrv.2009.05.003.
3. Camerota M, Propper CB, Teti DM. Intrinsic and extrinsic factors predicting infant sleep: Moving beyond main effects. *Dev Rev.* 2019;53:100871. Available at: https://doi.org/10.1016/j.dr.2019.100871.
4. El-Sheikh M, Sadeh A. I. Sleep and development: introduction to the monograph. *Monogr Soc Res Child Dev.* 2015;80(1):1-14. Available at: https://doi.org/10.1111/mono.12141.
5. Tikotzky L. Parenting and sleep in early childhood. *Curr Opin Psychol.* 2017;15:118-124. Available at: https://doi.org/10.1016/j.copsyc.2017.02.016.
6. Anders TF, Halpern LF, Hua J. Sleeping through the night: a developmental perspective. *Pediatrics.* 1992;90(4):554-560. Available at: https://doi.org/10.1542/peds.90.4.554.
7. Anders TF, Keener M. Developmental course of nighttime sleep-wake patterns in full-term and premature infants during the first year of life. *Sleep.* 1985;8(3):173-192. Available at: https://doi.org/10.1093/sleep/8.3.173.
8. Henderson JM, France KG, Blampied NM. The consolidation of infants' nocturnal sleep across the first year of life. *Sleep Med Rev.* 2011;15(4):211-220. Available at: https://doi.org/10.1016/j.smrv.2010.08.003.

9. Mindell JA, Owens AO. *A Clinical Guide to Pediatric Sleep: Diagnosis and Management of Sleep Problems.* 3rd ed. Wolters Kluwer; 2015.
10. Galland BC, Taylor BJ, Elder DE, Herbison P. Normal sleep patterns in infants and children: a systematic review of observational studies. *Sleep Med Rev.* 2012;16(3):213-222. Available at: https://doi.org/10.1016/j.smrv.2011.06.001.
11. Bruni O, Baumgartner E, Sette S, et al. Longitudinal study of sleep behavior in normal infants during the first year of life. *J Clin Sleep Med.* 2014;10(10):1119-1127. Available at: https://doi.org/10.5664/jcsm.4114.
12. Hysing M, Harvey AG, Torgersen L, Ystrom E, Reichborn-Kjennerud T, Sivertsen B. Trajectories and predictors of nocturnal awakenings and sleep duration in infants. *J Dev Behav Pediatr.* 2014;35(5):309-316. Available at: https://doi.org/10.1097/DBP.0000000000000064.
13. Tikotzky L, Sadeh A. The role of cognitive-behavioral therapy in behavioral childhood insomnia. *Sleep Med.* 2010;11(7):686-691. Available at: https://doi.org/10.1016/j.sleep.2009.11.017.
14. Wake M, Morton-Allen E, Poulakis Z, Hiscock H, Gallagher S, Oberklaid F. Prevalence, stability, and outcomes of cry-fuss and sleep problems in the first 2 years of life: Prospective community-based study. *Pediatrics.* 2006;117(3):836-842.
15. Meltzer LJ, Mindell JA. Systematic review and meta-analysis of behavioral interventions for pediatric insomnia. *J Pediatr Psychol.* 2014;39(8):932-948. Available at: https://doi.org/10.1093/jpepsy/jsu041.
16. Sadeh A, Sivan Y. Clinical practice: sleep problems during infancy. *Eur J Pediatr.* 2009;168(10):1159-1164. Available at: https://doi.org/10.1007/s00431-009-0982-4.
17. Byars KC, Yolton K, Rausch J, Lanphear B, Beebe DW. Prevalence, patterns, and persistence of sleep problems in the first 3 years of life. *Pediatrics.* 2012;129(2):E276-E284. Available at: https://doi.org/10.1542/peds.2011-0372.
18. Owens JA, Mindell JA. Pediatric insomnia. *Pediatr Clin North Am.* 2011;58(3):555-569. Available at: https://doi.org/10.1016/j.pcl.2011.03.011.
19. Bayer JK, Hiscock H, Hampton A, Wake M. Sleep problems in young infants and maternal mental and physical health. *J Paediatr Child Health.* 2007;43(1-2):66-73. Available at: http://www.ncbi.nlm.nih.gov/entrez/query.fcgi?cmd=Retrieve&db=PubMed&dopt=Citation&list_uids=17207059.
20. Gregory AM, Sadeh A. Sleep, emotional and behavioral difficulties in children and adolescents. *Sleep Med Rev.* 2012;16(2):129-136. Available at: https://doi.org/10.1016/j.smrv.2011.03.007.
21. Insana SP, Williams KB, Montgomery-Downs HE. Sleep disturbance and neurobehavioral performance among postpartum women. *Sleep.* 2013;36(1):73-81. Available at: https://doi.org/10.5665/Sleep.2304.
22. Sadeh A, Tikotzky L, Kahn M. Sleep in infancy and childhood: implications for emotional and behavioral difficulties in adolescence and beyond. *Curr Opin Psychiatry.* 2014;27(6):453-459. Available at: https://doi.org/10.1097/Yco.0000000000000109.
23. Sinai D, Tikotzky L. Infant sleep, parental sleep and parenting stress in families of mothers on maternity leave and in families of working mothers. *Infant Behav Dev.* 2012;35(2):179-186. Available at: https://doi.org/10.1016/j.infbeh.2012.01.006.
24. Tikotzky L, Sadeh A, Volkovich E, Manber R, Meiri G, Shahar G. Infant sleep development from 3 to 6 months postpartum: links with maternal sleep and paternal Involvement. *Monogr Soc Res Child Dev.* 2015;80(1):107-124. Available at: https://doi.org/10.1111/mono.12147.
25. Volkovich E, Bar-Kalifa E, Meiri G, Tikotzky L. Mother-infant sleep patterns and parental functioning of room-sharing and solitary-sleeping families: a longitudinal study from 3 to 18 months. *Sleep.* 2018;41(2):zsx207. Available at: https://doi.org/10.1093/sleep/zsx207.
26. Williamson AA, Mindell JA, Hiscock H, Quach J. Longitudinal sleep problem trajectories are associated with multiple impairments in child well-being. *J Child Psychol Psychiatry.* 2020. Available at: https://doi.org/10.1111/jcpp.13303.
27. Anders TF. Infant sleep, nighttime relationships, and attachment. *Psychiatry.* 1994;57(1):11-21. Available at: https://doi.org/10.1080/00332747.1994.11024664.
28. Adair R, Bauchner H, Philipp B, Levenson S, Zuckerman B. Night waking during infancy: role of parental presence at bedtime. *Pediatrics.* 1991;87(4):500-504. Available at: https://doi.org/10.1542/peds.87.4.500.
29. Burnham MM, Goodlin-Jones BL, Gaylor EE, Anders TF. Nighttime sleep-wake patterns and self-soothing from birth to one year of age: a longitudinal intervention study. *J Child Psychol Psychiatry.* 2002;43(6):713-725.

30. DeLeon CW, Karraker KH. Intrinsic and extrinsic factors associated with night waking in 9-month-old infants [Article]. *Infant Behav Dev.* 2007;30(4):596-605. Available at: https://doi.org/10.1016/j.infbeh.2007.03.009.

31. Goodlin-Jones BL, Burnham MM, Gaylor EE, Anders TF. Night waking, sleep-wake organization, and self-soothing in the first year of life. *J Dev Behav Pediatr.* 2001;22(4):226-233.

32. Messayke S, Franco P, Forhan A, Dufourg MN, Charles MA, Plancoulaine S. Sleep habits and sleep characteristics at age one year in the ELFE birth cohort study. *Sleep Med.* 2020;67:200-206. Available at: https://doi.org/10.1016/j.sleep.2019.11.1255.

33. Mindell JA, Sadeh A, Kohyama J, How TH. Parental behaviors and sleep outcomes in infants and toddlers: a cross-cultural comparison. *Sleep Med.* 2010;11(4):393-399. Available at: https://doi.org/10.1016/j.sleep.2009.11.011.

34. Morrell J, Cortina-Borja M. The developmental change in strategies parents employ to settle young children to sleep, and their relationship to infant sleeping problems, as assessed by a new questionnaire: The Parental Interactive Bedtime Behaviour Scale. *Infant Child Dev.* 2002;11(1):17-41.

35. Philbrook LE, Teti DM. Bidirectional associations between bedtime parenting and infant sleep: parenting quality, parenting practices, and their interaction. *J Fam Psychol.* 2016;30(4):431-441. Available at: https://doi.org/10.1037/fam0000198.

36. Sadeh A, Mindell JA, Luedtke K, Wiegand B. Sleep and sleep ecology in the first 3 years: a web-based study. *J Sleep Res.* 2009;18(1):60-73. Available at: https://doi.org/10.1111/j.1365-2869.2008.00699.x.

37. Schlarb AA, Seiler D, Werner A, Kater MJ. Modern strategies for settling infants to sleep A comparison between sleep-disturbed and non-sleep-disturbed infants. *Somnologie.* 2020;24(4):237-244. Availabe at: https://doi.org/10.1007/s11818-020-00279-0.

38. Tikotzky L, Sadeh A. Maternal sleep-related cognitions and infant sleep: a longitudinal study from pregnancy through the first year. *Child Dev.* 2009;80(3):860-874.

39. Yu XT, Sadeh A, Lam HS, Mindell JA, Li AM. Parental behaviors and sleep/wake patterns of infants and toddlers in Hong Kong, China. *World J Pediatr.* 2017;13(5):496-502. Available at: https://doi.org/10.1007/s12519-017-0025-6.

40. Zreik G, Asraf K, Tikotzky L, Haimov I. Sleep ecology and sleep patterns among infants and toddlers: a cross-cultural comparison between the Arab and Jewish societies in Israel. *Sleep Med.* 2020;75:117-127. Available at: https://doi.org/10.1016/j.sleep.2020.07.017.

41. St James-Roberts I, Roberts M, Hovish K, Owen C. Video evidence that parenting methods predict which infants develop long night-time sleep periods by three months of age. *Prim Health Care Res Dev.* 2017;18(3):212-226. Available at: https://doi.org/10.1017/S1463423616000451.

42. Henderson JMT, Blampied NM, France KG. Longitudinal study of infant sleep development: early predictors of sleep regulation across the first year. *Nat Sci Sleep.* 2020;12:949-957. Available at: https://doi.org/10.2147/NSS.S240075.

43. Voltaire ST, Teti DM. Early nighttime parental interventions and infant sleep regulation across the first year. *Sleep Med.* 2018;52:107-115. Available at: https://doi.org/10.1016/j.sleep.2018.07.013.

44. Teti DM, Crosby B. Maternal depressive symptoms, dysfunctional cognitions, and infant night waking: the role of maternal nighttime behavior. *Child Dev.* 2012;83(3):939-953. Available at: https://doi.org/10.1111/j.1467-8624.2012.01760.x.

45. Ball HL. Breastfeeding, bed-sharing, and infant sleep. *Birth.* 2003;30(3):181-188. Available at: http://www.ncbi.nlm.nih.gov/pubmed/12911801.

46. Galbally M, Lewis AJ, McEgan K, Scalzo K, Islam FA. Breastfeeding and infant sleep patterns: an Australian population study. *J Paediatr Child Health.* 2013;49(2):E147-E152. Available at: https://doi.org/10.1111/jpc.12089.

47. Huang XN, Wang HS, Chang JJ, et al. Feeding methods, sleep arrangement, and infant sleep patterns: a Chinese population-based study. *World J Pediatr.* 2016;12(1):66-75. Available at: https://doi.org/10.1007/s12519-015-0012-8.

48. Tikotzky L, De Marcas G, Har-Toov J, Dollberg S, Bar-Haim Y, Sadeh A. Sleep and physical growth in infants during the first six months. *J Sleep Res.* 2010;19:103-110.

49. Volkovich E, Ben-Zion H, Karny D, Meiri G, Tikotzky L. Sleep patterns of co-sleeping and solitary sleeping infants and mothers: a longitudinal study. *Sleep Med.* 2015;16(11):1305-1312. Available at: https://doi.org/10.1016/j.sleep.2015.08.016.

50. Baddock SA, Galland BC, Bolton DPG, Williams SM, Taylor BJ. Differences in infant and parent behaviors during routine bed sharing compared with cot sleeping in the home setting. *Pediatrics.* 2006;117(5):1599-1607.
51. Paul IM, Loken EE, Hohman EE, et al. Mother-infant room-sharing and sleep outcomes in the INSIGHT Study. *Pediatircs.* 2017;140(1):e20170122.
52. Teti DM, Shimizu M, Crosby B, Kim BR. Sleep arrangements, parent-infant sleep during the first year, and family functioning. *Dev Psychol.* 2016;52(8):1169-1181. Available at: https://doi.org/10.1037/dev0000148.
53. Mileva-Seitz VR, Bakermans-Kranenburg MJ, Battaini C, Luijk MP. Parent-child bed-sharing: the good, the bad, and the burden of evidence. *Sleep Med Rev.* 2017;32:4-27. Available at: https://doi.org/10.1016/j.smrv.2016.03.003.
54. Mindell JA, Williamson AA. Benefits of a bedtime routine in young children: sleep, development, and beyond. *Sleep Med Rev.* 2018;40:93-108. Available at: https://doi.org/10.1016/j.smrv.2017.10.007.
55. Fiese BH, Cai TY, Sutter C, Bost KK. Bedtimes, bedtime routines, and children's sleep across the first 2 years of life. *Sleep.* 2021;44(8):zsab045. Available at: https://doi.org/10.1093/sleep/zsab045.
56. Jones CH, Ball H. Exploring socioeconomic differences in bedtime behaviours and sleep duration in English preschool children. *Infant Child Dev.* 2014;23(5):518-531. Available at: https://doi.org/10.1002/icd.1848.
57. Mindell JA, Li AM, Sadeh A, Kwon R, Goh DY. Bedtime routines for young children: a dose-dependent association with sleep outcomes. *Sleep.* 2015;38(5):717-722. Available at: https://doi.org/10.5665/sleep.4662.
58. Wilson KE, Lumeng JC, Kaciroti N, et al. Sleep hygiene practices and bedtime resistance in low-income preschoolers: does temperament matter? *Behav Sleep Med.* 2015;13(5):412-423. Available at: https://doi.org/10.1080/15402002.2014.940104.
59. Koulouglioti C, Cole R, Moskow M, McQuillan B, Carno MA, Grape A. The longitudinal association of young children's everyday routines to sleep duration. *J Pediatr Health Care.* 2014;28(1):80-87. Available at: https://doi.org/10.1016/j.pedhc.2012.12.006.
60. Staples AD, Bates JE, Petersen IT. Bedtime routines in early childhood: prevalence, consistency, and associations with nighttime sleep. *Monogr Soc Res Child Dev.* 2015;80(1):141-159. Available at: https://doi.org/10.1111/mono.12149.
61. Mindell JA, Sadeh A, Kwon R, Goh DY. Relationship between child and maternal sleep: a developmental and cross-cultural comparison. *J Pediatr Psychol.* 2015;40(7):689-696. Available at: https://doi.org/10.1093/jpepsy/jsv008.
62. Adams EL, Savage JS, Master L, Buxton OM. Time for bed! Earlier sleep onset is associated with longer nighttime sleep duration during infancy. *Sleep Med.* 2020;73:238-245. Available at: https://doi.org/10.1016/j.sleep.2020.07.003.
63. Bowlby J. Attachment and loss. Volume 1. Attachment. London: Hogarth; 1969:24.
64. Bowlby J. Attachment and loss. Volume 2. Separation anxiety and anger. New York: Basic Books; 1973.
65. Dahl RE. The regulation of sleep and arousal: development and psychopathology. *Dev Psychopathol.* 1996;8(1):3-27.
66. Scher A. Attachment and sleep: a study of night waking in 12-month-old infants. *Dev Psychobiol.* 2001;38(4):274-285.
67. Simard V, Bernier A, Belanger ME, Carrier J. Infant attachment and toddlers' sleep assessed by maternal reports and actigraphy: different measurement methods yield different relations. *J Pediatr Psychol.* 2013;38(5):473-483. Available at: https://doi.org/10.1093/jpepsy/jst001.
68. Beijers R, Jansen J, Riksen-Walraven M, de Weerth C. Attachment and infant night waking: a longitudinal study from birth through the first year of life. *J Dev Behav Pediatir.* 2011;32(9):635-643. Available at: https://doi.org/10.1097/DBP.0b013e318228888d.
69. Pennestri MH, Moss E, O'Donnell K, et al. Establishment and consolidation of the sleep-wake cycle as a function of attachment pattern. *Attach Hum Dev.* 2015;17(1):23-42. Available at: https://doi.org/10.1080/14616734.2014.953963.
70. Perpetuo C, Diniz E, Verissimo M. A systematic review on attachment and sleep at preschool age. *Children-Basel.* 2021;8(10):895. Available at: https://doi.org/10.3390/children8100895.
71. Scher A, Asher R. Is attachment security related to sleep-wake regulation? Mothers' reports and objective sleep recordings. *Infant Behav Dev.* 2004;27(3):288-302.

72. Schwichtenberg AJ, Shah PE, Poehlmann J. Sleep and attachment in preterm infants. *Infant Ment Health J*. 2013;34(1):37-46. Available at: https://doi.org/10.1002/imhj.21374.

73. McNamara P, Belsky J, Fearon P. Infant sleep disorders and attachment: sleep problems in infants with insecure-resistant versus insecure-avoidant attachments to mother. *Sleep Hypnosis*. 2003;5(1):7-16.

74. Morrell J, Steele H. The role of attachment security, temperament, maternal perception, and care-giving behavior in persistent infant sleeping problems. *Infant Ment Health J*. 2003;24(5):447-468.

75. Belanger ME, Bernier A, Simard V, Bordeleau S, Carrier J. Viii. Attachment and sleep among toddlers: disentangling attachment security and dependency. *Monogr Soc Res Child Dev*. 2015;80(1):125-140. Available at: https://doi.org/10.1111/mono.12148.

76. Mileva-Seitz VR, Van Ijzendoorn MH, Bakermans-Kranenburg MJ, et al. Association between infant nighttime-sleep location and attachment security: no easy verdict. *Infant Ment Health J*. 2016;37(1): 5-16. Available at: https://doi.org/10.1002/imhj.21547.

77. Newland RP, Parade SH, Dickstein S, Seifer R. Goodness of fit between prenatal maternal sleep and infant sleep: Associations with maternal depression and attachment security. *Infant Behav Dev*. 2016;44:179-188. Available at: https://doi.org/10.1016/j.infbeh.2016.06.010.

78. Weinraub M, Bender RH, Friedman SL. Patterns of developmental change in infants' nighttime sleep awakenings from 6 through 36 months of age. *Dev Psychol*. 2012;48(6):1511-1528. Available at: https://doi.org/10.1037/a0027680.

79. Witte AM, de Moor MHM, Szepsenwol O, et al. Developmental trajectories of infant nighttime awakenings are associated with infant-mother and infant-father attachment security. *Infant Behav Dev*. 2021;65:101653. Available at: https://doi.org/10.1016/j.infbeh.2021.101653.

80. Field T. Postpartum depression effects on early interactions, parenting, and safety practices: a review. *Infant Behav Dev*. 2010;33(1):1-6. Available at: https://doi.org/10.1016/j.infbeh.2009.10.005.

81. Goodman SH, Simon HFM, Shamblaw AL, Kim CY. Parenting as a mediator of associations between depression in mothers and children's functioning: a systematic review and meta-analysis. *Clin Child Fam Psychol Rev*. 2020;23(4):427-460. Available at: https://doi.org/10.1007/s10567-020-00322-4.

82. Ross LE, Murray BJ, Steiner M. Sleep and perinatal mood disorders: a critical review. *J Psychiatry Neurosci*. 2005;30(4):247-256. Available at: http://www.ncbi.nlm.nih.gov/entrez/query.fcgi?cmd=Retrie ve&db=PubMed&dopt=Citation&list_uids=16049568.

83. Armitage R, Flynn H, Hoffmann R, Vazquez D, Lopez J, Marcus S. Early developmental changes in sleep in infants: the impact of maternal depression. *Sleep*. 2009;32(5):693-696. Available at: http://www.ncbi. nlm.nih.gov/entrez/query.fcgi?cmd=Retrieve&db=PubMed&dopt=Citation&list_uids=19480236.

84. Bat-Pitault F, Sesso G, Deruelle C, et al. Altered sleep architecture during the first months of life in infants born to depressed mothers. *Sleep Med*. 2017;30:195-203. Available at: https://doi.org/10.1016/j. sleep.2016.11.018.

85. Field T, Diego M, Hernandez-Reif M, Figueiredo B, Schanberg S, Kuhn C. Sleep disturbances in depressed pregnant women and their newborns. *Infant Behav Dev*. 2007;30(1):127-133. Available at: https://doi.org/10.1016/j.infbeh.2006.08.002.

86. Stein A, Pearson RM, Goodman SH, et al. Effects of perinatal mental disorders on the fetus and child. *Lancet*. 2014;384(9956):1800-1819. Available at: https://doi.org/10.1016/S0140-6736(14)61277-0.

87. Galbally M, Watson SJ, Teti D, Lewis AJ. Perinatal maternal depression, antidepressant use and infant sleep outcomes: exploring cross-lagged associations in a pregnancy cohort study. *J Affect Disord*. 2018;238:218-225. Available at: https://doi.org/10.1016/j.jad.2018.05.025.

88. Howard LM, Molyneaux E, Dennis CL, Rochat T, Stein A, Milgrom J. Non-psychotic mental disorders in the perinatal period. *Lancet*. 2014;384(9956):1775-1788. Available at: https://doi.org/10.1016/ S0140-6736(14)61276-9.

89. Karraker KH, Young M. Night waking in 6-month-old infants and maternal depressive symptoms. *J Appl Dev Psychol*. 2007;28(5-6):493-498.

90. Sharkey KM, Iko IN, Machan JT, Thompson-Westra J, Pearlstein TB. Infant sleep and feeding patterns are associated with maternal sleep, stress, and depressed mood in women with a history of major depressive disorder (MDD). *Arch Womens Ment Health*. 2016;19(2):209-218. Available at: https://doi. org/10.1007/s00737-015-0557-5.

91. Halal CS, Bassani DG, Santos IS, et al. Maternal perinatal depression and infant sleep problems at 1 year of age: subjective and actigraphy data from a population-based birth cohort study. *J Sleep Res*. 2021;30(2):e13047. Available at: https://doi.org/10.1111/jsr.13047.

92. Goldberg WA, Lucas-Thompson RG, Germo GR, Keller MA, Davis EP, Sandman CA. Eye of the beholder? Maternal mental health and the quality of infant sleep. *Soc Sci Med.* 2013;79:101-108. Available at: https://doi.org/10.1016/j.socscimed.2012.07.006.

93. Gress-Smith JL, Luecken LJ, Lemery-Chalfant K, Howe R. Postpartum depression prevalence and impact on infant health, weight, and sleep in low-income and ethnic minority women and infants. *Matern Child Health J.* 2012;16(4):887-893. Available at: https://doi.org/10.1007/s10995-011-0812-y.

94. Gueron-Sela N, Propper CB, Wagner NJ, Camerota M, Tully KP, Moore GA. Infant respiratory sinus arrhythmia and maternal depressive symptoms predict toddler sleep problems. *Dev Psychobiol.* 2017;59(2):261-267. Available at: https://doi.org/10.1002/dev.21480.

95. Hiscock H, Wake M. Infant sleep problems and postnatal depression: a community-based study. *Pediatrics.* 2001;107(6):1317-1322.

96. Hughes A, Gallagher S, Hannigan A. A cluster analysis of reported sleeping patterns of 9-month old infants and the association with maternal health: results from a population based cohort s tudy. *Matern Child Health J.* 2015;19(8):1881-1889. Available at: https://doi.org/10.1007/s10995-015-1701-6.

97. Morales-Munoz I, Saarenpaa-Heikkila O, Kylliainen A, et al. The effects of maternal risk factors during pregnancy on the onset of sleep difficulties in infants at 3 months old. *J Sleep Res.* 2018;27(5):e12696. Available at: https://doi.org/10.1111/jsr.12696.

98. Netsi E, van IMH, Bakermans-Kranenburg MJ, et al. Does infant reactivity moderate the association between antenatal maternal depression and infant sleep? *J Dev Behav Pediatr.* 2015;36(6):440-449. Available at: https://doi.org/10.1097/DBP.0000000000000181.

99. Pinheiro KA, Pinheiro RT, Silva RA, et al. Chronicity and severity of maternal postpartum depression and infant sleep disorders: a population-based cohort study in southern Brazil. *Infant Behav Dev.* 2011;34(2):371-373. Available at: https://doi.org/10.1016/j.infbeh.2010.12.006.

100. Toffol E, Lahti-Pulkkinen M, Lahti J, et al. Maternal depressive symptoms during and after pregnancy are associated with poorer sleep quantity and quality and sleep disorders in 3.5-year-old offspring. *Sleep Med.* 2019;56:201-210. Available at: https://doi.org/10.1016/j.sleep.2018.10.042.

101. Warren SL, Howe G, Simmens SJ, Dahl RE. Maternal depressive symptoms and child sleep: models of mutual influence over time. *Dev Psychopathol.* 2006;18(1):1-16.

102. Ystrom E, Hysing M, Torgersen L, Ystrom H, Reichborn-Kjennerud T, Sivertsen B. Maternal symptoms of anxiety and depression and child nocturnal awakenings at 6 and 18 months. *J Pediatr Psychol.* 2017;42(10):1156-1164. Available at: https://doi.org/10.1093/jpepsy/jsx066.

103. Ystrom H, Nilsen W, Hysing M, Sivertsen B, Ystrom E. Sleep problems in preschoolers and maternal depressive symptoms: an evaluation of mother- and child-driven effects. *Dev Psychol.* 2017;53(12): 2261-2272. Available at: https://doi.org/10.1037/dev0000402.

104. de Jong DM, Cremone A, Kurdziel LB, et al. Maternal depressive symptoms and household income in relation to sleep in early childhood. *J Pediatr Psychol.* 2016;41(9):961-970. Available at: https://doi.org/10.1093/jpepsy/jsw006.

105. Cook F, Giallo R, Petrovic Z, et al. Depression and anger in fathers of unsettled infants: a community cohort study. *J Paediatr Child Health.* 2017;53(2):131-135. Available at: https://doi.org/10.1111/jpc.13311.

106. Philpott LF, Corcoran P. Paternal postnatal depression in Ireland: prevalence and associated factors. *Midwifery.* 2018;56:121-127. Available at: https://doi.org/10.1016/j.midw.2017.10.009.

107. Ragni B, De Stasio S, Barni D, Gentile S, Giampaolo R. Parental mental health, fathers' involvement and bedtime resistance in infants. *Ital J Pediatr.* 2019;45(1):134. Available at: https://doi.org/10.1186/s13052-019-0731-x.

108. Bernier A, Belanger ME, Bordeleau S, Carrier J. Mothers, fathers, and toddlers: parental psychosocial functioning as a context for young children's sleep. *Dev Psychol.* 2013;49(7):1375-1384. Available at: https://doi.org/10.1037/a0030024.

109. Garthus-Niegel S, Horsch A, Graz MB, et al. The prospective relationship between postpartum PTSD and child sleep: a 2-year follow-up study. *J Affect Dis.* 2018;241:71-79. Available at: https://doi.org/10.1016/j.jad.2018.07.067.

110. Hodge D, Hoffman CD, Sweeney DP, Riggs ML. Relationship between children's sleep and mental health in mothers of children with and without Autism. *J Autism Dev Disord.* 2013;43(4):956-963. Available at: https://doi.org/10.1007/s10803-012-1639-0.

111. Petzoldt J, Wittchen HU, Einsle F, Martini J. Maternal anxiety versus depressive disorders: specific relations to infants' crying, feeding and sleeping problems. *Child Care Health Dev.* 2016;42(2):231-245. Available at: https://doi.org/10.1111/cch.12292.
112. Smith VC, Leppert KA, Alfano CA, Dougherty LR. Construct validity of the Parent-Child Sleep Interactions Scale (PSIS): associations with parenting, family stress, and maternal and child psychopathology. *Sleep Med.* 2014;15(8):942-951. Available at: https://doi.org/10.1016/j.sleep.2014.04.002.
113. Sorondo BM, Reeb-Sutherland BC. Associations between infant temperament, maternal stress, and infants' sleep across the first year of life. *Infant Behav Dev.* 2015;39:131-135. Available at: https://doi.org/10.1016/j.infbeh.2015.02.010.
114. O'Connor TG, Caprariello P, Blackmore ER, et al. Prenatal mood disturbance predicts sleep problems in infancy and toddlerhood. *Early Hum Dev.* 2007;83(7):451-458. Available at: https://doi.org/10.1016/j.earlhumdev.2006.08.006.
115. De Stasio S, Boldrini F, Ragni B, Gentile S. Predictive factors of toddlers' sleep and parental stress. *Int J Environ Res Public Health.* 2020;17(7):2494. Available at: https://doi.org/10.3390/ijerph17072494.
116. Millikovsky-Ayalon M, Atzaba-Poria N, Meiri G. The role of the father in child sleep disturbance: child, parent, and parent-child relationship. *Infant Mental Health J.* 2015;36(1):114-127. Available at: https://doi.org/10.1002/imhj.21491.
117. Tikotzky L, Volkovich E, Meiri G. Maternal emotional distress and infant sleep: a longitudinal study from pregnancy through 18 months. *Dev Psychol.* 2021;57(7):1111-1123. Available at: https://doi.org/10.1037/dev0001081.
118. Kim Y, Bird A, Peterson E, et al. Maternal antenatal depression and early childhood sleep: Potential pathways through infant temperament. *J Pediatr Psychol.* 2020;45(2):203-217. Available at: https://doi.org/10.1093/jpepsy/jsaa001.
119. Bei B, Coo S, Trinder J. Sleep and mood during pregnancy and the postpartum period. *Sleep Med Clin.* 2015;10(1):25-33. Available at: https://doi.org/10.1016/j.jsmc.2014.11.011.
120. Bhati S, Richards K. A systematic review of the relationship between postpartum sleep disturbance and postpartum depression. *J Obstet Gynecol Neonatal Nurs.* 2015;44(3):350-357. Available at: https://doi.org/10.1111/1552-6909.12562.
121. Swanson LM, Kalmbach DA, Raglan GB, O'Brien LM. Perinatal insomnia and mental health: a review of recent literature. *Curr Psychiatry Rep.* 2020;22(12):73. Available at: https://doi.org/10.1007/s11920-020-01198-5.
122. Tikotzky L, Bar-Shachar Y, Volkovich E, Meiri G, Bar-Kalifa E. A longitudinal study of the links between maternal and infant nocturnal wakefulness. *Sleep Health.* 2021;8(1):31-38. Available at: https://doi.org/10.1016/j.sleh.2021.09.003.
123. Hall WA, Clauson M, Carty EM, Janssen PA, Saunders RA. Effects on parents of an intervention to resolve infant behavioral sleep problems. *Pediatr Nurs.* 2006;32(3):243-250. Available at: http://www.ncbi.nlm.nih.gov/entrez/query.fcgi?cmd=Retrieve&db=PubMed&dopt=Citation&list_uids=16802683.
124. Hall WA, Hutton E, Brant RF, et al. A randomized controlled trial of an intervention for infants' behavioral sleep problems. *BMC Pediatr.* 2015;15:181. Available at: https://doi.org/10.1186/s12887-015-0492-7.
125. Hiscock H, Bayer J, Gold L, Hampton A, Ukoumunne OC, Wake M. Improving infant sleep and maternal mental health: a cluster randomised trial. *Arch Dis Child.* 2007;92(11):952-958. Available at: https://doi.org/10.1136/adc.2006.099812.
126. Ben-Zion H, Volkovich E, Meiri G, Tikotzky L. Mother-infant sleep and maternal emotional distress in solo-mother and two-parent families. *J Pediatr Psychol.* 2020;45(2):181-193. Available at: https://doi.org/10.1093/jpepsy/jsz097.
127. Bugental DB, Johnston C. Parental and child cognitions in the context of the family. *Annu Rev Psychol.* 2000;51:315-344. Available at: https://doi.org/10.1146/annurev.psych.51.1.315.
128. Golik T, Avni H, Nehama H, Greenfeld M, Sivan Y, Tauman R. Maternal cognitions and depression in childhood behavioral insomnia and feeding disturbances. *Sleep Med.* 2013;14(3):261-265. Available at: https://doi.org/10.1016/j.sleep.2012.10.025.
129. Johnson N, McMahon C. Preschoolers' sleep behaviour: associations with parental hardiness, sleep-related cognitions and bedtime interactions [Article]. *J Child Psychol Psychiatry.* 2008;49(7):765-773. Available at: https://doi.org/10.1111/j.1469-7610.2007.01871.x.

130. Sadeh A, Flint-Ofir E, Tirosh T, Tikotzky L. Infant sleep and parental sleep-related cognitions. *J Fam Psychol.* 2007;21(1):74-87. Available at: http://www.ncbi.nlm.nih.gov/entrez/query.fcgi?cmd=Retrieve &db=PubMed&dopt=Citation&list_uids=17371112.
131. Morrell J. The role of maternal cognitions in infant sleep problems as assessed by a new instrument, the maternal cognitions about infant sleep questionnaire. *J Child Psychol Psychiatry.* 1999;40(2):247-258. Available at: https://doi.org/10.1111/1469-7610.00438.
132. Scher A. Maternal separation anxiety as a regulator of infants' sleep. *J Child Psychol Psychiatry.* 2008;49(6):618-625. Available at: https://doi.org/10.1111/j.1469-7610.2007.01872.x.
133. Scher A, Blumberg O. Night waking among 1-year olds: a study of maternal separation anxiety. *Child.* 1999;25(5):323-334. Available at: https://doi.org/10.1046/j.1365-2214.1999.00099.x.
134. Sadeh A, Juda-Hanael M, Livne-Karp E, et al. Low parental tolerance for infant crying: an underlying factor in infant sleep problems? *J Sleep Res.* 2016. Available at: https://doi.org/10.1111/jsr.12401.
135. Kahn M, Bauminger Y, Volkovich E, Meiri G, Sadeh A, Tikotzky L. Links between infant sleep and parental tolerance for infant crying: longitudinal assessment from pregnancy through six months postpartum. *Sleep Med.* 2018;50:72-78. Available at: https://doi.org/10.1016/j.sleep.2018.05.014.
136. Kahn M, Livne-Karp E, Juda-Hanael M, et al. Behavioral interventions for infant sleep problems: the role of parental cry tolerance and sleep-related cognitions. *J Clin Sleep Med.* 2020;16(8):1275-1283. Available at: https://doi.org/10.5664/jcsm.8488.
137. Ragni B, De Stasio S, Barni D. Fathers and sleep: a systematic literature review of bidirectional links between paternal factors and children's sleep in the first three years of life. *Clin Neuropsychiatry.* 2020;17(6):349-360. Available at: https://doi.org/10.36131/cnfioritieditore20200604.
138. Teti DM, Crosby B, McDaniel BT, Shimizu M, Whitesell CJ. Marital and emotional adjustment in mothers and infant sleep arrangements during the first six months. *Monogr Soc Res Child Dev.* 2015;80(1):160-176. Available at: https://doi.org/10.1111/mono.12150.
139. McDaniel BT, Teti DM. Coparenting quality during the first three months after birth: the role of infant sleep quality. *J Fam Psychol.* 2012;26(6):886-895. Available at: https://doi.org/10.1037/a0030707.
140. Tikotzky L, Sadeh A, Glickman-Gavrieli T. Infant sleep and paternal involvement in infant caregiving during the first 6 months of life. *J Pediatr Psychol.* 2011;36:36-46. Available at: https://doi.org/10.1093/jpepsy/jsq036.
141. Covington LB, Patterson F, Hale LE, et al. The contributory role of the family context in early childhood sleep health: a systematic review. *Sleep Health.* 2021;7(2):254-265. Available at: https://doi.org/10.1016/j.sleh.2020.11.010.
142. Whitesell CJ, Crosby B, Anders TF, Teti DM. Household chaos and family sleep during infants' first year. *J Fam Psychol.* 2018;32(5):622-631. Available at: https://doi.org/10.1037/fam0000422.
143. Dahl RE, El-Sheikh M. Considering sleep in a family context: introduction to the special issue. *J Fam Psychol.* 2007;21(1):1-3. Available at: https://doi.org/10.1037/0893-3200.21.1.1.

Intrinsic Factors Associated With Infant Insomnia: The Impact of Temperament and Development

Melisa E. Moore ▓ Kelsey D. Csumitta ▓ Majalisa Dunnewald

Intrinsic Factors Associated With Infant Insomnia: The Impact of Temperament and Development

DEVELOPMENT OF INFANT SLEEP PROCESSES

The development of infant sleep processes occurs parallel to and in conjunction with physical and cognitive development. Sleep evolves rapidly in the first year of life and outcomes depend on both developmental and ecological factors. Nighttime sleep duration increases with age (generally nighttime sleep becomes consolidated and daytime sleep decreases in the first year of life) and becomes stable at 6 to 17 months.[1] Most variability occurs in the first 5 months, though sleep in the first year is highly variable overall.[2] This large variability may reflect differences in environmental factors[3]; however, the impact of intrinsic factors should also be highlighted.

The development of infant sleep processes occurs as biological rhythms including body temperature changes and hormones such as melatonin and cortisol reach mature levels. The coordination of these biological rhythms and their synchronization with the times of day develop rapidly over the first 6 months of life to develop the circadian system.[4] Infants are born with low levels of melatonin (transferred from the mother), which dissipate by 1 week, and infant melatonin secretion does not rise to detectable levels until approximately 6 weeks. Melatonin levels are still very low at 12 to 16 weeks, but by 6 months, they are a stable part of the sleep-wake cycle. Exposure to morning light decreases daytime melatonin production and is an important part of developing a consolidated sleep schedule. Temperature rhythms generally mature earlier at about 1 week. Early morning waking coordinates with increased body temperature by about 6 weeks, at approximately the time when melatonin first becomes detectable. Weeks later, nighttime sleep, sundown, and the decrease in body temperature become coordinated and the duration of nighttime sleep begins to increase. Cortisol secretion is also related to the sleep-wake cycle. Secretion peaks in the early morning and triggers an increase in glucose and metabolism during the day when energy demand is highest. Cortisol is at its lowest at about 12 to 4 a.m. when melatonin production is higher. Overall, the circadian pattern of sleeping at night and being awake during the day develops in the first 4 to 6 months of life.[5-8]

In addition to the biological development of sleep processes, the rapid acquisition of new skills and abilities during the first year of life can affect infant sleep.[6] Infants develop an understanding of object permanence and can experience separation anxiety, which generally peaks between 6 and 18 months. Separation anxiety can lead to increased sleep disruptions—both difficulty separating at bedtime and difficulty self-soothing and returning to sleep independently during nighttime arousals. Additionally, the development of new gross motor skills can negatively influence sleep, particularly sitting up, pulling to stand, and walking, as infants will often experiment with new skills during brief nighttime arousals leading to longer, more sustained arousals. As new motor skills begin to emerge, infants can get "stuck" until they have mastered a particular skill. For example, around 9 months of age, babies can often pull to stand but may have difficulty getting back to sitting or lying down without help.

INFANT INSOMNIA

Insomnia in infants is generally characterized by difficulty falling asleep independently as well as night wakings and is influenced by both developmental and behavioral/ecological factors. Because infants' feeding and sleep schedules are emerging, difficulty falling asleep and night wakings are generally not characterized as insomnia before age 6 months. As many as 20% to 30% of parents complain about night wakings.[9,10] A higher number of night wakings has been associated with ecological factors such as breastfeeding back to sleep, not sleeping in a separate room, giving a bottle during the night, bringing the child into the parents' bed, and an irregular bedtime routine.[1,3] In addition to the environmental factors that are typically modifiable, there are also intrinsic factors associated with infant insomnia including temperament, prematurity, and neurodevelopmental conditions. While other factors impact infant insomnia, including maternal factors, substance exposure, and sleep disorders such as obstructive sleep apnea, those are outside the scope of this chapter.

TEMPERAMENT AND INSOMNIA

Temperament is generalized as the individual differences in emotional reactivity and mood that are biologically determined and stable across the lifespan. Infant temperament can be categorized as easy, slow-to-warm-up, and difficult,[11] though these can also be understood as the level of inborn reactivity to stimuli. Certain inborn temperament traits may, to some extent, mediate infant sleep quality, for example, through the ability to "self-soothe." Infant sleep and temperament variables have notable effects on each other and on familial variables in an interactive way. As an infant's temperament becomes more reactive or "difficult," more disruptions in sleep can be observed.

Studies on infant sleep and temperament have found a correlation between infant sleep and reactivity. For example, infants with a negative reactivity type (also described as a negative mood) were found to have more symptoms of insomnia. Mindell and Lee assessed infant sleep and mood in a large sample ($n = 1351$) of mothers and infants (ages 3–13 months) in Brazil.[12] Significant relationships were identified between sleep and mood, as measured by the Brief Infant Sleep Questionnaire (BISQ).[13] Parental perception of infant mood was correlated with sleep outcomes, including night wakings, nighttime sleep duration, and parent reports of sleep problems. In addition, negative mood was related to increased sleep fragmentation and decreased sleep duration, including later bedtime, earlier wake times, and increased sleep problems. Another study by De Marcas et al. utilized objective measures of sleep (actigraphy) and infant reactivity (laboratory measures) at 3, 6, and 12 months of age.[14] An inverse effect was found, particularly in girls, wherein higher reactivity was associated with lower sleep quality. Both hyper- and hyporeactivity predicted poor quality sleep among infants at all time points. The authors suggested that these results may account for some inconsistencies in the relationship between infant temperament and sleep. An additional longitudinal study utilized maternal reports of infant sleep duration, night wakings, and temperament. Infants with more reactive temperaments, particularly boys, had shorter sleep duration and a greater number of night awakenings.[15]

Infant sleep has also been demonstrated to relate to the temperamental characteristics of approachability, adaptability, and emotion regulation. A longitudinal study that sought to assess the relationship between infant sleep/wake patterns, temperament, and development over the first year of life assessed infants at 3, 6, and 11 months via parental sleep diaries, actigraphy, the Early Infant Temperament Questionnaire[16] (EITQ), and the Revised Infant Temperament Questionnaire[11] (RITQ).[17] All three time points studied showed that nocturnal sleep was positively correlated with the temperamental trait of increased approachability. At 11 months, increased diurnal sleep was correlated with increased adaptability, and at 12 months, decreased daytime sleep was correlated with better levels of emotion regulation.

A more recent longitudinal study on infant temperament and sleep revealed some aspects of temperament measured at 6 months of age were related to greater sleep problems at 12 months. In this study, mothers of over 1000 infants rated infant temperament using The Infant Behavior Questionnaire-Revised Short Form (IBQ-R-SF)[18] and infant sleep using the BISQ at both 6 and 12 months of age. The authors found higher Negative Affectivity at 6 months of age was significantly related to greater sleep problems (increased night wakings, long sleep-onset latency, and ability to fall asleep independently) at 12 months after controlling for sleep quality at 6 months. Additionally, Regulation and Surgency traits at 6 months were associated with ability to fall asleep independently at 12 months.[19] These findings suggest temperament is related to later sleep problems in infants within the first year of life.

While temperament is understood to be set at birth, maternal and familial factors have been shown to affect temperament and infant sleep. One study examined the moderating link of infant temperament on mothers' emotional availability (EA) at bedtime and objectively assessed infant sleep development from 1 to 6 months via actigraphy. In a sample of 72 mother-infant dyads, infant sleep was assessed via actigraphy, and maternal EA and maternal reports of infant temperament were coded from bedtime videos at 3 and 6 months.[20] While little evidence was found to support the main effects of either infant temperament or maternal EA, the results indicate a strong effect of infant temperament, particularly surgency (the tendency to experience and maintain positive affect), moderating the link between maternal EA at bedtime and infant sleep duration.

Furthermore, infant sleep and temperament have been shown to be associated with both maternal depression and family functioning. In one longitudinal study, 131 families were assessed with temperament and sleep data collected at the 8-month time point and maternal depression data collected at 15 months.[21] Variability in infant sleep efficiency moderated the relationship between infant temperament and maternal depressive symptoms. Difficult temperament in the infant was associated with maternal depressive symptoms when infant sleep efficiency was variable, but not when infant sleep efficiency was consistent. These results highlight the complex links between infant sleep, temperament and maternal mental health.

Current research demonstrates that infants with more difficult temperament experience increased insomnia symptoms. While typical developmental processes and temperament relate to insomnia symptoms, other intrinsic factors such as prematurity and neurodevelopmental conditions also play a role.

PREMATURITY AND INSOMNIA

Many infants born preterm have sleep problems, altered sleep patterns, and increased insomnia symptoms as compared to term counterparts. For example, preterm newborns have been shown to spend 90% of each day sleeping as compared to term newborns, who spend about 70% of their day asleep.[22] Sleep disruptions often occur in preterm infants due to features of neonatal intensive care[23-25] including continuous light and sound which disrupt circadian rhythms, respiratory support,[26] and a variety of comorbidities.

Recent studies suggest that preterm birth impacts sleep duration and night wakings, possibly in contradictory ways. One cross-sectional study looked at the sleep characteristics of very low-birth-weight (birth weight <1500 g) infants compared to full-term infants at the age of 12 months to examine whether the sleep behaviors of preterm infants differed from those of full-term infants.[27] The authors found that at 1 year after preterm birth, preterm infants had a greater number of night wakings and slept less during the night than term counterparts. A successive study by the same authors found an overall reduction in overall sleep duration in preterm infants compared to term infants, when measured at 1 and 2 years of age.[28] Conversely, other studies have found that preterm infants had increased sleep duration as compared to term infants. Even with increased sleep duration, more night wakings were noted. One study found that compared to term controls, 6-month-old infants born preterm had longer nocturnal sleep duration, more night awakenings, and longer daytime sleep.[29]

Several studies have found no significant difference in the sleep of preterm and term infants. One study found no differences in parental reports of sleep duration, number of night wakings, or sleep-onset difficulties in preterm infants (median 34.1 weeks gestational age) and term controls.[30] Similarly, a study by Hoppenbrouwers and colleagues[31] found that beyond the neonatal period, preterm birth does not impact the development of sleep states, with a similar percentage of time spent in active sleep, quiet sleep, and wake time.

While there is variability among study results, many preterm infants have altered sleep patterns characterized by insomnia symptoms such as increased night wakings. It is clear that further studies are needed, given the lack of research on the impact of preterm sleep on sleep outcomes. This is especially true as several mediators may impact the relationship between gestational age at birth and sleep development, such as the degree of prematurity, growth restriction in the fetus, sleep-disordered breathing, occurrence of neurodevelopmental disorders, and chronic inflammation.[32,33]

NEURODEVELOPMENTAL CONDITIONS AND INSOMNIA

Neurodevelopmental disorders manifest in early development and cause specific or global deficits in learning and cognition which are evidenced across areas of functioning including sleep. Infants with certain neurodevelopmental conditions do not display the same trajectory of sleep as typically developing infants and are at a greater risk of having insomnia symptoms. While there are neurodevelopmental conditions that are associated with poor sleep (e.g., motor disorders), we limit our discussion to those conditions which can be diagnosed in infancy and which have evidence of sleep disruption. Namely, autism spectrum disorder, trisomy 21, intellectual disability, and other neurogenetic syndromes characterized by disrupted sleep (e.g., Smith-Magenis syndrome). Congenital blindness and visual impairment, which can cooccur with neurodevelopmental conditions, are also associated with insomnia symptoms due to the impact on the circadian system.

Autism spectrum disorder (ASD) is a neurodevelopmental disorder with a high rate of comorbid sleep problems. The prevalence rate of sleep problems is between 50% and 80% in children with ASD.[34] Insomnia symptoms in ASD typically include prolonged sleep onset, prolonged night wakings, early wakings, difficulty maintaining sleep, and daytime fatigue.[35-37] While symptoms of ASD may be present during infancy,[38-40] ASD is most commonly diagnosed after 3 years of age (e.g., van't Hof et al.).[41] As such, very little research has been conducted on infant sleep disturbance in ASD. A recent study of parent-reported sleep characteristics using the BISQ for over 1000 infants revealed the frequency of night wakings at 12 months old is associated with ASD screening scores at 24 months old. In contrast, ratings of nighttime and anytime sleep and sleep onset latency at 12 months were not found to relate to ASD screening scores at 24 months.[42] MacDuffie and colleagues[43] examined differences in parent-reported sleep onset difficulties using the Infant Behavior Questionnaire-Revised (IBQ-R) in infants at low and high risk of developing ASD, as well as infants at high risk who did and did not develop ASD. Sleep onset difficulty ratings and structural neuroimaging data were collected at 6, 12, and 24 months to examine the relation between sleep problems and subcortical brain volumes. Results of this study revealed sleep onset difficulties were more common in 6- and 12-month-old infants who were later diagnosed with ASD. This study also found a relationship between sleep onset problems in high-risk infants who developed ASD and hippocampal volume trajectories between 6 and 24 months. Though more research is needed, these preliminary findings suggest night wakings and sleep onset problems may precede ASD diagnosis.

Trisomy 21, also known as Down syndrome, is the most common genetic cause of intellectual disability (ID)[44] and is associated with sleep disorders. While obstructive sleep apnea (OSA) is known to be prevalent in infants with trisomy 21 (e.g., Goffinski et al.),[45] less is known about behavioral sleep disturbances in trisomy 21 within the first year of life. Studies that have examined behavioral sleep disturbances in children with trisomy 21 have included a large age range (e.g., birth to 18 years in Rosen et al.),[46] have not included a control group, or have used measures not validated for infants.[47-50] Very few studies have examined sleep in trisomy 21 with infant-only samples. McKay and Angulo-Barroso (2006) investigated sleeping patterns and leg activity overnight in infants 3 to 6 months with trisomy 21 using ankle activity monitors over 48 hours.[51] Infants with trisomy 21 had more sleep disturbances compared to TD infants, including less sleep, more night activity, and greater sleep fragmentation. In a recent study by Yau et al.[52] infant and toddler sleep habits in 104 individuals aged 6 to 36 months with trisomy 21 and 489 TD individuals of the same age range were measured with the BISQ. Parent-report of sleep habits revealed parents of infants and toddlers with trisomy 21 had more sleep problems, room sharing, and reduced night-time and total sleep over 24 hours. Parents in the trisomy 21 group were also more likely to be present when their child fell asleep. While snoring accounted for increased night waking, it did not account for reduced sleep time, whereas parental presence did. When controlling for snoring and parental presence during sleep onset, children with trisomy 21 had no significant difference in duration of sleep over a 24-hour period, as they slept less at night but more during the day.[52] These findings suggest signs of insomnia such as parental presence at bedtime, more night activity, and greater sleep fragmentation may also contribute to sleep loss in infants with trisomy 21 in addition to sleep-disordered breathing.

Insomnia symptoms such as long sleep onset latency, night and early morning wakings, and bedtime struggles are more common in children with intellectual disability (ID) than in typically developing children,[53] with prevalence rates varying between 23% and 86%.[54,55] Insomnia symptoms vary by neurodevelopmental condition, and many studies on children with ID include mixed groups with some having a specific genetic diagnosis and others not. As with research on other neurodevelopmental populations, very little sleep research has been conducted on infants with various forms of ID. Thus, while insomnia has been frequently documented in children with ID, more research is needed to determine whether insomnia symptoms emerge within the first year of life.

Smith-Magenis syndrome (SMS) is a genetic disorder characterized by neuropsychological and behavioral difficulties, as well as sleep disruptions typically related to inverted circadian rhythm of melatonin.[56,57] While sleep disruption related to inverted circadian rhythms has been documented in children and young adults with SMS,[56,57] very little is known about sleep in infants with this condition. Most research on the development of infants with SMS to date has been conducted using very small sample sizes using subjective descriptions, chart reviews, and retrospective observations.[58] Observations of infants with SMS have revealed reduced overall sleep,[59] lethargy, and placid behavior,[60,61] which could be related to insomnia and/or circadian rhythm problems. However, more research is needed to determine whether infants with SMS display symptoms of insomnia or whether inverted circadian rhythms are the primary sleep problem in this population.

Infants with congenital blindness and visual impairment (VI) are at greater risk of having sleep difficulties due to reduced light input which impacts melatonin production and sleep-wake patterns.[62-64] Parents of young children who are blind or VI have reported settling difficulties[65-67] as well as prolonged and more frequent night wakings[65] relative to TD children. Fazzi and colleagues' (2008) study included infants as young as 10 months and slightly over half the sample was under 20 months, suggesting insomnia symptoms of settling difficulties and night wakings may present before the toddler years in children with VI. Additionally, sleep behavior was not found to be related to the presence of associated disabilities (e.g., cortical visual impairment, epilepsy) within the VI group, suggesting sleep disturbance may be most related to circadian rhythm differences related to VI as opposed to other neurological pathologies.

In sum, neurodevelopmental conditions such as ASD and trisomy 21 as well as VI are associated with greater sleep difficulties in infancy and childhood. While more research is needed on insomnia symptoms in infants with developmental conditions, the current literature suggests insomnia symptoms may present within the first year of life in these populations. Insomnia symptoms documented in infants with neurodevelopmental and acquired conditions are variable, with sleep onset/settling difficulties and night wakings noted in ASD and VI as well as increased parental presence at bedtime, greater night activity, and greater sleep fragmentation noted in trisomy 21. While infants with SMS display sleep disturbances that could be related to insomnia such as reduced overall sleep and lethargy, more research is needed to parse insomnia symptoms from circadian rhythm differences in this population. Overall, greater attention to investigating insomnia symptoms in infants with developmental disorders and other disabilities is needed to inform targeted sleep interventions for these populations.

Conclusion

The development of biological rhythms such as body temperature, melatonin secretion, and cortisol secretion are needed for the development of the circadian system and mature rapidly during the first 4 to 6 months of life. In addition to typical developmental processes (e.g., the acquisition of new skills), intrinsic factors are associated with the development of infant insomnia symptoms such as night wakings and bedtime problems. These intrinsic factors include variability in reactivity and other temperamental traits as well as developmental differences (e.g., prematurity, ASD, trisomy 21, and VI). While ecological and familial factors related to the development of insomnia in infancy are well characterized, further investigations of intrinsic factors relating to infant insomnia are needed in order to identify avenues for future interventions.

Acknowledgement

This material is based upon work supported by the National Science Foundation Graduate Research Fellowship under Grant No. (1646737) to K.D.C.

References

1. Sadeh A, Mindell JA, Luedtke K, Wiegand B. Sleep and sleep ecology in the first 3 years: a web-based study. *J Sleep Res.* 2009;18(1):60-73. doi:10.1111/j.1365-2869.2008.00699.x.
2. Iglowstein I, Jenni OG, Molinari L, Largo RH. Sleep duration from infancy to adolescence: reference values and generational trends. *Pediatrics.* 2003;111:302-307.
3. Adair R, Bauchner H, Philipp B, Levenson S, Zuckerman B. Night waking during infancy: role of parental presence at bedtime. *Pediatrics.* 1991;87:500-504.
4. Bathory E, Tomopoulos S. Sleep regulation, physiology and development, sleep duration and patterns, and sleep hygiene in infants, toddlers, and preschool-age children. *Curr Probl Pediatr Adolesc Health Care.* 2017;47(2):29-42.
5. Coons S, Guilleminault C. Development of consolidated sleep and wakeful periods in relation to the day/night cycle in infancy. *Dev Med Child Neurol.* 1984;26:169-176.

6. Goodlin-Jones BL, Burnham MM, Gaylor EE, Anders TF. Night waking, sleep-wake organization, and self-soothing in the first year of life. *J Dev Behav Pediatr.* 2001;22:226-233.
7. Rivkees SA. Developing circadian rhythmicity in infants. *Pediatrics.* 2003;112(2):373-381.
8. Tham EK, Schneider N, Broekman BF. Infant sleep and its relation with cognition and growth: a narrative review. *Nat Sci Sleep.* 2017;9:135-149. doi:10.2147/NSS.S125992.
9. Zuckerman B, Stevenson J, Bailey V. Sleep problems in early childhood: continuities, predictive factors, and behavioral correlates. *Pediatrics.* 1987;80:664-671.
10. Lam P, Hiscock H, Wake M. Outcomes of infant sleep problems: a longitudinal study of sleep, behavior, and maternal well-being. *Pediatrics.* 2003;111:e203-e207.
11. Carey WB, McDevitt SC. Revision of the infant temperament questionnaire. *Pediatrics.* 1978;61(5):735-739.
12. Mindell JA, Lee C. Sleep, mood, and development in infants. *Infant Behav Dev.* 2015;41:102-107. Available at: https://doi.org/10.1016/j.infbeh.2015.08.004.
13. Sadeh A. A brief screening questionnaire for infant sleep problems: validation and findings for an internet sample. *Pediatrics.* 2004;113(6):e570-e577.
14. De Marcas GS, Soffer-Dudek N, Dollberg S, Bar-Haim Y, Sadeh A. Reactivity and sleep in infants: a longitudinal objective assessment. *Monogr Soc Res Child Dev.* 2015;80(1):49-69. Available at: https://doi.org/10.1111/mono.12144.
15. Netsi E, van IJzendoorn MH, Bakermans-Kranenburg MJ, et al. Does infant reactivity moderate the association between antenatal maternal depression and infant sleep? *J Dev Behav Pediatr.* 2015;36(6):440-449. Available at: https://doi.org/10.1097/DBP.0000000000000181.
16. Medoff-Cooper B, Carey WB, McDevitt SC. The early infancy temperament questionnaire. *J Dev Behav Pediatr.* 1993;14(4):230-235. Available at: https://doi.org/10.1097/00004703-199308010-00004.
17. Spruyt K, Aitken RJ, So K, Charlton M, Adamson TM, Horne RS. Relationship between sleep/wake patterns, temperament and overall development in term infants over the first year of life. *Early Hum Dev.* 2008;84(5):289-296. Available at: https://doi.org/10.1016/j.earlhumdev.2007.07.002.
18. Putnam SP, Helbig AL, Gartstein MA, Rothbart MK, Leerkes E. Development and assessment of short and very short forms of the Infant Behavior Questionnaire–revised. *J Pers Assess.* 2014;96(4):445-458. doi:10.1080/00223891.2013.841171.
19. Morales-Muñoz I, Nolvi S, Virta M, Karlsson H, Paavonen EJ, Karlsson L. The longitudinal associations between temperament and sleep during the first year of life. *Infant Behav Dev.* 2020;61:101485. Available at: https://doi.org/10.1016/j.infbeh.2020.101485.
20. Jian N, Teti DM. Emotional availability at bedtime, infant temperament, and infant sleep development from one to six months. *Sleep Med.* 2016;23:49-58. Available at: https://doi.org/10.1016/j.sleep.2016.07.001.
21. Parade SH, Wong K, Belair R, Dickstein S, Seifer R. Infant sleep moderates the effect of infant temperament on maternal depressive symptoms, maternal sensitivity, and family functioning. *Infant Behav Dev.* 2019;57:101343. Available at: https://doi.org/10.1016/j.infbeh.2019.101343.
22. Gaultier C. Cardiorespiratory adaptation during sleep in infants and children. *Pediatr Pulmonol.* 1995;19(2):105-117. Available at: https://doi.org/10.1002/ppul.1950190206.
23. Levy J, Hassan F, Plegue MA, et al. Impact of hands-on care on infant sleep in the neonatal intensive care unit. *Pediatr Pulmonol.* 2017;52(1):84-90. Available at: https://doi.org/10.1002/ppul.23513.
24. Liao JH, Hu RF, Su LJ, et al. Nonpharmacological interventions for sleep promotion on preterm infants in neonatal intensive care unit: a systematic review. *Worldviews Evid Based Nurs.* 2018;15(5):386-393. Available at: https://doi.org/10.1111/wvn.12315.
25. van den Hoogen A, Teunis CJ, Shellhaas RA, Pillen S, Benders M, Dudink J. How to improve sleep in a neonatal intensive care unit: a systematic review. *Early Hum Dev.* 2017;113:78-86. Available at: https://doi.org/10.1016/j.earlhumdev.2017.07.002.
26. Collins CL, Barfield C, Davis PG, Horne RS. Randomized controlled trial to compare sleep and wake in preterm infants less than 32 weeks of gestation receiving two different modes of non-invasive respiratory support. *Early Hum Dev.* 2015;91(12):701-704. Available at: https://doi.org/10.1016/j.earlhumdev.2015.09.011.
27. Asaka Y, Takada S. Activity-based assessment of the sleep behaviors of VLBW preterm infants and full-term infants at around 12 months of age. *Brain Dev.* 2010;32(2):150-155. Available at: https://doi.org/10.1016/j.braindev.2008.12.006.
28. Asaka Y, Takada S. Relation between sleep status of preterm infants aged 1-2 years and mothers' parenting stress. *Pediatr Int.* 2013;55(4):416-421. Available at: https://doi.org/10.1111/ped.12097.

29. Huang YS, Paiva T, Hsu JF, Kuo MC, Guilleminault C. Sleep and breathing in premature infants at 6 months post-natal age. *BMC Pediatr.* 2014;14:303. Available at: https://doi.org/10.1186/s12887-014-0303-6.
30. Iglowstein I, Latal Hajnal B, Molinari L, Largo RH, Jenni OG. Sleep behaviour in preterm children from birth to age 10 years: a longitudinal study. *Acta Paediatr.* 2006;95(12):1691-1693. Available at: https://doi.org/10.1080/08035250600686938.
31. Hoppenbrouwers T, Hodgman JE, Rybine D, et al. Sleep architecture in term and preterm infants beyond the neonatal period: the influence of gestational age, steroids, and ventilatory support. *Sleep.* 2005;28(11):1428-1436. Available at: https://doi.org/10.1093/sleep/28.11.1428.
32. Bennet L, Walker DW, Horne R. Waking up too early—the consequences of preterm birth on sleep development. *J Physiol.* 2018;596(23):5687-5708. Available at: https://doi.org/10.1113/JP274950.
33. Uchitel J, Vanhatalo S, Austin T. Early development of sleep and brain functional connectivity in term-born and preterm infants. *Pediatr Res.* 2022;91(4):771-786. Available at: https://doi.org/10.1038/s41390-021-01497-4.
34. Mannion A, Leader G. Sleep problems in autism spectrum disorder: a literature review. *Rev J Autism Dev Disord.* 2014;1:101-109. Available at: https://doi.org/10.1007/s40489-013-0009-y.
35. Krakowiak P, Goodlin-Jones B, Hertz-Picciotto I, Croen LA, Hansen RL. Sleep problems in children with autism spectrum disorders, developmental delays, and typical development: a population-based study. *J Sleep Res.* 2008. Available at: https://doi.org/10.1111/j.1365-2869.2008.00650.x.
36. Mayes SD, Calhoun SL. Variables related to sleep problems in children with autism. *Res Autism Spectr Disord.* 2009;3:931-941. Available at: https://doi.org/10.1016/j.rasd.2009.04.002.
37. Richdale AL, Schreck KA. Sleep problems in autism spectrum disorders: prevalence, nature, & possible biopsychosocial aetiologies. *Sleep Med Rev.* 2009;13(6):403-411. Available at: https://doi.org/10.1016/j.smrv.2009.02.003.
38. Martínez-Pedraza Fde L, Carter AS. Autism spectrum disorders in young children. *Child Adolesc Psychiatr Clin N Am.* 2009;18(3):645-663. Available at: https://doi.org/10.1016/j.chc.2009.02.002.
39. Osterling JA, Dawson G, Munson JA. Early recognition of 1-year-old infants with autism spectrum disorder versus mental retardation. *Dev Psychopathol.* 2002;14(2):239-251. Available at: https://doi.org/10.1017/s0954579402002031.
40. Ozonoff S, Iosif AM, Baguio F, et al. A prospective study of the emergence of early behavioral signs of autism. *J Am Acad Child Adolesc Psychiatry.* 2010;49(3):256-266.e1-e2. Available at: https://doi.org/10.1097/00004583-201003000-00009.
41. van't Hof M, Tisseur C, van Berckelear-Onnes I, et al. Age at autism spectrum disorder diagnosis: a systematic review and meta-analysis from 2012 to 2019. *Autism.* 2021;25(4):862-873. Available at: https://doi.org/10.1177/1362361320971107.
42. Nguyen AKD, Murphy LE, Kocak M, Tylavsky FA, Pagani LS. Prospective associations between infant sleep at 12 months and autism spectrum disorder screening scores at 24 months in a community-based birth cohort. *J Clin Psychiatry.* 2018;79(1):16m11127. Available at: https://doi.org/10.4088/JCP.16m11127.
43. MacDuffie KE, Shen MD, Dager SR, et al. Sleep onset problems and subcortical development in infants later diagnosed with autism spectrum disorder. *Am J Psychiatry.* 2020;177(6):518-525. Available at: https://doi.org/10.1176/appi.ajp.2019.19060666.
44. Parker SE, Mai CT, Canfield MA, et al. Updated national birth prevalence estimates for selected birth defects in the United States, 2004-2006. *Birth Defects Res A Clin Mol Teratol.* 2010;88(12):1008-1016. Available at: https://doi.org/10.1002/bdra.20735.
45. Goffinski A, Stanley MA, Shepherd N, et al. Obstructive sleep apnea in young infants with Down Syndrome evaluated in a Down Syndrome specialty clinic. *Am J Med Genet A.* 2015;167A(2):324-330. Available at: https://doi.org/10.1002/ajmg.a.36903.
46. Rosen D, Lombardo A, Skotko B, Davidson EJ. Parental perceptions of sleep disturbances and sleep-disordered breathing in children with Down syndrome. *Clin Pediatr.* 2011;50(2):121-125. Available at: https://doi.org/10.1177/0009922810384260.
47. Carter M, McCaughey E, Annaz D, Hill CM. Sleep problems in a Down syndrome population. *Arch Dis Child.* 2009;94(4):308-310. Available at: https://doi.org/10.1136/adc.2008.146845.
48. Edgin JO, Tooley U, Demara B, Nyhuis C, Anand P, Spanò G. Sleep disturbance and expressive language development in preschool-age children with Down syndrome. *Child Dev.* 2015;86(6):1984-1988. Available at: https://doi.org/10.1111/cdev.12443.

49. Bassell JL, Phan H, Leu R, Kronk R, Visootsak J. Sleep profiles in children with Down syndrome. *Am J Med Genet A*. 2015;167A(8):1830-1835. Available at: https://doi.org/10.1002/ajmg.a.37096.
50. Lukowski AF, Milojevich HM. Sleep problems and temperament in young children with Down syndrome and typically developing controls. *J Intellect Disabil Res*. 2017;61(3):221-232. Available at: https://doi.org/10.1111/jir.12321.
51. McKay SM, Angulo-Barroso RM. Longitudinal assessment of leg motor activity and sleep patterns in infants with and without Down syndrome. *Infant Behav Dev*. 2006;29(2):153-168. Available at: https://doi.org/10.1016/j.infbeh.2005.09.004.
52. Yau S, Pickering RM, Gringras P, et al. Sleep in infants and toddlers with Down syndrome compared to typically developing peers: looking beyond snoring. *Sleep Med*. 2019;63:88-97. Available at: https://doi.org/10.1016/j.sleep.2019.05.005.
53. Richdale A, Francis A, Gavidia-Payne S, Cotton S. Stress, behaviour, and sleep problems in children with an intellectual disability. *J Intellect Dev Disabil*. 2000;25(2):147-161. Available at: https://doi.org/10.1080/13269780050033562.
54. Didden R, Korzilius H, Van Aperlo B, Van Overloop C, De Vries M. Sleep problems and daytime problem behaviours in children with intellectual disability. *J Intellect Disabil Res*. 2002;46(Pt 7):537-547. Available at: https://doi.org/10.1046/j.1365-2788.2002.00404.x.
55. Bartlett LB, Rooney V, Spedding S. Nocturnal difficulties in a population of mentally handicapped children. *Br J Ment Subnorm*. 1985;31(60):54-59. Available at: https://doi.org/10.1179/bjms.1985.009.
56. Potocki L, Glaze D, Tan DX, et al. Circadian rhythm abnormalities of melatonin in Smith-Magenis syndrome. *J Med Genet*. 2000;37(6):428-433. Available at: https://doi.org/10.1136/jmg.37.6.428.
57. De Leersnyder H, De Blois MC, Claustrat B, et al. Inversion of the circadian rhythm of melatonin in the Smith-Magenis syndrome. *J Pediatr*. 2001;139(1):111-116. Available at: https://doi.org/10.1067/mpd.2001.115018.
58. Wolters PL, Gropman AL, Martin SC, et al. Neurodevelopment of children under 3 years of age with Smith-Magenis syndrome. *Pediatr Neurol*. 2009;41(4):250-258. Available at: https://doi.org/10.1016/j.pediatrneurol.2009.04.015.
59. Duncan WC, Gropman A, Morse RS, Krasnewich D, Smith ACM. Good babies sleeping poorly: insufficient sleep in infants with Smith-Magenis syndrome. *Am J Hum Genet*. 2003;73:A896.
60. Gropman A, Wolters P, Solomon B, Smith ACM. Neurodevelopmental assessment and functioning in five young children with Smith-Magenis syndrome (SMS). *Am J Hum Genet*. 1999;65:A151.
61. Gropman AL, Duncan WC, Smith ACM. Neurologic and developmental features of the Smith-Magenis syndrome (del 17p11.2). *Pediatr Neurol*. 2006;34(5):337-350. Available at: https://doi.org/10.1016/j.pediatrneurol.2005.08.018.
62. Leger D, Guilleminaul C, Defrance R, Domont A, Paillard M. Prevalence of sleep/wake disorders in persons with blindness. *Clin Sci*. 1999;97(2):193-199. Available at: https://doi.org/10.1042/CS19990004.
63. Okawa M, Nanami T, Wada S, et al. Four congenitally blind children with circadian sleep-wake rhythm disorder. *Sleep*. 1987;10(2):101-110. Available at: https://doi.org/10.1093/sleep/10.2.101.
64. Wee R, Van Gelder RN. Sleep disturbances in young subjects with visual dysfunction. *Ophthalmology*. 2004;111(2):297-302. Avalable at: https://doi.org/10.1016/j.ophtha.2003.05.014.
65. Fazzi E, Zaccagnino M, Gahagan S, et al. Sleep disturbances in visually impaired toddlers. *Brain Dev*. 2008;30(9):572-578. Available at: https://doi.org/10.1016/j.braindev.2008.01.008.
66. Kitzinger M, Hunt H. The effect of residential setting on sleep and behaviour patterns of young visWually-handicapped children. In: Stevenson J, ed. *Recent Research in Developmental Psychopathology*. Pergamon Press; 1985.
67. Jan JE, Freeman RD, Scott EP. *Visual Impairment in Children and Adolescents*. Grune & Stratton; 1977.

CHAPTER 13

Behavioral Sleep Assessment Methods

Graham J. Reid   ▤   Wendy A. Hall   ▤   Katarina N. A. McKenzie

Background/Rationale

It is important for care providers who are promoting healthy sleep for infants and toddlers to be familiar with empirical data to inform their areas of assessment. The background/rationale section provides information about the complexities of factors to consider when assessing sleep. Then, we review various methods of assessing sleep among infants and toddlers, providing suggestions for assessments in different contexts (e.g., primary care, sleep specialist).

SLEEP AND FEEDING

There is a complex relationship between feeding and sleep from the outset of infancy. Starting as early as 6 weeks post birth, infant-only night waking (i.e., waking but not signaling parents) increases over the first 24 weeks of life; the presence of infant-only wakes is associated with a faster rate of decline in infants' night-time feeds from 6 to 24 weeks.[1]

Breastfeeding tends to relate to shorter night sleep durations. Portuguese infants who were exclusively breastfed at 3 months had shorter longest sleep period at night when ages 3 and 6 months, compared to exclusively formula-fed infants.[2] In an Asia-Pacific region study,[3] breastfed infants at less than 6 months of age had increased number and duration of night waking and less consolidated sleep; however, breastfeeding at less than 6 months of age was related to longer duration of daytime sleep and more sleep overall.

A French longitudinal study examined feeding at 4 months, 8 months, and 1 year and sleep quantity and quality trajectories at ages 2, 3, and 5 to 6 years. There was no association between the use of thickened baby formula, or age of introduction of complementary foods or baby cereal, and persistent sleep onset difficulties.[4] Infants predominantly breastfed for more than 4 months were *less likely* to belong to the persistent sleep onset difficulties trajectory. Early introduction (<4 months) to complementary foods, excluding baby cereals, was related to lower risk of belonging to the short-sleepers trajectory.

A key issue is feeding at night. Night feeding, in infancy or at 2 years, has been associated with higher risk of persistent sleep-onset difficulties between 2 and 5 to 6 years old; night-feeding at 8 months was related to a higher risk of persistent night-waking over time and short-sleep between 2 and 5 to 6 years of age.[4] In a cross-sectional study, breastfed infants (6–12 months of age) who were also breastfed back to sleep during the night woke more frequently at night and had shorter continuous nighttime sleep periods.[3]

Conclusion

It is important to explore the type of infant feeding (e.g., breast, bottle) at the time of assessment including the timing of feeding before the start of nighttime sleep and timing of feeding during the night. The fit with feeding over 24 hours and the developmental stage of the infant needs to be considered. Pay particular attention to whether or not the child's sleep onset occurs during/at the end of a feeding.

SLEEP AND SAFETY

Highly developed countries around the world have guidelines about infant sleep position and safety practices to reduce sudden infant death (SID).[5] In particular, there is wide consensus around key preventive factors including: (1) supine positioning; (2) firm and flat sleep surfaces; (3) minimal coverings and clothing; (4) low room temperature; (5) nonexposure to smoking; (6) parental avoidance of alcohol, sedating medications, and illicit drugs; and (7) nonshared sleep surfaces.[5] In addition to SID, there is also sudden unexpected death in infancy: deaths of "well" infants for whom cause of death is not obvious, with external risk factors that may have contributed to the death.[6] Risk factors include: (1) suffocation due to soft bedding, (2) overlay, by another person, and (3) wedging.[7]

Considerable empirical data has indicated that many parents have difficulty adhering to safe sleep guidelines, in particular following supine positioning and avoiding bedsharing.[6,8,9] Those findings have resulted in some jurisdictions incorporating harm reduction strategies in guidelines for health care providers and parents, such as preparing a safe bed for healthy full term breastfeeding infants.[10]

In contrast to infants, there are limited data about toddlers and sleep safety. Scheers and colleagues (2019) reported maternal assessment of infant and toddler injuries associated with crib-bumpers and mesh liners, versus no barriers.[11] Injuries included face covered, climb-out and falls, slat entrapment, and hitting head. Crib bumpers had higher risks of face covering, breathing difficulties, and wedging. Climb-out and falls were not associated with any of the crib arrangements.[11] For toddlers who are walking, it is important for parents to consider gates on bedroom doors to avoid toddlers accessing stairs or other hazards during the night. Locking bedroom doors is *not* recommended due to safety hazards in the event of situations such as a fire.

Conclusion

It is important to incorporate questions about sleep safety when undertaking a sleep assessment, as is recommended by multiple organizations. For example, the Academy of Breastfeeding Medicine has recommended that health care providers counsel all families about children's safe sleep, including elements of safe bedsharing advice, hazardous circumstances during bedsharing, and risk minimization strategies for families where bedsharing is high risk (e.g., referral for smoking cessation and alcohol and/or drug treatment[12]). It is important for care providers to be open to listening to parents' difficulties following proscriptions and consider harm reduction principles.

SLEEP TIME

Total sleep time

Despite some controversy about recommending sleep duration ranges for children, two organizations have created documents with recommendations. Table 13.1 presents the recommendations from the National Sleep Foundation[13] and the American Academy of Sleep Medicine.[14] The National Sleep Foundation acknowledges that, although sleep and/or time-in-bed duration represents a major dimension for measuring sleep, other indices important to consider are sleep quality, sleep architecture, and the timing of sleep within the day.

Naps and sleep consolidation

A study of American children between birth and age 36 months, using an iPhone app, identified sleep consolidating into two naps of about 1.5 hours in length and a night-time sleep session of

TABLE 13.1 ■ Sleep Duration Recommendations by Age

Age		National Sleep Foundation[1]			American Academy of Sleep Medicine[2]	24-Hour Movement Guidelines (Canada)[3]
		Total Sleep—24 hours	Minimal	Maximal		
Newborns	0–3 months	14–17 hours	Not less than 11	19	No recommendation	14–17 hours
Infants	4–12 months	12–15 hours	Not less than 11	19	12–16 hours	12–16 hours
Toddlers	1–2 years	11–14 hours	Not less than 10	18	11–14 hours	11–14 hours

[1]Hirshkowitz M, Whiton K, Albert SM, et al. National Sleep Foundation's updated sleep duration recommendations: final report. *Sleep Health*. 2015;1(4):233–243.
[2]Paruthi S, Brooks LJ, D'Ambrosio C, et al. Recommended amount of sleep for pediatric populations: a consensus statement of the American Academy of Sleep Medicine. *J Clin Sleep Med*. 2016;12(6):785–786.
[3]Tremblay MS, Chaput JP, Adamo KB, et al. Canadian 24-hour movement guidelines for the early years (0–4 years): an integration of physical activity, sedentary behaviour, and sleep. *BMC Public Health*. 2017;17(Suppl 5):874.

about 10.5 hours occurred between 3 and 7 months of age.[15] Naps varied with age, decreasing between 1 and 5 months old and then increasing monotonically through 28 months. Between 12 and 24 months, only about 2.5% of children will cease napping and switch to monophasic (night only) sleep.[16] It is critical to reinforce the need for naps among young children.

Sleep duration varies across families

One study examined racial/ethnic and socioeconomic differences in objectively measured sleep-wake patterns between 1 and 6 months of age among American infants using actigraphy. Changes in nighttime sleep duration from age 1 to 6 months varied by race: White infants' sleep duration increased by 82 minutes, while Hispanic infants increased by 49 minutes and Black infants increased by 32 minutes.[17] In general, Hispanic/Latino, Asian, and Black infants or infants from lower SES families had less consolidated and shorter 24-hour sleep; for daytime sleep duration at 6 months of age, Hispanic-Latino, Asian, and Black infants had longer daytime sleep duration.[17] Nighttime sleep duration also varied, with lower maternal education and lower household income related to shorter sleep. In addition, after adjusting for maternal education and household income, Asian infants had more frequent wakes and reduced nighttime sleep at 6 months.[17]

Conclusion

Sleep time varies considerably based on individual differences. Nevertheless, it is important to consider if an infant/toddler is sleeping outside of the range of recommended sleep times.

SLEEP ASSOCIATIONS AND ROUTINES

Sleep associations are particularly important for infants and toddlers. Sleep associations refer to the conditions present at sleep onset, including presence of parents, toys, other objects, playing music, etc. When sleep onset is paired with a specific set of conditions, children can quickly become dependent on having these conditions in order to sleep, which can contribute to signaled night waking. Thus, when an infant is fed or rocked to sleep and then put in the crib, they will struggle to fall asleep independently when they wake at night.

In contrast to negative sleep associations, sleep hygiene refers to behaviors conducive to adequate sleep duration and quality, including sleep schedules, sleep habits, and sleep environment. A systematic review examined sleep hygiene for infants, toddlers, and older children.[18] For infants and toddlers, bedtime routines (regular activities such as reading and brushing teeth) and independently falling asleep (self-soothing) are related to increased sleep duration, decreased sleep onset latency, and reduced night waking.

Another systematic review examined sleep-wake behavior in the first 12 months of life.[19] Lack of bedtime routines and more television and media exposure before bedtime related to poorer sleep, that is, shorter nighttime sleep duration and more night wakes. Establishing positive routines when children are young sets a foundation for good sleep as children develop. For example, a longitudinal study of American children[20] found positive activities in the hour before bed (e.g., reading a story, cuddle with a caregiver) at 3 months predicted longer sleep duration at 12 months of age; these bedtime activities at 12 months of age predicted fewer sleep problems at 18 months.

Conclusion

Whenever a health care provider is assessing infant and toddler sleep it is critical to examine sleep associations. Assess both negative sleep associations and positive routines and behaviors that facilitate sleep.

SLEEP ENVIRONMENT

Light levels are an important consideration when assessing infant and toddler sleep. Light is considered one of the most powerful factors in synchronizing the circadian sleep/wake rhythm to the 24-hour day and particularly important for infants developing this synchronization between 2 and 10 weeks of age.[21] Tsai and colleagues (2012) found that 2- to 10-week-old infants spent the majority of their time in low light settings and had only brief exposure to bright light settings over 7 days. Harrison (2004) found that 6- to 12-week-old infants who slept more during the night were exposed to significantly more light during the afternoon.[22]

Data on light and infant sleep are limited. Among preschool age children (3–5 years), bright light (>1000 lux; considered bright outdoor light) exposure in the hour before bed induced a 90% suppression of melatonin assessed by saliva, and melatonin suppression remained high for 50 minutes following exposure.[23,24] Melatonin suppression would tend to delay nighttime sleep onset. Further, children may be more sensitive than adults to light before bed,[25] although no data are available for infants.

Artificial light at night (ALAN) may also play a role in night-time sleep,[26] although research is limited and mixed.[27-30] Higher levels of ALAN may be related to later bedtimes and complaints of disrupting sleep in older samples (ages 8–18).[28-30] No studies of infants or preschool-aged children have been identified.

Mold and water damage are risk factors for wheezing in infants, even after controlling for dust mite exposure, and wheezing may impair sleep.[31] For infants prone to allergies, risk of wheezing when mold or water damage was present was five times greater (compared to no mold/water damage). Given the amount of time infants spend in their sleep environments, assessment of environmental exposures is critical.[32] Due to lower weight and smaller size, contaminant exposures (from mattresses, sheets, cribs, etc.) may pose a heightened health risk to infants compared to older children and adults.

Noise in the home and neighborhood (e.g., traffic, sirens) may also impact children's sleep.[33-35] A number of qualitative studies have investigated parent-identified barriers to infant and preschool sleep in multiethnic samples.[34-36] For example, Sanler and colleagues[35] interviewed parents of infants (aged 3–36 months) and pediatric health care and childcare providers. Neighborhood and in-home noise were noted as barriers to sleep by all reporters. A longitudinal study by Blume and colleagues[33] investigated the relationship between night-time transportation noise and infant sleep (via actigraphy) over an 11-day period at ages 3, 6, and 12 months. Overall, night-time transportation noise did *not* significantly predict sleep outcomes (i.e., sleep duration, activity, and variability). However, there was a significant interaction between having siblings in the home and transportation noise; infants without siblings were more sensitive to transportation noise than infants with siblings who have habituated to louder conditions.

Material hardship: Environmental factors associated with poor sleep tend to cooccur. Thus, socio-economic factors are also important to note when assessing sleep in infants. A longitudinal study by Duh-Leong and colleagues (2020)[37] investigated the relationship between financial difficulty, food insecurity, housing disrepair and multiple hardships and sleep duration in a sample of Hispanic families. Financial difficulties, multiple hardships and housing disrepair were associated with poorer sleep duration in 3-month-old infants. Mechanisms linking hardship and child sleep also include psychosocial factors. Increased stress in the household as a result of financial difficulties, multiple hardships or housing disrepair may disrupt parent night-time sleep and shorten night sleep in infants.

Conclusion

Health care providers should incorporate environmental considerations in their assessments of infant and toddler sleep; there is a need to move beyond the focus on individual child- and parent/family-factors to consider how the immediate (e.g., bedroom) and housing (e.g., neighborhood) environment may enhance or interfere with sleep. Many of these factors can be targeted with interventions (e.g., black out curtains, use of a fan for white noise), so assessing the impact of these factors on sleep may be important.

Sleep and Screen Exposure

Attention is increasingly being directed to the relationship between children's screen exposure and sleep. There are four aspects of sleep and screen time to consider.

(a) **Screen time is common:** Among Singaporean children between 0 and 2 years, 53% had daily screen viewing, with a higher prevalence of TV viewing (44.3%) and mobile device viewing (30.1%) than computer time.[38] Children were exposed to a median of 1 hour of screen viewing per day; TV median time was 0.98 hours per day and mobile devices and computer viewing 0.50 hours per day.[38]

(b) **Screen time increases with age:** Among older children (7–24 months), 73% had some screen viewing within a 24-hour period, compared to 28% of children 6 months or younger.[38]

(c) **More screen time is linked to more sleep problems:** Moorman and colleagues (2019)[39] conducted a systematic review of effects of screen time on children's sleep between 1 and 5 years of age. They reported that greater consumption of, access and exposure to, and engagement with screen media were associated with shorter nighttime and total sleep duration, poorer sleep quality, later bed times and wake times, and longer time for sleep onset.[39] Similar findings exist for infants.

For 3-month-old infants, 5 minutes of daytime touchscreen exposure was associated with an average decrease of 13 minutes in daytime sleep, while about 34 minutes of TV exposure was associated with a 20-minute decrease in daytime sleep duration. TV exposure also impacted 24-hour sleep duration. On average, 34 minutes of TV exposure was linked to a 22-minute decrease in 24-hour sleep duration.[40] Among children aged 6 months or less, compared with no screen viewing time, screen viewing up to 1 hour related to 1.5 hours shorter total sleep duration, and viewing of 2 or more hours per day was associated with almost 3 hours of shorter sleep duration.[40] In addition, more daytime touchscreen exposure was associated with fewer night wakes for infants, but was associated with *more* night wakes for 13 month olds.[40] Increased evening/nighttime touchscreen exposure was also associated with increased daytime sleep duration in younger infants.[40] Similarly, a study by Chen and colleagues (2019) found that for every hour of screen time in Singaporean children (aged 0–2), sleep duration was significantly decreased by approximately 16 minutes.[38] Among 7 to 24 month olds, screen times of 1 to 2 hours were associated with 0.84 hours less sleep, and 2 or more hours was related to 0.91 hours less total sleep duration.[38]

   (d) **Screen time varies across families, as does its impact:** In a systematic review, more robust associations between screen media use and negative sleep outcomes occurred for: (1) boys and (2) racial and ethnic minorities.[39] Similar associations were found among children with families characterized by: (1) larger size, (2) parents who work long hours, (3) lower income, (4) less educated parents, (5) single parent households, (6) and urban residence.[39]

On the other hand, lower daytime and evening/nighttime screen exposure occurred among younger infants who (1) shared a room with parents, (2) were breastfed, and (3) had highly educated parents.[39] Black infants also tend to have longer evening/nighttime screen exposures.[40] A Canadian study recruited children from daycare settings (as such children had no/minimal exposure to screens during this time) and found that parents' higher education and income related to longer sleep duration.[41] Even though children were in childcare during the day, an increase of 1 minute per day in total screen time (e.g., TV, video game) was associated with a decrease of 0.2 minutes per day in nighttime sleep duration.[41]

Conclusion

The ubiquity of children's exposure to screens and relationships between infants' and toddlers' exposure to screens and sleep problems emphasizes the importance of health care providers' incorporation of questions about the nature and duration of screen time in assessments of infants' and toddlers' sleep.

BEDSHARING

Parents' and infants' bedsharing, defined as sharing a sleeping surface, remains a controversial area of sleep research. In a narrative review, Mileva-Seitz et al. (2017) distinguished between proactive (or intentional) and reactive (in response to child distress, protests) bedsharing.[42] Families who proactively bedshare tend to take into account safety (e.g., pay attention to potential risks associated with bedding). In contrast, reactive bedsharing involves spontaneous introduction of an infant to the parental bed and safety issues that may result.[42] Volpe and Ball (2015) argued that parents intentionally bedsharing attended to potential risks.[43] Mileva-Seitz et al.'s review indicated that bedsharing was widely associated with older infant and child sleep problems including frequent night-waking and/or time spent awake at night, nighttime crying, requests for comfort and getting out of bed at night, nightmares, and less nighttime sleep.[42] For example, a large Norwegian study of nocturnal sleep duration and waking in infants from 6 to 18 months of age found bedsharing at 6 months predicted more frequent night waking and short nighttime sleep duration at 18 months of age.[44]

Conclusion

Health care providers' awareness of empirical evidence about bedsharing should inform assessments of children's sleep problems. In particular, inquiry about proactive versus reactive bedsharing and attention to safe sleep conditions are important considerations for effects on caregivers and children.

Parent Factors

Sleep behaviors

Parent sleep behaviors (e.g., sleep duration, sleep schedules) have been linked to child sleep in a number of studies of school-age and adolescent children.[45-47] These behaviors include attention to children's sleep hygiene, as well as timing and duration of children's sleep. Research on infant sleep has examined how sleep architecture (such as persistent, regular, and lengthy night waking) in infants impacts maternal/parental sleep. Lack of extensive empirical work about effects of parents' sleep on infants represents an important gap in our understanding of infant sleep.

Parents' mental health

Parents' mental health has largely been linked to parental perceptions of infant sleep problems, rather than infant sleep per se. There is difficulty, however, in determining whether parents' mental distress precedes infants' and toddlers' sleep problems, *or* whether children's sleep problems produce parental distress. For example, Tikotzky and colleagues (2021)[98] studied Israeli mothers longitudinally from the third trimester of pregnancy to 18 months post birth. High maternal distress related to perceptions of children's sleep as problematic.[48] However, from pregnancy to 18 months, changes in maternal emotional distress did not predict changes in infants' objective sleep.

Nevertheless, parents' distress and perceptions of their child's sleep are linked with parents' perceptions of sleep problems.[49] In mediation analyses, Teti and Crosby (2012) found maternal depressive symptoms and dysfunctional cognitions about infant sleep behavior (worries about infant physical/emotional needs) led to maternal presence during the night and in turn higher levels of infant night waking.[50] A study of Canadian mothers and 6-month-old infants found that mothers with higher levels of depressive symptoms and who perceived their infants as having more negative affect reported the most problematic infant sleep.[51] An Israeli intervention study[52] found parents' reactivity to infant crying affected responses to using camping out (i.e., parents sitting in child's sleep space without contact) or checking in (i.e., parents entering the child's sleep space briefly). Higher parental tolerance for crying at baseline predicted larger reductions in the number of infants' nighttime awakenings and greater improvement in parent-reported sleep.[52]

Conclusion

Any assessment of children's sleep requires an understanding of the family context and dynamics. In particular, attention should be paid to how parents create conditions for children's sleep and the psychological effects of children's sleep on parents.

FAMILY FACTORS: FAMILY STRUCTURE/COPARENTING/ MARITAL CONFLICT

The literature specifically examining differences in family structure on sleep among infants and toddlers is sparse. An Israeli study found no differences in infants' or mothers' sleep (by actigraphy and diaries) between single mothers by choice and two-parent families.[53] Studies have examined whether infant sleep predicts coparenting (i.e., how parents work together,[54,55] but not whether coparenting predicts infant sleep. An important contribution of these studies has been to document how disagreements between parents regarding responding to infant night-waking leads to worse perceptions of coparenting over time. Similarly, children's sleep problems have been shown to predict poorer marital relationship.[56,57] Reciprocal effects are also evident; that is, marital conflict is predictive of children's sleep problems.[58,59]

Conclusion

Although data are limited, a basic understanding of family structure/dynamics is essential in any assessment. Attention to how parents work together, or have conflict, with respect to their infant's sleep is also important, as is an understanding of how infant sleep may be affecting coparenting and the parents' relationship.

Assessment Methods

Recommendations for assessment methods are presented first for situations in which a brief assessment is needed; these methods may be relevant for primary care physicians/nurse practitioners or other general health/mental health providers. For example, when a child is being assessed for possible mental health or developmental issues, a provider may wish to screen for sleep-related issues. Second, we provide recommendations for more detailed assessments, which might be relevant when a family is seeking help specifically for their child's sleep issues or when screening suggests more detailed assessment is warranted. Finally, we provide suggestions for a sequenced approach to an in-depth assessment. A recent review[60] noted that there is currently a very limited evidence base when it comes to specific measurement tools for sleep in young children. As such, our recommendations are based on the extant literature and our clinical and research expertise.

BRIEF-SCREENING METHODS

Items assessing parent perceptions of a sleep problem

If clinicians are using brief questionnaires as part of an assessment, there are some sleep-related items that may be useful to include. Parental endorsement of one or two items related to sleep issues would warrant further screening questions.

A recent study of parents of young children (5–19 months) in a pediatric primary care setting examined the utility of using screening items asking about parental perceptions of sleep problems and night waking.[61] However, they were unable to develop an optimal set of items that was both sensitive and specific compared to the Brief Infant Sleep Questionnaire (BISQ).[62] Items asking about parent perceptions of a sleep concern/problem ("Do you think [child's name] has a sleep problem") identified about a third of cases who had a clinically significant score on the BISQ. In contrast, items about night waking ("Does [child's name] often wake up one or more times in the night and does an adult go to [HIM/HER]?") appear to identify too many children (68%) as having sleep problems.

One widely used screening item is from the BISQ. The item asks, "Do you consider your child's sleep a problem?" with four response options: 0 (*no*), 1 (*yes, mild*), 2 (*yes, moderate*), to 3 (*yes, severe*). This item has been used in numerous studies (e.g., Mindell et al., 2010[63]). In light of findings from the Honaker et al. (2021) study,[61] we recommend this single item as a good screening item. It may also be helpful to have an item related to the duration of sleep problems. For example, "How long have your child sleep problems been going on?" ___ Months.

Interview screening questions

Frequently, clinicians need to conduct brief screening for sleep issues, rather than using a full interview. We were unable to identify specific screening questions for infants or toddlers. We propose the following as means of capturing the issues that impact sleep in children of this age. These questions address the factors that have substantial evidence supporting their relationship to sleep issues among infants and toddlers.

SNOOSIE	*Infants (0–2 Years)*
Sleep hygiene	Any screens in rooms or use before bed?
	Any sleep schedules?
	Any sleep routines?
	Attention to sleep safety?
Night-waking	How often, and for how long is child waking?
	Can child get back to sleep independently?
Only back on bed	Is child placed on back in crib or bed?

SNOOSIE	*Infants (0–2 Years)*
Only breastfeeding or bottle feeding 15 minutes before bed	(For infants 5 months or more) Does feeding end before child begins sleep?
Sleep duration	Is child getting enough sleep, including naps?
Independent settling to sleep	Are there any negative sleep associations (e.g., rocking to sleep or feeding to sleep)?
Environment	How much screen time in 24 hours? Any signs of mold in the bedroom? Is there dim light in bedroom? Is there much noise in the neighborhood?

For children age 2 to 5 years old, the BEARS is a widely recommended mnemonic.[64]

BEARS	*Toddler/Preschool (2–5 years)*
Bedtime problems	Does your child have any problems going to bed? Falling asleep?
Excessive daytime sleepiness	Does your child seem overtired or sleepy a lot during the day? Does she still take naps?
Awakenings during the night	Does your child wake up a lot at night?
Regularity and duration of sleep	Does your child have a regular bedtime and wake time? What are they?
Snoring	Does your child snore a lot or have difficult breathing at night?

Questionnaires

The Patient-Reported Outcome Measurement Information System (PROMIS®) instrument development process was recently used to create measures for early childhood (1–5 years olds; PROMIS-EC).[65] The PROMIS-EC sleep disturbance measure assesses: delayed sleep, sleep onset, sleep continuity, and sleep quality; there are 4- and 8-item versions. Parents are asked to report on the child's sleep in the past week on a 5-point Likert scale (1 = Never; 5 = Always). There are also 4- and 8-item versions of the sleep-related impairment scale, which assesses impact on daytime functioning, routines, and mood. Although recently developed, these measures are very promising and have numerous strengths including application of a well-defined process of measure development and norms. A Spanish translation is currently available. Free versions are available at www.healthmeasures.net. In addition, there are multiple ways of deploying the measures including: Electronic Health Record systems, PROMIS® iPad App, REDCap, etc.

In Depth Assessment Methods

Interviews

There are no well-established interviews designed specifically to assess sleep in young children. We briefly review how sleep has been assessed within longer established interviews.

The Preschool Age Psychiatric Assessment (PAPA https://devepi.duhs.duke.edu/measures/the-preschool-age-psychiatric-assessment-papa/[66]) is a structured diagnostic interview to assess psychopathology among 2 to 5 years olds. It includes a section on sleep that captures sleep arrangements, bedtime resistance and rituals, behaviors interfering with sleep initiation, night waking, nap history, etc. It is informed by the work of Anders and colleagues.[67,68]

The Diagnostic Infant and Preschool Assessment (DIPA https://www.michaelscheeringa.com/tools.html) is another diagnostic interview designed to assess "*Diagnostic and Statistical Manual of Mental Disorders,*" Fourth Edition (DSM-IV) disorders in children age 1 to 6.[69] Apart

TABLE 13.2 ■ Summary of Byars et al. (2012) Interview for Infants and Toddlers

Instructions for infants are: "Now I'm going to ask you some questions about (infant's name)'s sleeping habits over the past month. Please think about the past month when answering these questions."
Instructions for 24 to 36 months olds are: "The following statements are about your child's sleep habits and possible difficulties with sleep. Think about the past week. Was this a typical week for your child's sleep or was there something that made it unusual? If typical, then think about this past week when you answer the questions. If last week was unusual for a specific reason, choose the most recent typical week."

Domain	6–12 Months Olds	24–36 Months Olds
	# of Items	# of Items
Overall sleep problem perception	1	1
Sleep onset latency	2	4
Sleep maintenance	2	2
24-hour sleep duration	2	1
Naps	2	1
Sleep location	2	2
Restlessness and vocalizations	2	2
Nightmares/night terrors	1	2
Snoring	1	1
TOTAL	15	16

Structured response options are provided for each item and vary depending on the item.
For example, the napping items for 6 to 12 months olds are:
On average, over the past month, how many days per week has (name) napped during the day?
On average, over the past month, how many naps has (name) taken per day?
For 24 to 36 months olds the item is "How often does (name) nap during the day?" Responses coded as 0 to 1 times per week, 2 to 4 times per week, 5 to 7 times per week.
From Byars, KC, et al. "Prevalence, patterns, and persistence of sleep problems in the first 3 years of life." *Pediatrics*. 2012;129(2):e276–e284.

from sleep items related to specific disorders (e.g., nightmares and trauma), it has items to assess sleep onset disorder and night waking disorder.

Study-specific interviews have also been developed. Gaylor and colleagues[70,71] developed a detailed interview (about 30 minutes) based on the Sleep Habits Questionnaire (a precursor to the Children's Sleep Habits Questionnaire; CSHQ). Mindell and Owens' (2015) textbook includes a "Sleep Evaluation Questionnaire" which is set up in an interview format and provides detailed questions for multiple aspects of sleep.[72]

Similarly, Byars et al. (2012) developed two interviews, one for 6 to 12 months olds (26 items) and another for 24 to 36 months olds (53 items), to assess developmentally relevant domains of sleep; items were adapted from the CSHQ. The interviews assess: sleep onset latency, sleep maintenance; 24-hour sleep duration; naps; sleep location; restlessness and vocalizations; nightmares and night terrors, and snoring. Table 13.2 presents a brief description and the number of items per domain for each age group. We suggest the 6- to 12-month items would be appropriate for children up to age 2 years. If a shorter interview is needed, an 11-item version could be used by excluding the less common issues (i.e., restlessness and vocalizations; nightmares and night terrors; snoring). Coding of responses could be done using the response options provided by Byars et al. (2012),[73] or simply recorded as parents respond.

Diaries

There is no agreement about standards for a sleep diary for young children. The Infant Sleep Chronogram is a sleep diary that has been used in multiple studies.[74] A sleep diary initiated by

Sadeh et al.[75] for assessing sleep in infants includes: (1) lights-off time; (2) morning rise time; (3) sleep duration (from lights-off to waking-up time); (4) number of night wakes; (5) sleep quality, rated on a 4-point scale ranging from 0 (very good) to 3 (bad); (6) duration to fall asleep, rated on a 4-point scale ranging from 0 (less than 5 minutes) to 3 (more than 30 minutes); (7) evening sleepiness, rated on a 3-point scale ranging from 0 (very alert) to 2 (very sleepy); (8) morning drowsiness, rated on a 3-point scale ranging from 0 (very alert) to 2 (very sleepy); and (9) sleep duration/naps during the day. Table 13.3 presents the Tikotzky and Sadeh sleep diary (2009).[76]

TABLE 13.3 ■ Daily Sleep/Activity Log for Infants and Toddlers

Date: dd mm yy **Day:** ☐ Monday ☐ Tuesday ☐ Wednesday ☐ Thursday ☐ Friday ☐ Saturday ☐ Sunday

Person completing the questionnaire: ☐ Father ☐ Mother ☐ Other; Specify →

Were both parents at home during bedtime? ☐ Yes ☐ No; Specify →

Evening Report (when child is going to sleep):
Daytime

Compared to regular days this day was for the child: ☐ A low-activity ☐ An average activity ☐ A high-activity

During the day the child was: ☐ Healthy ☐ Not so healthy ☐ Sick; Specify: →

Daytime Naps: 1) From: ___ To: ___ 2) From: ___ To: ___ 3) From: ___ To: ___ 4) From: ___ To: ___

Bedtime
Exact time of lights-off and getting into bed **for the night**

Upon going to bed the child appeared: ☐ Not sleepy ☐ Somewhat sleepy ☐ Very sleepy

Were there any difficulties with getting into bed (bedtime resistance)? ☐ Not at all ☐ A little ☐ A lot

How long did it take the child to fall asleep: ___

Where did the child fall asleep? ☐ In his/her crib ☐ In parent(s)' bed ☐ Stroller ☐ Parent's arms/lap ☐ Other; Specify: →

How did the child fall asleep? (You can mark more than one option)
☐ In his/her crib, by himself/herself without a caregiver's help.
☐ In his/her crib with parent's active help limited to 2 minutes or less.
☐ In his/her crib with parent's active help for more than 2 minutes.
☐ In his crib with parent's passive presence (without talking, touching, etc.).
☐ Outside the crib, while feeding.
☐ Outside the crib, with a caregiver's active help, other than feeding.
☐ After being moved from his crib (to parent's bed, being rocked, etc.').

TABLE 13.3 ▦ **Daily Sleep/Activity Log for Infants and Toddlers** (Continued)

Night Report (during the night): Please write down all your infant's night wakings, their time and duration. If you had to help your infant fall asleep again, please write down your soothing techniques (feeding, rocking, etc.)

	Time Awoke:	Duration:	Soothing Technique	Parent	
1)				mother, father, other →	
2)				mother, father, other →	
3)				mother, father, other →	
4)				mother, father, other →	
5)				mother, father, other →	
6)				mother, father, other →	

Morning Report (Immediately After the Child Wakes Up)

Morning Rising Time: ☐

Overall Total Sleep Time: ☐ Hours ☐ Minutes

Number of night-wakings ☐ Length of nighttime wakefulness ☐ (total minutes)

The child's sleep was: ☐ Excellent ☐ Good ☐ Somewhat disturbed ☐ Very disturbed

In the morning, the child woke up: ☐ Spontaneously ☐ By noise or disturbance ☐ By an alarm clock ☐ By parents

In the morning the child ☐ Very alert ☐ Slightly tired ☐ Very tired

Special events, phenomena or remarks regarding day or night: ☐

Tikotzky and Sadeh Sleep Diary (used with permission).
Tikotzky L, Sadeh A. Maternal sleep related cognitions and infant sleep: a longitudinal study from pregnancy through the first year. *Child Development.* 2009;80(3):860–874.

Questionnaires

There are few questionnaires designed specifically to assess sleep among infants and young children. Some measures are focused on specific issues, such as safe sleep environment[77]; other studies have included infants but focus on assessment of specific sleep issues (e.g., sleep apnea[78]) or specific populations (e.g., intellectual disabilities; Maas et al.[79]). Recent reviews suggest two measures are widely used and have reasonable psychometric properties[60,80]: The Brief Infant Sleep Questionnaire[62] and the Children's Sleep Habit Questionnaire.[81] It should be noted that the above cited reviews do differ in their appraisal of the literature; for example, Phillips and colleagues[60] recommend the Sleep Habits Questionnaire,[82] which is not part of the review by Sen and Spruyt.[80]

The *Brief Infant Sleep Questionnaire (BISQ)* is one of the most widely used parent-report measures of sleep among young children.[62] In the original version parents complete 10 items regarding their child's sleep. Criteria for defining "poor" versus "good" sleepers was proposed as: waking >3 times per night, waking > 1 hour at night, and total sleep time <9 hours. The measure has good psychometric properties and has been used with infants and toddlers; it has also been used with preschool-age children up to age 6 years.[83,84] A revised version, the BISQ-R,[85] has 3 subscales: Infants' sleep (5 items), Parent perceptions (3 items), and Parent behavior (11 items) and a total score can also be computed. Normative data are available based on multiple US samples; age-referenced norms and scoring instructions are available, upon completion of a terms of use agreement (see https://www.babysleep.com/bisq/). It is important to note that norms for clinical populations are not available.

The *Children's Sleep Habit Questionnaire (CSHQ)* has 33 items that are grouped into 8 subscales: Bedtime Resistance, Sleep-onset Delay, Sleep Duration, Sleep Anxiety, Night Wakings, Parasomnias, Sleep-Disordered Breathing, and Daytime Sleepiness.[81] Scales were formed based on concordance with the International Classification of Sleep Disorders-1 (ICSD-1) system. The measure has good internal consistency and test-retest reliability (0.62–0.79) and differentiates samples of children in the community and children with a sleep disorder. Parent reports of sleep duration are highly related ($r = .80+$) with objective measures such as actigraphs.[86] A short-form of the scale (23 items) omitted "medically-related" items (i.e., parasomnias, sleep disordered breathing) and demonstrated good concordance with the full version in a sample as young as 24 months of age.[87] There have been numerous translations of the scale (e.g., Chinese, Spanish; see Bonuck et al.,[87] for citations). An infant version of the scale was recently developed[88] and tested in Portuguese sample. Data on its use in English-speaking countries is not yet available. Copies of the measure are available online or through ResearchGate (https://www.researchgate.net/publication/12184585).

Sleep assessment incorporated in other early childhood assessments

Given the importance of sleep to infant and child health and the struggles many parents have with their child's sleep, it is not surprising that sleep is noted within the context of child health and preventive health care.

The Rourke Baby Record (https://www.rourkebabyrecord.ca) is widely used by family physicians in Canada for monitoring and preventive health for infants and young children.[89] Items for assessment and advice vary for specific ages (e.g., 0–1; 2, 4, 6 months) to align with well-baby visits. Creating a safe sleep environment is a focus for young infants, which includes sleep position, bedsharing, and other SIDS-related risk factors (e.g., maternal smoking). For older children, recommendations are provided for determining sleep duration and night waking and minimizing screen time.

In the Bright Futures recommendations by the American Academy of Pediatrics for preventive pediatric health care, sleep is not specifically listed (https://downloads.aap.org/AAP/PDF/periodicity_schedule.pdf). However, within the context of anticipatory guidance, it is recommended that parents limit screen time in general, with no screen in the hour before bed given links to sleep issues; sleep safety with respect to SIDS is also noted.[90] There are no specific recommendations for how clinicians should assess these sleep-related issues.

DEVICES

Actigraphy and videosomnography

Actigraphy refers to assessments measured through a small watch-like device that records movement and is typically placed on infants' wrists or ankles.[91,92] The devices record continuously for a set duration and can be scored by hand or by algorithms to get sleep outcomes (e.g., sleep duration, sleep quality). Importantly, actigraphy is a cost-efficient method (compared to polysomnography) most suited for use by specialized sleep professionals. It allows for acquiring data on sleep over long durations (e.g., a week) and can be recorded in real-life settings (e.g., clients' homes), as opposed to polysomnography, which is usually a lab-based assessment method.[91] Actigraphy has demonstrated validity for use with infants when compared to polysomnography and direct observation.[93-95] There are, however, important discrepancies. Camerota et al.[91] compared actigraphy with videosomnography and sleep diaries in sample of 3-month-old infants. Actigraphy was highly related to sleep diary measures of sleep onset time, rise time, and sleep period (r's ranged from .84 to .90), but not night waking (r = .51). Actigraphy showed low agreement with videosomnography for night waking, longest sleep period, wake time and sleep time (r's ranged from .38 to .59). Similarly, actigraphy was observed to have poor specificity (24%) for night-waking in comparison to videosomnography in a sample of neurotypical and neurodivergent children (aged 2–6[96]). Sadeh[97] reviewed the role and validity of actigraphy in sleep medicine; he suggested that actigraphy be used in concert with complementary objective and subjective methods to reduce uncertainties and that the validity of actigraphy be assessed based on reasonable sensitivity (not below .60) in the epoch-by-epoch PSG-actigraphy comparisons and Kappa estimates of reliability, correlations between actigraphy and PSG-derived measures.

In summary, actigraphy is a useful means of obtaining detailed sleep metrics for young children, when such detailed information is needed. There are costs related to the device itself and scoring time. When using actigraphy with young children, it is important to measure sleep across 24 hours (to capture naps), and scoring requires calibration with sleep diaries (to properly code sleep onset). A key limitation is that actigraphy is not be the best method of capturing aspects of sleep that are distressing for parents such as bedtime conflicts. Actigraphy data and parent ratings of night waking have poor agreement, which increases as children age.[96,98] This is primarily because normal night waking, which occurs when infants self-soothe and return to sleep without signaling parents, occurs outside of parents' awareness. However, from a clinical perspective, non-signaled night waking is rarely of concern.

Of note, actigraphy-like devices are also being directly marketed to parents outside of research and clinical contexts. Clinicians may encounter parents who seek care based on the data from these types of devices. The reliability and validity of these devices are often untested.[99,100] There may also be potentially harmful consequences from relying on these devices including parents having a false sense of security or false alarms that increase parents' anxiety about infant's health.[100]

Electronic and smart devices

Parents also have access to smart devices marketed as promoting infant sleep, called Consumer Sleep Technology (CST).[101] Devices such as video baby monitors offer parents the ability to record video examples of problematic sleep (e.g., night waking) and parent-child night-waking interactions at home.[101] Health professionals may elect to use such information to formulate case-by-case interventions for families, if such data are available; however, the American Academy of Sleep Medicine highlights important considerations for their use (see Khosla et al.[101]). Briefly, it is imperative that clinicians understand the capabilities and limitations of CST. Secondly, health data gathered from these devices should be considered in the context of a sleep evaluation by validated measures.

There are other devices marketed for sleep in young children. These include cribs with motion, cribs with built-in white noise machines, and devices that track infant breathing and notify parents of apnea. The efficacy of promoting sleep for many of these devices has not been tested. Further, use of these devices could have detrimental effects on infant sleep or parent anxiety about infant sleep. Clinicians may consider asking parents if they have any sleep-related devices for their infants.

A Sequenced Approach to Detailed Sleep Assessment

When there is time permitting and appointments are scheduled in advance, it is good to have parents' complete questionnaires prior to the initial meeting. When possible and in two-parent families, having both parents/caregivers complete forms may be useful. We recommend using both the PROMIS-EC and either the BISQ-R or CSHQ, depending on the child's age. The CSHQ does not have an item on parental perception of a sleep problem, which we would recommend including. Neither measure inquires about the duration of any sleep problems. As such, we would recommend adding an item to capture parent perceptions of the duration of sleep problems, immediately following the sleep problem perception item. Completion of measures before the first meeting allows for scoring to be completed and highlights areas/issues that may require more in-depth assessment. The PROMIS-EC measures can be administered following treatment recommendations to provide monitoring of outcomes. Outcome monitoring has become the standard of care in the treatment of mental health issues and we encourage adoption of similar practice in pediatric sleep field.[102,103]

Second, a clinical interview can then be used to obtain a better understanding of the child's sleep behaviors, sleep environment, parents' behavior, and family context. As noted, the interview by Byers et al.[38] provides a set of questions related to the child's sleep that could use, with or without, coding responses in a standardized manner. Additional questions can be added in a way that flows directly from these standard questions. For example, the item on sleep onset latency for 6 to 12 months olds is "Some parents have a routine that they follow to prepare their children for bed at night. This may include a bath, reading a book, or other activities. Thinking about the period of time that occurs after this routine has been finished, over the past month, how long has it usually taken to get (name) to sleep at night, on average?" A natural follow-up to understand any bedtime routines would be: "What do you to prepare your child for bed at night?" Similarly, for older infants the items on sleep maintenance are: "On average, over the past month, how many nights a week has (name) woken when he or she sleeps?" "On average, over the past month, how many times has (name) woken each night?." A natural follow-up to understand parents' responses to night waking would be: "What do you do when your child wakes at night?"

Finally, if there is a need for more details on the child's sleep, a sleep diary can be added. We recommend that parents be asked to complete a sleep diary for 2 weeks. The 2-week time frame ensures that both weekdays and weekends are captured. Furthermore, it will provide insight into variation from week to week.

References

1. Adams EL, Master L, Buxton OM, Savage JS. Patterns of infant-only wake bouts and night feeds during early infancy: an exploratory study using actigraphy in mother-father-infant triads. *Pediatr Obes.* 2020;15(10):e12640. Available at: https://doi.org/10.1111/ijpo.12640.
2. Figueiredo B, Dias CC, Pinto TM, Field T. Exclusive breastfeeding at three months and infant sleep-wake behaviors at two weeks, three and six months. *Infant Behav Dev.* 2017;49:62-69. Available at: https://doi.org/10.1016/j.infbeh.2017.06.006.

3. Ramamurthy MB, Sekartini R, Ruangdaraganon N, Huynh DH, Sadeh A, Mindell JA. Effect of current breastfeeding on sleep patterns in infants from Asia-Pacific region. *J Paediatr Child Health*. 2012;48(8): 669-674. Available at: https://doi.org/10.1111/j.1440-1754.2012.02453.x.
4. Murcia L, Reynaud E, Messayke S, et al. Infant feeding practices and sleep development in pre-schoolers from the EDEN mother–child cohort. *J Sleep Res*. 2019;28(6):e12859. Available at: https://doi.org/10.1111/jsr.12859.
5. Doering JJ, Salm Ward TC, Strook S, Campbell JK. A comparison of infant sleep safety guidelines in nine industrialized countries. *J Community Health*. 2019;44(1):81-87. Available at: https://doi.org/10.1007/s10900-018-0556-3.
6. Cole R, Young J, Kearney L, Thompson JMD. Infant care practices and parent uptake of safe sleep messages: a cross-sectional survey in Queensland, Australia. *BMC Pediatr*. 2020;20(1):27. Available at: https://doi.org/10.1186/s12887-020-1917-5.
7. Erck Lambert AB, Parks SE, Cottengim C, Faulkner M, Hauck FR, Shapiro-Mendoza CK. Sleep-related infant suffocation deaths attributable to soft bedding, overlay, and wedging. *Pediatrics*. 2019;143(5):e20183408. Available at: https://doi.org/10.1542/peds.2018-3408.
8. Cole R, Young J, Kearney L, Thompson JMD. Challenges parents encounter when implementing infant safe sleep advice. *Acta Paediatr*. 2021;110(11):3083-3093. Available at: https://doi.org/10.1111/apa.16040.
9. Lau A, Hall W. Safe sleep, day and night: Mothers' experiences regarding infant sleep safety. *J Clin Nurs*. 2016;25(19-20):2816-2826. Available at: https://doi.org/10.1111/jocn.13322.
10. Perinatal Services BC and The Provincial Health Services Authority. *Safer Infant Sleep: Practice Resource for Health-Care Providers*. Perinatal Services BC and The Provincial Health Services Authority; 2022. Available at: http://www.perinatalservicesbc.ca/Documents/Resources/HealthPromotion/Sleep/PSBC_Safer_Infant_Sleep_Practice_Resource.pdf.
11. Scheers NJ, Dayton C, Batcher M, Thach BT. Reports of injury risks and reasons for choice of sleep environments for infants and toddlers. *Matern Child Health J*. 2019;23(12):1613-1620. Available at: https://doi.org/10.1007/s10995-019-02803-7.
12. Blair PS, Ball HL, McKenna JJ, et al. Bedsharing and breastfeeding: The Academy of Breastfeeding Medicine Protocol# 6, Revision 2019. *Breastfeed Med*. 2020;15(1):5-16.
13. Hirshkowitz M, Whiton K, Albert SM, et al. National Sleep Foundation's sleep time duration recommendations: methodology and results summary. *Sleep Health*. 2015;1(1):40-43. Available at: https://doi.org/10.1016/j.sleh.2014.12.010.
14. Paruthi S, Brooks LJ, D'Ambrosio C, et al. Consensus Statement of the American Academy of Sleep Medicine on the Recommended Amount of Sleep for Healthy Children: Methodology and Discussion. *J Clin Sleep Med*. 2016;12(11):1549-1561. Available at: https://doi.org/10.5664/jcsm.6288.
15. Mindell JA, Leichman ES, Composto J, Lee C, Bhullar B, Walters RM. Development of infant and toddler sleep patterns: real-world data from a mobile application. *J Sleep Res*. 2016;25(5):508-516. Available at: https://doi.org/10.1111/jsr.12414.
16. Staton S, Rankin PS, Harding M, et al. Many naps, one nap, none: a systematic review and meta-analysis of napping patterns in children 0-12 years. *Sleep Med Rev*. 2020;50:101247. Available at: https://doi.org/10.1016/j.smrv.2019.101247.
17. Yu X, Quante M, Rueschman M, et al. Emergence of racial/ethnic and socioeconomic differences in objectively measured sleep–wake patterns in early infancy: results of the Rise & SHINE study. *Sleep*. 2021;44(3):zsaa193. Available at: https://doi.org/10.1093/sleep/zsaa193.
18. Hall WA, Nethery E. What does sleep hygiene have to offer children's sleep problems? *Paediatr Respir Rev*. 2019;31:64-74. Available at: https://doi.org/10.1016/j.prrv.2018.10.005.
19. Dias CC, Figueiredo B. Sleep-wake behaviour during the first 12 months of life and associated factors: a systematic review. *Early Child Dev Care*. 2020;190(15):2333-2365. Available at: https://doi.org/10.1080/03004430.2019.1582034.
20. Fiese BH, Cai T, Sutter C, Bost KK. Bedtimes, bedtime routines, and children's sleep across the first 2 years of life. *Sleep*. 2021;44(8):zsab045. Available at: https://doi.org/10.1093/sleep/zsab045.
21. Tsai S, Thomas KA, Lentz MJ, Barnard KE. Light is beneficial for infant circadian entrainment: an actigraphic study. *J Adv Nurs*. 2012;68(8):1738-1747. Available at: https://doi.org/10.1111/j.1365-2648.2011.05857.x.
22. Harrison Y. The relationship between daytime exposure to light and night-time sleep in 6–12-week-old infants. *J Sleep Res*. 2004;13(4):345-352. Available at: https://doi.org/10.1111/j.1365-2869.2004.00435.x.

23. Akacem LD, Wright KP, LeBourgeois MK. Bedtime and evening light exposure influence circadian timing in preschool-age children: a field study. *Neurobiol Sleep Circadian Rhythms*. 2016;1(2):27-31. Available at: https://doi.org/10.1016/j.nbscr.2016.11.002.
24. Akacem LD, Wright KP, LeBourgeois MK. Sensitivity of the circadian system to evening bright light in preschool-age children. *Physiol Rep*. 2018;6(5):e13617. Available at: https://doi.org/10.14814/phy2.13617.
25. Hartstein LE, Behn CD, Akacem LD, Stack N, Wright Jr KP, LeBourgeois MK. High sensitivity of melatonin suppression response to evening light in preschool-aged children. *J Pineal Res*. 2021;72(2):e12780. Available at: https://doi.org/10.1111/jpi.12780.
26. Jackson CL, Gaston SA. The impact of environmental exposures on sleep. In: Grandner MA, ed. *Sleep and Health*. Academic Press; 2019:85-103. Available at: https://doi.org/10.1016/B978-0-12-815373-4.00008-3.
27. Côté-Lussier C, Knudby A, Barnett TA. A novel low-cost method for assessing intra-urban variation in night time light and applications to public health. *Soc Sci Med*. 2020;248:112820. Available at: https://doi.org/10.1016/j.socscimed.2020.112820.
28. Paksarian D, Rudolph KE, Stapp EK, et al. Association of outdoor artificial light at night with mental disorders and sleep patterns among US adolescents. *JAMA Psychiatry*. 2020;77(12):1266-1275. Available at: https://doi.org/10.1001/jamapsychiatry.2020.1935.
29. Spilsbury JC, Frame J, Magtanong R, Rork K. Sleep environments of children in an urban U.S. setting exposed to interpersonal violence. *Behav Sleep Med*. 2016;14(6):585-601. Available at: https://doi.org/10.1080/15402002.2015.1048449.
30. Vollmer C, Michel U, Randler C. Outdoor light at night (LAN) is correlated with eveningness in adolescents. *Chronobiol Int*. 2012;29(4):502-508. Available at: https://doi.org/10.3109/07420528.2011.635232.
31. Cho SH, Reponen T, LeMasters G, et al. Mold damage in homes and wheezing in infants. *Ann Allergy Asthma Immunol*. 2006;97(4):539-545. Available at: https://doi.org/10.1016/S1081-1206(10)60947-7.
32. Boor BE, Spilak MP, Laverge J, Novoselac A, Xu Y. Human exposure to indoor air pollutants in sleep microenvironments: a literature review. *Build Environ*. 2017;125:528-555. Available at: https://doi.org/10.1016/j.buildenv.2017.08.050.
33. Blume C, Schoch SF, Vienneau D, et al. Association of transportation noise with sleep during the first year of life: a longitudinal study. *Environ Res*. 2021;203:111776. Available at: https://doi.org/10.1016/j.envres.2021.111776.
34. Martin-Biggers J, Spaccarotella K, Hongu N, Alleman G, Worobey J, Byrd-Bredbenner C. Translating it into real life: a qualitative study of the cognitions, barriers and supports for key obesogenic behaviors of parents of preschoolers. *BMC Public Health*. 2015;15:189. Available at: https://doi.org/10.1186/s12889-015-1554-3.
35. Sadler LS, Banasiak N, Canapari C, et al. Perspectives on sleep from multiethnic community parents, pediatric providers, and childcare providers. *J Dev Behav Pediatr*. 2020;41(7):540-549. Available at: https://doi.org/10.1097/DBP.0000000000000799.
36. Lindsay AC, Moura Arruda CA, Tavares Machado MM, De Andrade GP, Greaney ML. Exploring Brazilian immigrant mothers' beliefs, attitudes, and practices related to their preschool-age children's sleep and bedtime routines: a qualitative study conducted in the United States. *Int J Environ Res Public Health*. 2018;15(9):1923. Available at: https://doi.org/10.3390/ijerph15091923.
37. Duh-Leong C, Messito MJ, Katzow MW, et al. Material hardships and infant and toddler sleep duration in low-income Hispanic families. *Acad Pediatr*. 2020;20(8):1184-1191. Available at: https://doi.org/10.1016/j.acap.2020.07.003.
38. Chen B, van Dam RM, Tan CS, et al. Screen viewing behavior and sleep duration among children aged 2 and below. *BMC Public Health*. 2019;19(1):1-10. Available at: https://doi.org/10.1186/s12889-018-6385-6.
39. Moorman JD, Morgan P, Adams TL. The implications of screen media use for the sleep behavior of children ages 0–5: a systematic review of the literature. *Curr Sleep Med Rep*. 2019;5(3):164-172.
40. Kahn M, Barnett N, Glazer A, Gradisar M. Sleep and screen exposure across the beginning of life: deciphering the links using big-data analytics. *Sleep*. 2021;44(3):zsaa158. Available at: https://doi.org/10.1093/sleep/zsaa158.
41. Zhang Z, Adamo KB, Ogden N, et al. Longitudinal correlates of sleep duration in young children. *Sleep Med*. 2021;78:128-134. Available at: https://doi.org/10.1016/j.sleep.2020.12.023.
42. Mileva-Seitz VR, Bakermans-Kranenburg MJ, Battaini C, Luijk MP. Parent-child bed-sharing: the good, the bad, and the burden of evidence. *Sleep Med Rev*. 2017;32:4-27. Available at: https://doi.org/10.1016/j.smrv.2016.03.003.

43. Volpe LE, Ball HL. Infant sleep-related deaths: why do parents take risks? *Arch Dis Child*. 2015;100(7): 603-604. Available at: https://doi.org/10.1136/archdischild-2014-307745.

44. Hysing M, Harvey AG, Torgersen L, Ystrom E, Reichborn-Kjennerud T, Sivertsen B. Trajectories and predictors of nocturnal awakenings and sleep duration in infants. *J Dev Behav Pediatr*. 2014;35(5): 309-316. Available at: https://doi.org/10.1097/DBP.0000000000000064.

45. Kouros CD, El-Sheikh M. Within-family relations in objective sleep duration, quality, and schedule. *Child Dev*. 2017;88(6):1983-2000. Available at: https://doi.org/10.1111/cdev.12667.

46. Meltzer LJ, Mindell JA. Relationship between child sleep disturbances and maternal sleep, mood, and parenting stress: a pilot study. *J Fam Psychol*. 2007;21(1):67-73. Available at: https://doi.org/10.1037/0893-3200.21.1.67.

47. Urfer-Maurer N, Weidmann R, Brand S, et al. The association of mothers' and fathers' insomnia symptoms with school-aged children's sleep assessed by parent report and in-home sleep-electroencephalography. *Sleep Med*. 2017;38:64-70. Available at: https://doi.org/10.1016/j.sleep.2017.07.010.

48. Tikotzky L, Volkovich E, Meiri G. Maternal emotional distress and infant sleep: a longitudinal study from pregnancy through 18 months. *Dev Psychol*. 2021;57(7):1111-1123. Available at: https://doi.org/10.1037/dev0001081.

49. Hall WA, Moynihan M, Bhagat R, Wooldridge J. Relationships between parental sleep quality, fatigue, cognitions about infant sleep, and parental depression pre and post-intervention for infant behavioral sleep problems. *BMC Pregnancy Childbirth*. 2017;17(1):1-10.

50. Teti DM, Crosby B. Maternal Depressive symptoms, dysfunctional cognitions, and infant night waking: the role of maternal nighttime behavior. *Child Dev*. 2012;83(3):939-953. Available at: https://doi.org/10.1111/j.1467-8624.2012.01760.x.

51. Burdayron R, Butler BP, Béliveau MJ, Dubois-Comtois K, Pennestri MH. Perception of infant sleep problems: the role of negative affectivity and maternal depression. *J Clin Sleep Med*. 2021;17(6): 1279-1285. Available at: https://doi.org/10.5664/jcsm.9188.

52. Kahn M, Livne-Karp E, Juda-Hanael M, et al. Behavioral interventions for infant sleep problems: the role of parental cry tolerance and sleep-related cognitions. *J Clin Sleep Med*. 2020;16(8):1275-1283. Available at: https://doi.org/10.5664/jcsm.8488.

53. Ben-Zion H, Volkovich E, Meiri G, Tikotzky L. Mother–infant sleep and maternal emotional distress in solo-mother and two-parent families. *J Pediatr Psychol*. 2020;45(2):181-193. Available at: https://doi.org/10.1093/jpepsy/jsz097.

54. McDaniel BT, Teti DM. Coparenting quality during the first three months after birth: the role of infant sleep quality. *J Fam Psychol*. 2012;26(6):886-895. Available at: https://doi.org/10.1037/a0030707.

55. Reader JM, Teti DM, Cleveland MJ. Cognitions about infant sleep: interparental differences, trajectories across the first year, and coparenting quality. *J Fam Psychol*. 2017;31(4):453-463. Available at: https://doi.org/10.1037/fam0000283.

56. Martin J, Hiscock H, Hardy P, Davey B, Wake M. Adverse associations of infant and child sleep problems and parent health: an Australian population study. *Pediatrics*. 2007;119(5):947-955. Available at: https://doi.org/10.1542/peds.2006-2569.

57. Meijer AM, van den Wittenboer GLH. Contribution of infants' sleep and crying to marital relationship of first-time parent couples in the 1st year after childbirth. *J Fam Psychol*. 2007;21(1):49-57. Available at: https://doi.org/10.1037/0893-3200.21.1.49.

58. Bernier A, Bélanger MÈ, Bordeleau S, Carrier J. Mothers, fathers, and toddlers: Parental psychosocial functioning as a context for young children's sleep. *Dev Psychol*. 2013;49(7):1375-1384. Available at: https://doi.org/10.1037/a0030024.

59. Kelly RJ, El-Sheikh M. Marital conflict and children's sleep: reciprocal relations and socioeconomic effects. *J Fam Psychol*. 2011;25(3):412-422. Available at: http://dx.doi.org.proxy1.lib.uwo.ca/10.1037/a0023789.

60. Phillips SM, Summerbell C, Ball HL, Hesketh KR, Saxena S, Hillier-Brown FC. The validity, reliability, and feasibility of measurement tools used to assess sleep of pre-school aged children: a systematic rapid review. *Front Pediatr*. 2021;9:770262. Available at: https://doi.org/10.3389/fped.2021.770262.

61. Honaker SM, McQuillan ME, Mindell JA, Downs SM, Slaven JE, Schwichtenberg AJ. Screening for problematic sleep in a diverse sample of infants. *J Pediatr Psychol*. 2021;46(7):824-834. Available at: https://doi.org/10.1093/jpepsy/jsab050.

62. Sadeh A. A brief screening questionnaire for infant sleep problems: validation and findings for an internet sample. *Pediatrics*. 2004;113(6):e570-e577. Available at: https://doi.org/10.1542/peds.113.6.e570.

63. Mindell JA, Sadeh A, Wiegand B, How TH, Goh DY. Cross-cultural differences in infant and toddler sleep. *Sleep Med.* 2010;11(3):274-280. Available at: https://doi.org/10.1016/j.sleep.2009.04.012.

64. Owens JA, Dalzell V. Use of the "BEARS" sleep screening tool in a pediatric residents' continuity clinic: a pilot study. *Sleep Med.* 2005;6(1):63-69. Available at: https://doi.org/10.1016/j.sleep.2004.07.015.

65. Blackwell CK, Wakschlag L, Krogh-Jespersen S, et al. Pragmatic health assessment in early childhood: the PROMIS® of developmentally based measurement for pediatric psychology. *J Pediatr Psychol.* 2020;45(3):311-318. Available at: https://doi.org/10.1093/jpepsy/jsz094.

66. Egger HL, Angold A, Small B, Copeland W. The Preschool Age Psychiatric Assessment: a structured parent interview for assessing psychiatric symptoms and disorders in preschool children. In: Carmen-Wiggins R, Carter AS, eds. *The Oxford Handbook of Infant, Toddler, and Preschool Mental Health Assessment.* 2nd ed. Oxford University Press; 2019:227-243.

67. Anders TF, Goodlin-Jones B, Sadeh A. Sleep disorders. In: Zeanah CH, ed. *Handbook of Infant Mental Health.* Guilford Press, New York; 2000;326-338.

68. Anders TF, Eiben LA. Pediatric sleep disorders: a review of the past 10 years. *J Am Acad Child Adolesc Psychiatry.* 1997;36(1):9-20. Available at: https://doi.org/10.1097/00004583-199701000-00012.

69. Scheeringa MS, Haslett N. The reliability and criterion validity of the Diagnostic Infant and Preschool Assessment: a new diagnostic instrument for young children. *Child Psychiatry Hum Dev.* 2010;41(3):299-312. doi:10.1007/s10578-009-0169-2.

70. Gaylor EE, Goodlin-Jones BL, Anders TF. Classification of young children's sleep problems: a pilot study. *J Am Acad Child Adolesc Psychiatry.* 2001;40(1):61-67. doi:10.1097/00004583-200101000-00017.

71. Gaylor EE, Burnham MM, Goodlin-Jones BL, Anders TF. A longitudinal follow-up study of young children's sleep patterns using a developmental classification system. *Behav Sleep Med.* 2005;3(1):44-61. Available at: https://doi.org/10.1207/s15402010bsm0301_6.

72. Mindell JA, Owens AO. *A Clinical Guide to Pediatric Sleep: Diagnosis and Management of Sleep Problems.* 3rd ed. Wolters Kluwer; 2015.

73. Byars KC, Yolton K, Rausch J, Lanphear B, Beebe DW. Prevalence, patterns, and persistence of sleep problems in the first 3 years of life. *Pediatrics.* 2012;129(2):e276-e284. Available at: https://doi.org/10.1542/peds.2011-0372.

74. Figueiredo B, Dias CC, Pinto TM, Field T. Infant sleep-wake behaviors at two weeks, three and six months. *Infant Behav Dev.* 2016;44:169-178. Available at: https://doi.org/10.1016/j.infbeh.2016.06.011.

75. Sadeh A, Lavie P, Scher A, Tirosh E, Epstein R. Actigraphic home-monitoring sleep-disturbed and control infants and young children: a new method for pediatric assessment of sleep-wake patterns. *Pediatrics.* 1991;87(4):494-499. Available at: https://doi.org/10.1542/peds.87.4.494.

76. Tikotzky L, Sadeh A. Maternal sleep-related cognitions and infant sleep: a longitudinal study from pregnancy through the 1st year. *Child Dev.* 2009;80(3):860-874. Available at: https://doi.org/10.1111/j.1467-8624.2009.01302.x.

77. Whiteside-Mansell L, Nabaweesi R, Caballero AR, Mullins SH, Miller BK, Aitken ME. Assessment of safe sleep: validation of the Parent Newborn Sleep Safety Survey. *J Pediatr Nurs.* 2017;35:30-35. Available at: https://doi.org/10.1016/j.pedn.2017.02.033.

78. Bertran K, Mesa T, Rosso K, Krakowiak MJ, Pincheira E, Brockmann PE. Diagnostic accuracy of the Spanish version of the Pediatric Sleep Questionnaire for screening of obstructive sleep apnea in habitually snoring children. *Sleep Med.* 2015;16(5):631-636. Available at: https://doi.org/10.1016/j.sleep.2014.10.024.

79. Maas AP, Didden R, Korzilius H, et al. Psychometric properties of a sleep questionnaire for use in individuals with intellectual disabilities. *Res Dev Disabil.* 2011;32(6):2467-2479. Available at: https://doi.org/10.1016/j.ridd.2011.07.013.

80. Sen T, Spruyt K. Pediatric sleep tools: an updated literature review. *Front Psychiatry.* 2020;11:317. Available at: https://www.frontiersin.org/article/10.3389/fpsyt.2020.00317.

81. Owens JA, Spirito A, McGuinn M. The Children's Sleep Habits Questionnaire (CSHQ): Psychometric properties of a survey instrument for school-aged children. *Sleep.* 2000;23(8):1043-1051.

82. Sekine M, Chen X, Hamanishi S, Wang H, Yamagami T, Kagamimori S. The validity of sleeping hours of healthy young children as reported by their parents. *J Epidemiol.* 2002;12(3):237-242. Available at: https://doi.org/10.2188/jea.12.237.

83. Bruni O, Melegari MG, Esposito A, et al. Executive functions in preschool children with chronic insomnia. *J Clin Sleep Med.* 2020;16(2):231-241. Available at: https://doi.org/10.5664/jcsm.8172.

84. Hysing M, Sivertsen B, Garthus-Niegel S, Eberhard-Gran M. Pediatric sleep problems and social-emotional problems. A population-based study. *Infant Behav Dev.* 2016;42:111-118. Available at: https://doi.org/10.1016/j.infbeh.2015.12.005.
85. Mindell JA, Gould RA, Tikotzy L, Leichman ES, Walters RM. Norm-referenced scoring system for the Brief Infant Sleep Questionnaire—Revised (BISQ-R). *Sleep Med.* 2019;63:106-114. Available at: https://doi.org/10.1016/j.sleep.2019.05.010.
86. Tikotzky L, Sadeh A. Sleep patterns and sleep disruptions in kindergarten children. *J Clin Child Adolesc Psychol.* 2001;30(4):581-591. Available at: https://doi.org/10.1207/S15374424J CCP3004_13.
87. Bonuck KA, Goodlin-Jones BL, Schechter C, Owens J. Modified Children's sleep habits questionnaire for behavioral sleep problems: a validation study. *Sleep Health.* 2017;3(3):136-141. Available at: https://doi.org/10.1016/j.sleh.2017.03.009.
88. Dias CC, Figueiredo B, Pinto TM. Children's sleep habits questionnaire-infant version. *J Pediatr.* 2018;94(2):146-154.
89. Li P, Rourke L, Leduc D, Arulthas S, Rezk K, Rourke J. Rourke Baby Record 2017: clinical update for preventive care of children up to 5 years of age. *Can Fam Physician.* 2019;65(3):183-191.
90. Turner K. Well-child visits for infants and young children. *Am Fam Physician.* 2018;98(6):347-353.
91. Camerota M, Tully KP, Grimes M, Gueron-Sela N, Propper CB. Assessment of infant sleep: how well do multiple methods compare? *Sleep.* 2018;41(10):zsy146. Available at: https://doi.org/10.1093/sleep/zsy146.
92. Schoch SF, Kurth S, Werner H. Actigraphy in sleep research with infants and young children: current practices and future benefits of standardized reporting. *J Sleep Res.* 2021;30(3):e13134. Available at: https://doi.org/10.1111/jsr.13134.
93. Gnidovec B, Neubauer D, Zidar J. Actigraphic assessment of sleep–wake rhythm during the first 6 months of life. *Clin Neurophysiol.* 2002;113(11):1815-1821. Available at: https://doi.org/10.1016/S1388-2457(02)00287-0.
94. Meltzer LJ, Montgomery-Downs HE, Insana SP, Walsh CM. Use of actigraphy for assessment in pediatric sleep research. *Sleep Med Rev.* 2012;16(5):463-475. Available at: https://doi.org/10.1016/j.smrv.2011.10.002.
95. So K, Buckley P, Adamson TM, Horne RS. Actigraphy correctly predicts sleep behavior in infants who are younger than six months, when compared with polysomnography. *Pediatr Res.* 2005;58(4):761-765. Available at: https://doi.org/10.1203/01.PDR.0000180568.97221.56.
96. Sitnick SL, Goodlin-Jones BL, Anders TF. The use of actigraphy to study sleep disorders in preschoolers: some concerns about detection of nighttime awakenings. *Sleep.* 2008;31(3):395-401.
97. Sadeh A. The role and validity of actigraphy in sleep medicine: an update. *Sleep Med Rev.* 2011;15(4):259-267. Available at: https://doi.org/10.1016/j.smrv.2010.10.001.
98. Tikotzky L, Volkovich E. Infant nocturnal wakefulness: a longitudinal study comparing three sleep assessment methods. *Sleep.* 2019;42(1):zsy191. Available at: https://doi.org/10.1093/sleep/zsy191.
99. Bonafide CP, Jamison DT, Foglia EE. The emerging market of smartphone-integrated infant physiologic monitors. *JAMA.* 2017;317(4):353-354. Available at: https://doi.org/10.1001/jama.2016.19137.
100. Stiefel A. At-home cardiorespiratory monitors for newborns: helping or hurting parents' peace of mind. *Pediatr Nurs.* 2021;47(1):11-16.
101. Khosla S, Deak MC, Gault D, et al. Consumer sleep technology: an American Academy of Sleep Medicine Position Statement. *J Clin Sleep Med.* 2018;14(5):877-880. Available at: https://doi.org/10.5664/jcsm.7128.
102. Dozois DJA, Mikail SF, Alden LE, et al. The CPA Presidential Task Force on evidence-based practice of psychological treatments. *Can Psychol.* 2014;55(3):153-160. Available at: https://doi.org/10.1037/a0035767.
103. Wolpert M, Ford T, Trustam E, et al. Patient-reported outcomes in child and adolescent mental health services (CAMHS): Use of idiographic and standardized measures. *J Mental Health.* 2012;21(2):165-173. Available at: https://doi.org/10.3109/09638237.2012.664304.

Behavioral Interventions for Infant Sleep Problems: Efficacy, Safety, Predictors, Moderators, and Future Directions

Michal Kahn ■ Hannah Whittall ■ Liat Tikotzky

Introduction

Pediatric insomnia is highly prevalent, with an estimated 15% to 30% of infants and toddlers having difficulties initiating and maintaining sleep, prolonged nighttime wakefulness, and high dependency on external regulation to assume sleep.[1,2] When untreated, such sleep problems tend to persist and cause considerable disruption in the family context. It is thus unsurprising that they constitute one of the most common concerns presented to pediatricians and other health care professionals. Furthermore, sleep problems have been associated with a myriad of negative short- and long-term outcomes, including child physiological, emotional, cognitive, and behavioral difficulties, and poor parent health and well-being.[3-9] Given these adverse consequences, adequate assessment and intervention are clearly required to alleviate the burden of insomnia in young children.

Behavioral interventions have been the most widely researched treatment approach for pediatric insomnia. These interventions include a broad spectrum of modules and techniques to address fragmented or insufficient sleep in infants. Systematic reviews and meta-analyses have consistently demonstrated the benefits of behavioral sleep interventions. In a canonical review paper and companion practice parameter paper, an American Academy of Sleep Medicine task force found that 94% of the 52 treatment studies available at the time yielded clinically significant improvement, with 82% of participating infants and young children deriving benefit.[10,11] Further support was found in a meta-analysis of controlled clinical trials, demonstrating that behavioral interventions for children 0 to 5 years old yield significant reductions in sleep onset latency, night waking frequency, and nocturnal wakefulness, with small to medium effect sizes for each of these metrics.[12] Most recently, Meltzer et al.[13] published a scoping review, encompassing a broad range of studies evaluating behavioral treatments for pediatric insomnia, including various study designs and populations (e.g., typically and atypically developing children). Sixty-one studies were identified as focusing on young children's sleep, and these generated moderate to strong empirical evidence of efficacy.

Despite this wealth of evidence, many questions continue to keep researchers in this field up at night, along with many infants and their parents. While behavioral interventions are efficacious, they do not benefit all families, and many parents are deterred from implementing them.[14] Clinical trials have reported attrition rates of 10% to 30%,[15,16] partly due to difficulties adhering to treatment. Correspondingly, behavioral sleep interventions have generated heated debates among academics, clinicians, and parents, rendering many unsure as to how to manage issues with their infant's sleep.

This chapter aims to address the existing key questions concerning behavioral interventions for infant sleep problems. First, we address the "what" and "which" questions, by presenting the main available intervention approaches, evidence for their efficacy and effectiveness, and comparisons between them. Second, we focus on the "when" and "for whom," discussing factors that may predict and moderate these interventions' outcomes. We then examine the controversy around the use of some of these approaches (represented by the provoking "which side are you on" question), including evidence for safety versus "side-effects," and suggest a middle ground through which these interventions can be perceived. Finally, we pinpoint gaps in the existing literature and address the question of "where to next" by proposing directions for future research in this field.

The "What" and "Which"—Existing Behavioral Interventions for Infant Sleep Problems and How Well They Compare With One Another

The term "behavioral sleep interventions" encompasses various techniques, all of which are based to some extent on learning principles and target infant or parent behavior to improve sleep. While pharmacological treatments for pediatric insomnia are available, and melatonin specifically has recently received increased research attention (e.g., Esposito et al.[17]), synthesizing findings regarding pharmacological interventions exceeds the scope of the present chapter. Also noteworthy is our focus on behavioral insomnia, diagnosed after adequate assessment has been carried out, ruling out other possible medical issues (e.g., obstructive sleep apnea). In the following section we present behavioral approaches starting with preventative, low-intensity methods (that usually entail less infant distress) and concluding with the more intensive extinction-based techniques.

SLEEP EDUCATION

Psychoeducation about sleep has been one of the fundamental and most common approaches to address infant sleep problems. It is usually the main modality in prevention programs, delivered during pregnancy or in the first months postpartum.[18] It is also often incorporated in treatment programs aimed at alleviating existing infant sleep problems, typically in infants aged >6 months (e.g., Gradisar et al.[19]). Sleep education may cover a broad spectrum of topics, including typical sleep development, circadian rhythms, the effects of light exposure, sleep homeostatic pressure, sleep architecture and spontaneous awakenings between sleep cycles, sleep hygiene, constructive sleep associations, links between sleep and feeding, and parental involvement in the sleep context. The potential benefits of preventing sleep problems before they occur are vast, given the considerable physiological, emotional, and economic costs of such problems. Due to the low intensity of many sleep education interventions, they also have the potential for high cost-effectiveness and can be used as a first step in stepped care approaches.[20]

In the AASM's 2006 practice parameter paper,[11] parent education/prevention was deemed a *Standard* treatment approach for young children, based on modified Sackett criteria. This indicated a generally accepted patient care strategy, with high-quality evidence. Still, the recommendation was based on four studies that were available at the time. A 2010 Cochrane review found that postnatal parental education programs resulted in increased infant sleep duration, but not increased sleep consolidation.[18] This review was based on randomized controlled trials (RCTs) alone, yet only four studies were identified, precluding any exhaustive conclusions regarding the efficacy of prevention programs. A meta-analysis published in 2016 identified nine RCTs that examined the efficacy of sleep-focused interventions administered in the perinatal period.[21] Consistent with Bryanton and Beck,[18] benefits were observed for infant sleep nighttime duration but not for nighttime awakenings.[21] Small improvements in maternal mood were also detected in this meta-analysis, although the authors suggested that this result was not definitive, due to a potential risk for publication bias.

Since then, several additional investigations into the effects of psychoeducation on infant sleep have been conducted, generally yielding null to small effects. Galland and colleagues[22] conducted a large ($N = 802$) RCT to test the effects of group sleep education delivered antenatally and a home visit at 3 weeks postpartum. These authors found that parent-reported infant sleep problems at 6 months of age were equivalent between groups that received sleep education and those that did not. Moreover, no significant differences were found between groups in infant self-settling and benefits were not documented for parent depression, nor for parent fatigue or sleep. Actigraphic infant nighttime awakenings were significantly less frequent in the intervention group, yet this difference was not deemed clinically meaningful.

Santos et al.[23] evaluated the impact of sleep education delivered at 3 months postpartum on infants' sleep duration (assessed using actigraphy and parent reports) compared to a feeding education control group. This too was a large-scale RCT ($N = 586$) and included follow-up assessments at 6, 12, and 24 months of age. The intervention was delivered in two home visits and two telephone calls when infants were 3 months old. In line with Galland et al.'s[22] findings, no significant differences were found between groups following the intervention, despite some trends in the expected direction (e.g., longer nighttime sleep duration in infants whose parents received sleep education). A third RCT assessed whether a two-session group psychoeducation intervention delivered during the third trimester to first-time mothers would prevent postpartum sleep problems.[24] Mothers who received the intervention and mothers who only received information booklets did not differ significantly in ratings of infant sleep quality. At 4 months postpartum, maternal sleep quality was higher in the intervention group, and insomnia symptoms were lower, yet these effects were small and not apparent at 6 weeks or 10 months postpartum.

The null or very modest effects detected in these three recent large and well-controlled RCTs may be due to several factors, such as low adherence, the exclusion of fathers from prevention programs, and the high potential for floor effects when psychoeducation is provided to educated mothers of typically developing infants.[25] Preventative interventions addressing infant sleep may be more beneficial when delivered beyond the antenatal or newborn period, once parents have gotten to know their infant better and got through the "fourth trimester."[22] Moreover, given these latest RCTs, it has been suggested that resources such as home visits and face-to-face counseling may be more wisely invested in delivering interventions to families at risk or to those that already report infant sleep problems.[25]

When provided to parents who already perceive their infant's sleep as a problem, psychoeducation has usually been offered in conjunction with other treatment modalities (e.g., graduated extinction), making it difficult to evaluate its therapeutic effect as a standalone treatment. Sleep education is often used as a control group for other intervention strategies (e.g., Gradisar et al.[19]), but to the best of our knowledge, has not been compared to a nonactive control when treating infants with insomnia. Moreover, the topics covered may vary significantly between studies and protocols, possibly rendering psychoeducation a "catchall category." For example, some educational interventions have guided parents to wait a few minutes before attending to the infant when they wake at night,[23,26] resembling extinction-based approaches. Additionally, many educational interventions emphasize the importance of a consistent structured bedtime routine.[24,27,28] This overlap in content blurs the distinction between psychoeducation and other intervention approaches, making the specific benefit of psychoeducation unclear. More research is needed to determine which topics should be covered in sleep education interventions, perhaps by developing standardized protocols.

In summary, almost all forms of behavioral interventions for infant sleep problems include a psychoeducation module of some kind. Within the context of prevention programs, these have generated null to small benefits for infants and parents. Providing the education after the first few months, when parents have gotten to know their infant, may lead to superior outcomes. When provided later on in development, in families who report problems with their infant's sleep, psychoeducation usually forms the basis for other treatment components (e.g., education about sleep homeostatic pressure to provide a rationale for bedtime fading). Despite its modest efficacy, psychoeducation could be used as a low-intensity, low-cost, first-step approach to address mild to moderate cases of infant insomnia. Future work is warranted to determine the efficacy of psychoeducation approaches for diverse and at-risk populations, which content modules should be included in these interventions, what would be the optimal timing of delivery, and whether low-cost highly accessible delivery modes (e.g., digital programs) yield equally beneficial effects.

BEDTIME ROUTINES

Implementing consistent and appropriate bedtime routines is a highly ubiquitous pediatric sleep health recommendation. Bedtime routines may include 2 to 4 activities, such as bathing and reading stories, lasting no longer than 30 to 40 minutes, followed by lights out time.[29] Consistency is key, and parents are advised to repeat the same activities at the same time each night, for as many nights a week as possible. Building on stimulus control therapy techniques,[30] and accordant with the idea of "sleep hygiene," bedtime routines aim to strengthen associations between sleep-promoting stimuli (e.g., a massage) and sleep onset and to avoid stimuli that may interfere with sleep onset (e.g., technology devices). Sleep then becomes an anticipated and rewarding experience, rather than an unpredictable and potentially unpleasant occurrence. Consistent routines hold the potential to regulate not only behavioral and emotional responses to the sleep context but also the child's circadian rhythms, provided that bedtimes are consistent across nights.[29]

The links between consistent implementation of bedtime routines and young children's sleep have been demonstrated in multiple studies. Cross-sectional and longitudinal investigations have identified associations between bedtime routines and earlier bedtimes, shorter sleep onset latencies, longer nighttime sleep duration, and more consolidated sleep.[31-34] Benefits extend beyond the sleep domain, and include reduced bedtime resistance, and improved child and parent mood, emotion regulation, and child literacy outcomes.[35-37]

Intervention studies have further established the role of bedtime routines in pediatric sleep. A recent scoping review of behavioral treatments for pediatric insomnia found that bedtime/positive routines were the most commonly studied approach, included in 29 (61.7%) of the 47 studies investigating treatments for insomnia in young children.[13] Most of these studies examined the use of bedtime routines as part of multicomponent behavioral sleep interventions, not allowing for evaluation of their individual therapeutic potency. Yet, the efficacy of bedtime routines or individual prebedtime activities as independent interventions has been demonstrated in a few studies.[38-40] Mindell and colleagues[38] randomly assigned mothers of children aged 7 to 36 months old with perceived sleep problems to either a bedtime routine or to a control condition. Instructions for the bedtime routine group included implementing the following three steps over approximately 30 minutes: (1) bathing; (2) massage or lotion; and (3) quiet activities, such as cuddling or singing a lullaby. Mothers in the control group were instructed to continue their child's usual routine. Two weeks following the intervention, significant reductions in maternal reports of sleep onset latency and in the frequency and duration of nighttime awakenings were found in the bedtime routine group, but not in the control group. Mothers who implemented bedtime routines also reported having improved mood and decreased child bedtime resistance.

Studies into the effects of prebedtime massage have also found beneficial effects. In a study of 23 infants and toddlers, a 15-minute massage before lights out time resulted in lower bedtime resistance and shorter sleep onset latencies compared to reading a bedtime story.[40] In a later study, massage with lotion was found to be superior to massage without lotion and to a no massage condition, in reducing mother-reported nighttime awakenings and increasing sleep duration in newborn infants.[41] The mechanisms by which prebedtime massage may exercise its benefits may include positive parent-child interactions, muscle relaxation, and circadian regulation. Evidence for the latter is indicated in a study by Ferber et al.,[42] revealing that 30-minute prebedtime "massage therapy" for 2 weeks, starting when infants were 10 days old, led to higher levels of nocturnal melatonin secretion (6-sulfatoxymelatonin excretions) at 12 weeks of age, compared to control. These authors concluded that the massage served as a zeitgeber, facilitating the alignment of infants' circadian rhythms to the 24-hour day. While these findings provide preliminary evidence for a physiological pathway through which bedtime routines may promote sleep, further investigations are warranted to establish these effects and examine them in infants with pediatric insomnia. Furthermore, more research is needed to explore other potential mechanisms of bedtime routines and their individual components, and so are studies examining diverse infant populations (e.g., infants with neurodevelopmental conditions and diverse cultural backgrounds).

BEDTIME FADING

In the late 1980s Sleep Restriction Therapy (SRT) was developed as a behavioral intervention for chronic insomnia in adults.[43] SRT involves implementing a prescribed time-in-bed that matches the individual's baseline average total sleep time. This new restricted schedule is intended to regularize and entrain circadian rhythms and assure that homeostatic sleep pressure is sufficiently elevated when sleep is attempted, so that time in bed is mostly spent asleep rather than awake.[44] This in turn reconditions sleep-related associations, so that the bed and bedroom environment are more closely associated with feeling sleepy and falling asleep.

In the early 1990s, a pediatric variation of this treatment was introduced as "bedtime fading" by Piazza and Fisher.[45] Using a similar technique, in which the sleep window is restricted and titrated (by first delaying bedtimes and subsequently "fading" them earlier by 15 minutes at a time), these authors successfully treated insomnia in two young children in an inpatient unit. Bedtime fading has since yielded promising results in several other case reports in both typically and nontypically developing preschool children.[46-48] Still, the efficacy of this intervention remained unsubstantiated due to the relatively limited number of investigations assessing its effects, many of which were of poor quality. Importantly, most of these reports used multicomponential treatment packages, in which bedtime fading was delivered together with other treatment modules (e.g., positive routines), making it impossible to evaluate the specific contribution of each technique. Consequently, the 2006 AASM practice parameters recommended bedtime fading as a *Guideline* treatment, indexing only a moderate level of clinical evidence for this treatment.[11]

In contrast to the increasing recognition and popularity of this approach in the treatment of adult insomnia,[49] bedtime fading has remained a rather overlooked approach in pediatric sleep research and practice. This is quite surprising, given the considerable advantages this intervention may have in lowering the probability of child distress and bedtime resistance.[45] These advantages may be particularly important when treating infants and toddlers, whose parents often seek gentle intervention approaches.

Two more recent investigations have reinstituted the efforts to establish an evidence base for bedtime fading in young children. In an open trial, Cooney et al.[50] provided two group sessions to mothers of 1- to 4-year-old children with behavioral insomnia. Treatment included basic sleep education and a bedtime fading protocol. Following treatment, large reductions were observed in children's sleep onset latency, nighttime wakefulness, and the frequency of bedtime tantrums. Gradisar and colleagues[19] tested the efficacy of bedtime fading for infant sleep problems in an RCT. Infants aged 6 to 16 months were randomized to receive either bedtime fading, graduated extinction, or sleep education control. Treatment was delivered in one individualized session, with the option of subsequent phone call support. At posttreatment, parents of infants who received bedtime fading reported large reductions in sleep onset latency, which were comparable to graduated extinction and greater than those observed in the control group. Bedtime fading also generated reductions in maternal stress compared to control, but not in nighttime awakenings. This study provided the first high-quality evidence for the efficacy of bedtime fading to improve the sleep of infants. Additional RCTs are warranted to replicate these findings and potentially form a sound evidence base for the routine use of this intervention in clinical practice.

SCHEDULED AWAKENINGS AND DREAM FEEDING

The scheduled awakenings procedure was developed to enhance sleep consolidation in infants. In this approach, parents wake their child 15 to 30 minutes prior to the timing of their typical spontaneous awakening to soothe, feed, or facilitate the onset of a new sleep cycle. When spontaneous awakenings diminish, parent-induced awakenings are faded out by gradually increasing the time increments between them. This technique was first introduced in 1980,[51] and was subsequently evaluated in a series of small studies.[52-54] While benefits were documented, not all parents adhered to the technique, and the latency to see improvement, as well as its extent, were found to be inferior to extinction.[54] Based on this evidence, scheduled awakenings were considered "probably efficacious" and regarded as a *Guideline* treatment by the AASM 2006 task force.[11] This approach has received very limited research attention since and is seldom recommended in clinical practice.[55] The reasons for this may include the lack of consistently timed awakenings in infants, making it difficult for parents to time their induced awakenings. In addition, parents may prefer not to disrupt their infant's and their own sleep, in case spontaneous awakenings do not occur.

Despite the dearth of studies into scheduled awakenings over the past three decades, a derivative of this technique—"dream feeding"—seems to have accrued much more popularity. In this method, parents initiate a nighttime feed before going to bed themselves.[56] As opposed to the original scheduled awakenings protocol, the timing of the "dream feed" is determined by the parents' sleep schedule, aiming to reduce the chance of infant awakenings while parents are asleep. Moreover, parents are not advised to wake their infants per se, but rather feed them while asleep. This technique is meant to reduce awakenings triggered by hunger, especially in young infants who still need to be fed throughout the night.

Dream feeding is commonly suggested in self-help books, websites, and colloquial advice for infant sleep problems.[57,58] Yet, scientific evidence for its efficacy is lacking. To date, two controlled trials have incorporated dream feeding for young infants (aged <4 months) as part of a multicomponent treatment.[59,60] While both studies documented benefits for infants receiving intervention, the use of comprehensive "package" treatments did not allow conclusions regarding the efficacy of dream feeding as a standalone component in enhancing sleep consolidation. Hence, given its apparent ubiquity, systematic research is clearly warranted to determine the efficacy of this technique for improving infant sleep.

EXTINCTION-BASED METHODS

Based heavily on classical and operant conditioning principles, extinction-based interventions aim to provide parents with skills on how to modify and reduce their involvement in the infant's sleep context. These changes are expected to foster children's ability to fall asleep independently at bedtime and after waking up at night (i.e., to self-soothe), thus promoting consolidated sleep. To that effect external regulation—such as feeding, holding, or rocking the baby to attain sleep—is targeted and decreased. Extinction-based approaches correspond with evidence for concurrent and longitudinal links between increased parental involvement in the infant's sleep context and infant sleep fragmentation and disruption[61-63] (see Chapter 12 for a comprehensive description of these links). Infants usually require similar conditions to initiate sleep at the start of the night and throughout it.[64] Hence, given that spontaneous awakenings frequently occur in the first year of life,[65] facilitating the development of self-soothing to sleep has the potential to reduce nocturnal wakefulness and allow more consolidated sleep for both infants and parents.

Several variations of extinction-based approaches have been developed and studied. The three most common variations are unmodified extinction, modified (or gradual) extinction, and extinction with parental presence. These will be described in the following sections.

Unmodified Extinction

Unmodified extinction (or simply "extinction") is one of the earliest interventions to be investigated in young children with sleep problems. Also termed "cry it out" or "systematic ignoring," it was first suggested for preschool children[66] and subsequently for infants with disrupted sleep.[54,67] The technique involves parents putting the infant to bed drowsy but awake at a set bedtime and then ignoring any crying or signaling until a set morning wake-up time. Parents remain attentive, making sure that the child is not ill, hurt, or in danger, but otherwise refrain from intervening throughout the entire night. Based on the 19 studies available at the time, 17 of which showed beneficial effects, the 2006 AASM Task Force judged unmodified extinction to be a *Standard* treatment approach for infants and young children.[11]

Consistent with this recommendation, a recent survey found that unmodified extinction was a common technique, attempted by 34.9% of parents who have used behavioral sleep interventions.[68] Moreover, unmodified extinction was reported to have a very high first attempt success rate, with 89.5% of parents reporting improvement in infant sleep parameters on their first implementation. Participants in this survey, however, were recruited through a social media peer support group for parents using behavioral sleep interventions; thus findings may not be representative of the general parent population. In fact, while its greatest advantage may be the short latency to see improvement, the greatest drawback of unmodified extinction is the distress entailed in its implementation due to the advice to delay response to the infant's cry, making many parents deterred from trying it with their infants.[10] Moreover, extinction bursts may occur, in which there is a relapse of the dependency on parents for sleep, and parents may find it difficult to repeat the procedures on more than one occasion. Given its high intensity but immediate impact, it is not surprising that unmodified extinction has been one of the most controversial intervention approaches for infant sleep.[69-72] This vehement controversy will be discussed later in this chapter.

Modified Extinction

Modified extinction was developed in the mid-1980s as a gentler alternative to the original extinction approach.[73,74] Instead of delaying parental response for the entire night, this approach prescribes a schedule in which parents wait for a few minutes before briefly checking in on their infant for as long as the crying or distress continues. Waiting periods are intended to allow the child an opportunity to explore and practice ways to self-regulate to sleep. Parents are usually advised to keep visits between waiting periods brief and minimize interactions that may stimulate the child or reinforce dependence on external care.[10] Many variations of this technique have been proposed, some employing a fixed schedule (e.g., responding every 3 minutes), and some progressively increasing intervention delays (e.g., every 3 minutes, then every 5 minutes, and so on, either within the same night or across consecutive nights). Some variations suggest implementing the technique only at the start of the night (e.g., Eckerberg[75]), and some throughout the entire night or 24-hour day. These approaches have received various titles throughout the years, including "graduated extinction," "the Ferber method," "checking in," "controlled crying," "controlled comforting," and "sleep training."

Modified extinction was already considered a *Standard* treatment approach for young children based on the evidence available in 2006.[11] Since then, it has continued to be widely used and investigated in clinical and research settings. Several RCTs have further demonstrated the efficacy of graduated extinction for infants aged ≥6 months in reducing sleep onset latency, the frequency of nighttime awakenings, wakefulness after sleep onset, and the severity of parent-perceived infant sleep problems, as well as improving parental sleep and mood.[15,19,76,77] Importantly, gains have been shown to sustain over time. For example, Hiscock and colleagues[78] showed superior outcomes of graduated extinction compared to control at a 2-year follow-up assessment. Still, despite its solid evidence for efficacy, and more gradual approach, graduated extinction protocols may also be difficult to follow through, and some parents experience substantial barriers to implementation.[14] Like its unmodified predecessor, this intervention has also been subject to considerable criticism and debate, as will be discussed in subsequent sections.

Extinction With Parental Presence

Extinction with parental presence similarly aims to facilitate the development of infant self-soothing to sleep by reducing parental involvement in the sleep context, however—parental proximity to the child is maintained in this approach. Also termed "Camping out," this method is based on the premise that parent-infant separation may provoke stress in both parents and infants, thus exacerbating infants' difficulty to initiate and remain asleep.[79] In extinction with parental presence, parents stay next to their child throughout the night, often feigning sleep, and not responding to the infant until a set morning time. This approach may have the benefit of being better accepted by parents, as many of them do not wish to be away from their child while they are distressed. Based on four research studies showing evidence for efficacy, the 2006 AASM Task Force deemed extinction with parental presence to be a *Standard* treatment.[11]

Analogous to the evolution of the gentler "graduated extinction" from "extinction," variations emerged adding a *gradual* aspect to extinction with parental presence. In these versions, parents remain at close proximity to the infant (e.g., lie on a mattress near the crib) and increasingly delay their responses to infant signaling or crying. Namely, rather than refraining from soothing the infant throughout the entire night, they wait a few minutes before responding to their signaling, while staying close by the entire time. The benefits of this approach were documented in a small uncontrolled trial of infants aged 6 to 23 months old,[80] as well as in two more recent randomized trials.[15,81]

HOW WELL DO BEHAVIORAL INTERVENTIONS COMPARE?

The various behavioral sleep intervention approaches described above were presented as separate standalone entities, yet in clinical trials and practice they are often combined or delivered in succession. In their recent scoping review, Meltzer and colleagues[13] reported that in roughly 82% of the investigations into these treatments, a combination of multiple treatment approaches was used. Furthermore, Honaker et al.[68] found that approximately 25% of parents using extinction-based techniques start with one approach and then switch to another, with the most common transition occurring from modified to unmodified extinction. Thus, the treatment of infant sleep problems is rarely unidimensional, and optimal efficacy might require flexibility, and a willingness to try various components.

Several studies have compared the efficacy or effectiveness of behavioral sleep interventions, aiming to gauge whether some methods are superior to others. Most of the RCTs that compared the efficacy of techniques found null to small differences between methods. For example, in a trial of 36 young children, Adams and Rickert[16] found that delaying bedtimes in addition to positive routines was as beneficial in reducing young children's bedtime tantrums as modified extinction, both of which were more beneficial than the nonactive control. However, improvements were achieved more quickly following bedtime fading with positive bedtime routines. Moreover, the latter approach yielded improvements in marital satisfaction, which did not occur in the other two groups. The authors attributed these gains to the additional opportunity for family "quality time" when bedtimes are delayed and routines include positive parent-child activities, as opposed to the distress that is often involved in modified extinction.

As mentioned earlier, the RCT conducted by Gradisar and colleagues[19] compared the efficacy of modified extinction, bedtime fading, and a sleep education control. Here too benefits were demonstrated following both intervention groups compared to control, yet there were some indications of superior benefits for infants undergoing modified extinction. Specifically, while sleep onset latency was similarly reduced in both intervention groups, sleep consolidation metrics (nocturnal wakefulness and the number of awakenings) indexed greater improvement in graduated extinction compared to bedtime fading (which did not differ from control). In their conclusions, the authors proposed that these two intervention approaches could be delivered in succession, with bedtime fading increasing sleepiness, shortening the procedure of parents checking in and out, and thus facilitating the learning of more independent sleep associations.

Different variations of extinction-based approaches were compared in three randomized trials.[15,79,81,82] Matthey and Črnčec[81] compared modified extinction with and without parental presence in 16 infants aged 6 to 18 months and found that equal proportions of infants had reductions in the number of nighttime awakenings in both groups. Sadeh[79] conducted an RCT to compare the efficacy of modified extinction ("checking") and unmodified extinction with parental presence in 50 infants aged 9 to 24 months with sleep disturbances, using actigraphy in addition to parent-reported infant sleep. Both assessment methods revealed equivalent improvement in infant sleep between both intervention groups at posttreatment. Kahn et al.[15,82] similarly used multimethod assessment in an RCT comparing modified extinction ("checking-in") and modified extinction with parental presence ("camping out"). This trial had a larger sample ($N = 91$) and included a 6-month follow-up assessment. Corresponding with Sadeh's[79] findings, benefits were indexed for actigraphic and parent-reported infant sleep following both extinction-based approaches, with no significant group by time interaction effects.[15,82] Of note, these two RCTs revealed a similar pattern, in which benefits were greater and more robust according to parent-reports compared to actigraphic monitoring.[15,79,82] This pattern points to the mechanistic pathway by which benefits are exercised, suggesting that during "sleep training" with or without parental presence, infants acquire self-regulatory capabilities, and are thus less inclined to signal to their parents when waking at night.

Comparisons between extinction-based approaches were also examined in Honaker et al.'s[68] retrospective survey of parents who had used these interventions with their infants. Here too, differences were not found between approaches on most of the assessed outcomes. Specifically, unmodified extinction, modified extinction, and each of these combined with parental presence did not differ in reported improvements in infant sleep-wake patterns and parental stress, nor did they differ in infant age, the amount and intensity of infant crying, or parental stress at time of implementation. However, differences were found in the rates of parent satisfaction, with only 76% of parents who used modified extinction with parental presence reporting being satisfied, compared to 94%, 91%, and 87% in the three other groups. Furthermore, parents using unmodified extinction reported the greatest first-attempt success rate. Yet, the sample for this study was recruited via social media peer support groups for parents using behavioral sleep intervention, and thus findings may not be representative of the general parent population.

While small differences in efficacy and effectiveness have been found in the studies described above, several factors make it difficult to draw conclusions regarding their relative effects. First, different studies have used different treatment protocols, including varying checking-in schedules (e.g., length of waiting periods, implementation including bedtime only versus nighttime and naps as well), different bedtime fading schedules, and varying content covered in psychoeducation interventions. While real-world implementation of these interventions requires flexibility and pragmatism, developing standardized protocols that entail certain degrees of freedom would allow more careful evaluation of their comparative effects. Similarly, the use of different designs, populations, and outcome measures across studies limits the ability to assess the relative efficacy of these interventions. In particular, only a few studies have included objective assessment of sleep in addition to parent reports. Given the risk of recall bias when it comes to nighttime events, and considering the potential for objective measures such as actigraphy and auto-videosomnography to evaluate sleep-related events that parents were not aware of,[71,83] including these measures provide a much more comprehensive account of the infant's sleep-wake patterns. Future investigations should thus use standardized protocols and standardized multimethod assessment of outcomes. This would allow future meta-analytic studies to draw more accurate conclusions regarding efficacy that would better inform clinical practice guidelines.

Notwithstanding these suggestions, it might be the case that focusing on the "horse race" question might not be the best use of research resources. Namely, instead of directing our efforts at identifying which interventions work best, we might have more to gain by attempting to identify *how*, *for whom*, and *under what circumstances* do they work best. Scientific knowledge regarding predictors, moderators, and mediators of treatment has advanced considerably in the realm of behavioral interventions for various child psychopathologies.[84,85] However, pediatric sleep research has only recently begun to address these questions. The following section reviews findings from these preliminary attempts and outlines a path for further investigations in these directions.

The "When" and "For Whom"—Predictors and Moderators of Outcome

AT WHAT INFANT AGE ARE (WHICH) BEHAVIORAL SLEEP INTERVENTIONS MOST EFFICACIOUS?

One of the most important questions regarding behavioral interventions for infant sleep has to do with timing. Parents often ask whether there is a youngest appropriate age to intervene and what approach is suitable for different stages in development. Despite the gravity and ubiquity of this question, there is limited evidence to answer it. The dramatic development of sleep-wake patterns and underlying physiology during infancy[86,87] has led many to doubt the value of intervening at an early age. As discussed at length later in this chapter, it has been argued that behavioral sleep interventions "pathologize" the normal developmental trajectories of infant sleep, particularly in the early stages of development. A systematic review focusing on interventions implemented during the first 6 months of life indicated that despite evidence for increased self-regulated sleep following these interventions, they do not improve other infant or mother outcomes.[88] Other systematic reviews and meta-analyses found increases in infant sleep duration, as well as benefits for maternal mood, yet these included studies of sleep in the first 12 months[21] and beyond.[12]

Importantly, most studies of behavioral interventions implemented during the first 6 months have evaluated either psychoeducation, bedtime routines, or a combination of both. In their meta-analysis of RCTs conducted within the first year of life, Kempler et al.[21] note that none of the interventions administered within the first 6 months employed extinction-based approaches. We have identified only one prospective investigation of such methods which included infants aged <6 months. Middlemiss et al.[89] assessed the effects of unmodified extinction in 4- to 10-month-old infants, finding that by the third intervention day all 25 participating infants settled to sleep independently without signaling distress. Other studies of extinction-based approaches have included infants who were either ≥6 or ≥9 months old. Hence, it seems that while preventative programs—focusing mostly on educating parents about realistic expectations and positive routines—have been shown to be beneficial early on, the efficacy of extinction-based methods has been demonstrated primarily from the second half of the infant's first year.

Importantly, to the best of our knowledge no study has yet to examine whether infant age acts as a *predictor* or *moderator* of treatment outcomes. Namely, it has not been tested whether older infants derive more benefit from a certain intervention compared to younger infants (potentially confirmed using infant age-by-time interaction effects in repeated measure designs), nor has it been tested whether this potential age effect might vary as a function of the specific intervention implemented (potentially confirmed using infant age-by-time-by-intervention type interaction effects in repeated measure designs). Given the widespread use of these interventions with young infants,[68] and the dearth of studies examining their effects on this age group, research is warranted assessing whether infant age predicts and/or moderates outcomes of behavioral sleep interventions.

FOR WHOM ARE (WHICH) BEHAVIORAL SLEEP INTERVENTIONS MOST EFFICACIOUS?

Other child-related factors may also impact the outcomes of behavioral interventions for insomnia. For example, since extinction-based methods usually entail a certain degree of separation from the parents, heightened infant separation anxiety might impede compliance to these interventions, as infants may express increased distress when left on their own, making it more difficult for parents to delay their response to the infant. Indeed, in an RCT of 91 infants aged 9 to 18 months old focusing on predictors and moderators of modified extinction versus camping out, Kahn et al.[15] found that infant separation anxiety moderated treatment efficacy. While significant reductions in nighttime wakefulness were documented for low-anxiety infants in both intervention groups, and for high-anxiety infants in the camping-out group, no significant reductions were observed for infants with high separation anxiety in the modified extinction group. This moderation effect was found for both parent-reported and actigraphic nighttime wakefulness. Other sleep metrics, such as sleep onset latency and the frequency of nighttime awakenings, were reduced following both interventions, regardless of infant separation anxiety. Still, these findings suggest that interventions involving a smaller "dose" of separation from parents may be more beneficial for infants who exhibit heightened separation anxiety.

Parent factors were also examined in this RCT, considering the important part parents play in the development of infant sleep, and given that behavioral interventions for infant insomnia primarily target parent behaviors. Two related parent factors were examined in this trial: parental cry tolerance and sleep-related cognitions.[82] These constructs have previously been implicated in infant sleep problems both concurrently and longitudinally.[63,90,91] In this RCT, both low cry tolerance and distress attributions predicted inferior treatment outcomes.[82] Namely, reductions in the frequency of nighttime awakenings and in parent-reported sleep problems were greater when parents exhibited higher tolerance for crying and lower distress-attribution cognitions at baseline. These effects were demonstrated across modified extinction and camping-out groups, with no evidence for one treatment to be more beneficial than the other for parents with a certain baseline profile of cry tolerance or sleep-related cognitions. Given that both extinction-based methods require parents to refrain from providing immediate comfort and tolerate some extent of infant distress, parents who are highly sensitive to these stimuli may be less able to successfully implement the intervention. Interestingly, following the intervention, cry tolerance significantly increased, and distress-attribution cognitions decreased. This suggests that a positive feedback loop may have emerged, in which the increased ability to tolerate distress and the reciprocal increase in child independent sleep were mutually reinforcing.

Findings from this trial represent a first step in the transition to a precision medicine paradigm in the field of behavioral infant sleep interventions. They inform clinicians by indicating which parent populations may require more intensive support when attempting these interventions. They also advise practice guidelines as to which infant and parent factors should be taken into account when recommending a certain treatment method. As opposed to the one-treatment-fits-all approach, this knowledge can be used to personalize treatment so that it meets the needs of specific patient populations. More research is clearly needed to identify further parent and infant factors that may predict and/or moderate treatment success. Specifically, factors that have been shown to be associated with infant sleep problems should be considered, including infant temperament, physiological reactivity, atypical development, breastfeeding, cosleeping, as well as parent culture and ethnicity, health literacy, emotional availability, and psychopathology.[92,93] These factors should be examined within RCTs that include multiple types of interventions to determine which approach would most likely be appropriate and beneficial for each specific treatment-seeking family.

The "Which Side Are You on"—From Polarized Controversy to a Middle-Ground

As alluded to previously in this chapter, behavioral sleep interventions for infants—and extinction-based approaches in particular—have triggered tempestuous debates during the past decades. The critique focuses on the safety of these interventions, as well as their fundamental justification. Namely, it has been argued that extinction-based methods could be harmful and that they are in fact an unnecessary solution to a "made-up" problem. These claims have been voiced in the academic literature (e.g., Blunden et al.[72] and Douglas and Hill[88]), yet they are also echoed in social media outlets, websites, and colloquial sleep advice (e.g., "sleep coaches" or "influencers"; Alpha[94] and McKay[95]). While expressing divergent views has the potential to advance the field by inspiring new theories and paradigms, we recently seem to be witnessing quite the opposite process. A concerning dynamic of echo chambers is developing, where shared narratives are reinforced and amplified, remaining insulated from rebuttal.[96] This polarization may be in part due to the increasing engagement of parents in social media and the reliance on these platforms as a source of parenting information.[97] Social media discussions regarding other controversial topics, such as vaccination, have been shown to be dominated by echo chambers, making it easier for questionable information to proliferate and for "identity politics" to emerge.[98-100]

In our clinical work with parents, these "identity politics" are becoming more and more apparent. Parents may convey their identification with a certain side of this debate, while fiercely rejecting its "dangerous" approaches. We are seeing more parents concerned that their infants are not sleeping through the night at the newborn stage on the one hand, and on the other hand, meet more and more parents who are worried that if they allow their child to cry for a few minutes they are rendering them to a fate of "learned helplessness." While these concerns should be respected and addressed at the individual level, it is also important to understand the sociopolitical developments occurring in this field and examine which information is propagated and how much of it is backed up by systematic evidence. It is always a family's personal choice how to manage their child's sleep, and every choice is legitimate as long as proper measures are taken to secure the safety of the child. However, we worry that on top of the misinformation, the need to "choose sides" in itself is highly detrimental, as it deprives parents of a more free and open-minded choice. We thus believe that it is our responsibility as pediatric sleep researchers and clinicians to present a balanced account of the arguments as well as the existing evidence, aiming to promote a reconstruction of the two "camps" into one broad spectrum.

IS THERE ACTUALLY SUCH A THING AS "INFANT SLEEP PROBLEMS"?

Firstly, we wish to address the argument that there might not be a need for behavioral interventions for infant insomnia at all, but rather that normal infant sleep is culturally constructed and pathologized into an unwarranted diagnostic category.[72,101,102] These claims stem from biological and anthropological theories of development. From a biological standpoint, human infants are born at the most immature neurological stage compared to all other primates[103] and are completely dependent on external care for many months. More specifically, the physiological processes governing sleep (i.e., the homeostatic and circadian processes) gradually mature over the first year of the infant's life.[86,87] Thus, sleep in newborn infants is typically fragmented into multiple brief sleep episodes distributed around the 24-hour day and gradually consolidates into one major nocturnal sleep episode over the course of the first year.[104] Studies of typically developing infants indicate that although the number of night-wakings gradually declines and most infants develop self-soothing skills during the first year, nighttime awakenings do not entirely disappear. In fact, they are the norm throughout this year and beyond, with most infants presenting an average of approximately 1 to 3 awakenings between the ages of 3 and 18 months.[61,105,106] Thus, from a biological standpoint, one could argue that the expectation that babies "sleep through the night" is not realistic and discounts their normal biological developmental progression.

Sociocultural and anthropological arguments augment these claims by stating that prior to the 19th century, infant sleep was not considered a major concern for parents.[101] Families would cosleep in communal beds, and infants would be attended to quickly upon awakening.[107] Similar perceptions of and practices around infant sleep have been documented in modern times in non-industrial nonwestern settings.[108] The evolution of cultural norms around infant sleep was shaped by expansive developments, such as the strengthening of individualistic values, the industrial revolution, the increasing entrance of women into the work force, the emergence of human milk substitute formulas, the sexualization of the parents' bed, and the adoption of "scientific motherhood" according to which medical professionals became a more trusted authority regarding child rearing than parents themselves.[72,101,102] It is thus argued that "infant sleep problems" are a modern invention, whereas the real problem lies in holding unrealistic expectations and trying to force a 21st-century Western industrialized lifestyle on an infant brain which has failed to evolve at the same pace. According to this viewpoint, infant-parent cosleeping with responsive breastfeeding should be recommended, and parents should allow their children's sleep to become consolidated in their own time.

When contemplating these arguments, we believe there are a few points on which agreement could easily be achieved. These include the fragmented nature of infant sleep, especially during the first months of life, making it inherently misaligned with the sleep-wake patterns of most adults in contemporary modern society. They also include the dramatic evolution of cultural norms around sleep in these societies in the past centuries and the acknowledgment that there are infinite ways in which infant sleep can be perceived and constructed. We should, however, be wary not to over-romanticize the past. Historically, cosleeping was practiced for reasons such as assuring appropriate body temperature, as well as protection from predators that nighttime crying may attract. Moreover, historic evidence indicates that it was a widespread practice to drug babies to sleep, with indications of opium use in infants dating back to the 16th century BCE and continuing well into the 20th century.[109,110] Infants who were "sleepless," "restless," or displayed "fits of crying" were regularly provided opiate "soothers," to the point that opium intoxication was one of the main causes of infant mortality.[109] Therefore, it seems that the perception of infant sleep as a problem should not be treated as a modern invention since parents in ancient times were sometimes willing to use life-endangering measures to get their infants to sleep.

Furthermore, we must pose the question—would recommending practices that are harmonious with 16th-century social norms, necessarily do justice with parents living in capitalistic, industrialized 21st-century settings? Infant sleep problems are a source of major difficulty for present-day parents. They are the most common issue for which professional assistance is sought in the first 12 months of the infant's life.[111] Mounting evidence associates infant sleep problems with a multitude of parent adverse consequences, including depression, anxiety, stress, poor physical health, and reduced quality of life.[9,93,112] Parent sleep disturbances in the postpartum period have been associated with negative caregiving emotions and behaviors.[113-116] In extreme cases, these problems have been associated with child neglect and abuse, such as infant shaking, and even filicide.[117,118] Behavioral sleep interventions have been shown to significantly reduce maternal depression and benefit parental well-being.[21,77] The mechanisms through which these benefits are achieved are evident, given the vast literature demonstrating the devastating consequences of sleep deprivation and fragmentation in adults.[119-121] Thus, helping parents obtain sufficient consolidated sleep may benefit both themselves and—indirectly—their infants, who gain more rested, contented, and regulated caregivers.[122] Of course, infants also stand to gain *direct* benefit from behavioral sleep interventions, given that sleep problems in infancy have been shown to predict later cognitive, behavioral, and emotional difficulties, as well as the incidence of obesity.[4,6,123,124]

Therefore, while infant sleep problems may indeed be a culturally constructed notion, they nevertheless may cause substantial adverse consequences, and thus call for attention and intervention. In addressing these issues, we argue for a middle ground in which parents are offered education regarding the "fourth trimester," the normal progression of infant sleep, realistic expectations, and the potential influences of their specific cultural context. For those who experience these issues as burdensome and distressing, the full spectrum of available treatment approaches should be proposed.

ARE BEHAVIORAL SLEEP INTERVENTIONS FOR INFANTS SAFE?

The second major argument against extinction-based interventions focuses on their safety. Concerns have been raised as to whether these interventions generate undue stress, compromising parent-infant attachment and the infant's long-term emotional well-being. At the basis of these claims stands the notion that crying is a universal form of early communication, which promotes parental proximity and fulfillment of the infant's needs.[125,126] At the preverbal stage of their development, crying is the most effective means by which infants can communicate their distress and call for external support. Crying is also considered by attachment theorists to be part of a biological system that activates the attachment system and establishes a stable reciprocal bond of trust between infant and parent.[125,127] Parents are thus biologically primed to infant cry signals, as demonstrated in neuroimaging studies of "parental-brain network" activation in response to infant crying stimuli.[128,129]

Attachment researchers have claimed that ignoring an infant's cry means defying fundamental evolutionary drives and disregarding the infant's invitation to develop a shared relationship of trust and understanding with their parent. Extinction-based methods in which parents do not immediately respond to their infant's crying at night are thus seen as unnatural, unethical, and harmful in that they may cause unnecessary stress in the short term and hinder the development of secure attachment between infant and parent in the long term.[72,101,130] Notably, the argument here is not that extinction-based methods do not improve infants'—and by proxy parents'—nighttime sleep consolidation and duration for the majority of families who implement them. Rather, whether these improvements should be the criteria by which treatment "success" is determined and whether they outweigh the potential "side-effects" is called into question.

The links between parental responsiveness and infant behavior and development have stimulated vast theoretical and scientific discussions over the past decades. In their classical longitudinal Baltimore study of 26 infants during their first year of life, Bell and Ainsworth[127] reported that nonresponsive parenting early on predicted more crying in subsequent months. This was viewed as evidence to support the attachment-based approach, endorsing immediate parental responsiveness to crying. Approximately 30 years later, van IJzendoorn and Hubbard[131] attempted to replicate and extend this study, using a larger sample ($N = 50$) and more sophisticated methodology (e.g., measuring crying bouts objectively via audio recordings, and statistically controlling for important intervening variables). Astoundingly, not only did these authors fail to replicate Bell and Ainsworth's Baltimore findings,[127] but rather the direction of relationship between responsiveness and later crying was reversed. More frequent ignoring of infant crying early on predicted *less* crying later on. Pure behaviorists would presumably interpret this finding in terms of operant conditioning, arguing that immediate and frequent parents' responsiveness reinforces crying behavior, subsequently making it more recurrent and persistent.[132] van IJzendoorn and Hubbard,[131] on the other hand, suggested a more intricate interpretation, according to which "Benign neglect" of crying and fussing may stimulate infants' emergent abilities to self-regulate and cope with distress.[131] Further evidence for these findings was reported in a recent longitudinal study of 178 infants followed from birth throughout the age of 18 months.[133] Maternal reports of the use of "leaving the infant to cry it out" were associated with subsequent lower frequency and shorter duration of crying. Moreover, no adverse impact of occasionally or even frequently leaving infants to cry in the first 6 months was documented on observed infant behavior (e.g., attention, social referencing, aggression) or infant-mother attachment at 18 months of age.

Bilgin and Wolke[133] justly emphasize that their results neither suggest that leaving infants to cry it out should be generically recommended nor that it should be avoided. Instead, they embrace the concept of "differential responsiveness"[134] to convey the complexity of the relationship between parental responsiveness and infant emotion regulation. From this standpoint, greater and prompter parental responsiveness is not always better. Rather, parents are required to constantly adapt to the ever-changing infant needs and abilities and the ever-changing external circumstances, intuitively providing both high levels of emotional warmth and appropriate limits and challenges. These perceptions are in line with several psychodynamic theories of child development, including Donald Winnicott's concepts of the "good enough mother"[135] and the "capacity to be alone,"[136] as well as Heinz Kohut's idea of "optimal frustration."[137] It is hence the delicate, dynamic balance between fulfillment and nonfulfillment of the child's urges that provides the foundation for self-regulation. Studies demonstrating the associations between authoritative parenting and positive child outcomes provide evidence for this viewpoint.[138,139] Furthermore, the natural progression of parents' responsiveness throughout infant development suggests that different stages in development require differential responsiveness. For example, Bilgin and Wolke[133] report that the "leaving infant to crying" was uncommon at term, yet it increased across the next 18 months of the infant's life. Correspondingly, parental tolerance for infant crying has been shown to be lower in parents of infants compared to childless controls[91] and to significantly decrease from pregnancy to 6 months postpartum.[90]

Coming back to behavioral sleep interventions, to date, systematic investigations have failed to find support for negative impact on infant-parent attachment or child behavior and emotion at posttreatment or up to 5 years later.[15,19,78,140] Thus, interpretations according to which the infant-parent relationship is harmed, or that infants acquire "learned helplessness" in the process of behavioral sleep interventions lack any scientific foundation to date.

With regard to potential short-term harm, two studies have assessed infants' salivary cortisol levels before and after undergoing an extinction-based sleep intervention. The first study assessed the effects of a 5-day inpatient unmodified extinction program in 25 infants aged 4 to 10 months.[89] Salivary cortisol levels were sampled from mothers and infants on days 1 and 3 of the intervention, both before initiation of the nighttime sleep routine and 20 minutes after infant sleep onset. Results revealed that infant cortisol levels did not change significantly following unmodified extinction on either day. Namely, the expected increase in stress hormones following the intervention was not observed. Similarly, mothers' cortisol levels did not change from before to after the intervention on day 1, whereas on day 3 there was a significant decrease in their cortisol levels following the intervention. Authors attribute this decrease to the reduction in infant crying on the third day, in which all infants settled to sleep independently without signaling distress. In line with these patterns of results, the associations between infant and mother cortisol levels were significant on day 1, and nonsignificant on day 3, which was interpreted as asynchrony between mother's and infant's stress levels.[89] Noteworthy is that a lack of correlation between infant and mother cortisol levels has not been associated with any negative child or parent outcome in research work performed thus far. Moreover, the authors conclude that infants' cortisol levels "remained elevated" during unmodified extinction; however, at the time there was no normative data to describe normal infant cortisol levels over the course of a day.[141] Since then, reports have been published demonstrating normal cortisol levels (e.g., Ivars et al.[142]), suggesting that cortisol levels of babies in Middlemiss et al.'s[89] investigation were high (i.e., above the 75th percentile) at baseline. This could be explained by the fact that infants were transitioned to the inpatient unit and nurses—rather than mothers—implemented the interventions, which could be stressful in itself. Nevertheless, and most importantly, infant cortisol levels were not affected by unmodified extinction, which is arguably the most intense extinction-based approach.

Gradisar and colleagues[19] also investigated the effect of behavioral sleep interventions on infant salivary cortisol levels in their aforementioned RCT. These authors randomized 43 infants aged 6 to 16 months to either graduated extinction, bedtime fading, or education control. Salivary samples were collected at baseline, and again at 1 week, 1 month, and 12 months following treatment. While infant sleep latency and fragmentation significantly diminished in both intervention groups, no significant increases were found in infant cortisol levels from baseline to the 1-week assessment in any of the groups. Thus, in line with Middlemiss et al.'s findings,[89] infant stress levels remained unchanged following behavioral sleep interventions. Moreover, at the 12-month follow-up no differences were apparent between groups in parent-reported infant emotional and behavioral problems, or in infants' attachment style, as assessed using the strange situation procedure.[19]

In conclusion, research to date has not provided any indication of short- or long-term harm resulting from behavioral interventions for infant sleep problems. Consistent high-quality evidence demonstrates the efficacy and effectiveness of these treatments. This evidence should be made clear to parents, and efforts should be made to revise any communications of misinformation. At the same time, we should clearly acknowledge that behavioral interventions for infant insomnia may not be appropriate for everyone. Many parents feel that they do not fit well with their emotional resources, belief systems, or life circumstances at that time. Clinicians should make parents aware of the broad range of evidence-based treatments available and respect their choice to implement any or none of them, as research continues to refine existing interventions and develop novel approaches. Importantly, we should all be wary not to let ourselves get caught in a "Judgement of Solomon" scenario, wherein amid our attempts to prove that we are the righteous authority, we are willing to risk rendering parents torn between two sides of a highly polarized and depleting dispute.

The "Where to Next"—Future Directions in Behavioral Infant Sleep Intervention Research

Knowledge regarding behavioral interventions for infant insomnia has vastly broadened over the past decades. Yet, as suggested throughout this chapter, many questions still require further exploration. First, while some treatment approaches have a sound evidence base (e.g., bedtime routines, extinction-based interventions), others require further data to support their efficacy and effectiveness. Specifically, research is needed to establish the short- and long-term effects of bedtime fading protocols and dream feeding in alleviating infant sleep problems. Second, future studies would do well to utilize standardized protocols and standardized measures that would facilitate metaanalytic evaluation of these interventions' effects relative to control and to each other. Future work should also aim to use objective (i.e., actigraphy, videosomnography, autovideosomnography) as well as subjective (i.e., parent report) measures of infant sleep, as well as measures of other aspects of infant and parent well-being (e.g., emotion, behavior), to encompass the multifaceted phenomena and consequences of sleep-wake patterns.

As the field of psychotherapy research evolves from a generic to a personalized medicine approach, pediatric sleep researchers should also examine not only what works or what works better—but rather what works better for whom and under which circumstances. Attempts to identify predictors and moderators of treatment outcomes in this field are currently in their infancy[15,82] and may hold great promise in optimizing the care we provide. Specifically, assessing whether treatment efficacy differs as a function of infant age is critical and should be investigated across various treatment approaches. Similarly, evidence pointing to mechanistic pathways by which certain treatment components exercise their benefits has been scarce. Ferber et al.[42] demonstrated better circadian entrainment following prebedtime massage compared to control, suggesting an underlying mechanism through which this part of the bedtime routine may consolidate sleep. Similar research endeavors could be attempted to understand whether circadian alignment and/or improved infant-parent bonding mediate the outcomes of other bedtime routine components, whether changes in parent sleep-related cognitions and practices mediate the effects of psychoeducation, whether increases in sleep EEG slow wave activity mediate the effects of bedtime fading, and whether improvement in infant self-regulatory skills mediate the impact of extinction-based approaches.

Another important direction for future research is the effort to increase accessibility of behavioral interventions for infant insomnia. Given the progressively growing treatment gap in mental health, making evidence-based interventions available to more families in need of treatment is a high priority. Throughout the past decade, web-based and mHealth adaptations of behavioral sleep interventions have shown promise in improving multiple aspects of infant sleep, as well as parent sleep and mood.[143,144] The value of such highly accessible, low-cost interventions for sleep disturbances cannot be overrated, considering their high prevalence and adverse consequences in young children. More work is therefore needed to develop and test treatment adaptations that can be accessible to broad populations at a low cost, such as app-based interventions.

An additional research gap has at its core the role of fathers in behavioral sleep interventions. Investigations into infant sleep and interventions for infant insomnia have traditionally tended to focus on mothers, neglecting the role of fathers in the development, maintenance, and resolution of sleep problems. This is quite surprising, given that early theories have suggested that fathers may be one of the most potent facilitators in the development of child regulation and autonomy (e.g., Mahler[145]). Father involvement has been associated with positive child well-being in general,[146] as well as with better infant sleep.[147] Yet, father involvement in the treatment of pediatric sleep problems has not been examined thus far. Future investigations should address this gap by systematically assessing and/or manipulating the part each parent plays in treatment, as well as assessing outcome, moderating, and mediating factors for each parent (e.g., paternal, as well as maternal depression). Importantly, this line of inquiry should be extended to include other family structures, such as dual-father and multiple-parent families.

While research into interventions for older children has addressed special populations, the literature concerning treatment of infant sleep has focused mostly on typically developing children. Moreover, the majority of studies have been conducted with primarily White/Caucasian families, despite evidence to show that cultural factors may be closely related to sleep-wake patterns.[148] To date, very few intervention studies have been conducted in Asia and the Middle East, and no studies have been conducted in Africa, Eastern Europe, or South America.[13] A recent study found that Black non-Hispanic mothers, compared to mothers from other racial-ethnic backgrounds, were more likely to retrospectively report they had stopped using behavioral infant sleep interventions prior to completion.[149] However, other aspects of intervention implementation, barriers, and outcomes were equivalent across racial-ethnic groups. Prospective controlled studies are needed to evaluate behavioral interventions within diverse samples, including in infants with developmental problems and disabilities, and families from heterogeneous socioeconomic backgrounds, residing in various parts of the world.

To conclude, several behavioral intervention approaches exist for infants with insomnia. The efficacy and safety of these interventions have been demonstrated in multiple investigations, systematic reviews, and meta-analyses. Further systematic research is needed to evaluate the effects of these interventions within diverse populations, using standardized protocols and measures, while taking into account the role of fathers, increasing accessibility, and attempting to identify factors that may predict, moderate, and mediate outcomes. Findings that will emerge in the coming years will help elucidate which treatment could be most appropriate for which family, and substantially refine our best practice recommendations. In the meantime, we must be aware of the polarized debate regarding behavioral infant sleep interventions and their maladaptive rippling effects. Avid discussions have the potential to inspire new ideas, and we are clearly not suggesting that it is time to "put the controversy to bed." Rather, sleep researchers, clinicians, and parents should strive to avoid a judgmental stance, present a less polarized and emotionally charged account of these interventions, and allow each family to make a **free and informed** decision, without having to "choose sides." Helping parents consider the broad range of options, while balancing the specific needs of the family within the very dynamic process of infant development, may help empower parents and bring them and their infants more restful and healthy nights and days.

References

1. Honaker SM, Meltzer L. Sleep in pediatric primary care: a review of the literature. *Sleep Med Rev.* 2016;25:31-39. Available at: https://doi.org/10.1016/j.smrv.2015.01.004.
2. Williamson AA, Mindell JA, Hiscock H, Quach J. Child sleep behaviors and sleep problems from infancy to school-age. *Sleep Med.* 2019;63:5-8. Available at: https://doi.org/10.1016/j.sleep.2019.05.003.
3. Winsper C, Wolke D. Infant and toddler crying, sleeping and feeding problems and trajectories of dysregulated behavior across childhood. *J Abnorm Child Psychol.* 2014;42:831-843. Available at: https://doi.org/10.1007/s10802-013-9813-1.
4. Hemmi MH, Wolke D, Schneider S. Associations between problems with crying, sleeping and/or feeding in infancy and long-term behavioural outcomes in childhood: a meta-analysis. *Arch Dis Child.* 2011;96:622-629.
5. Mindell JA, Leichman ES, Dumond C, Sadeh A. Sleep and social-emotional development in infants and toddlers. *J Clin Child Adolesc Psychol.* 2017;46:236-246. Available at: https://doi.org/10.1080/15374416.2016.1188701.
6. Sadeh A, Tikotzky L, Kahn M. Sleep in infancy and childhood: implications for emotional and behavioral difficulties in adolescence and beyond. *Curr Opin Psychiatry.* 2014;27:453-459. Available at: https://doi.org/10.1097/YCO.0000000000000109.
7. Miller MA, Kruisbrink M, Wallace J, JI C, Cappuccio FP. Sleep duration and incidence of obesity in infants, children, and adolescents: a systematic review and meta-analysis of prospective studies. *Sleep.* 2018;41:zsy018. Available at: https://doi.org/10.1093/sleep/zsy018.
8. Petzoldt J, Wittchen HU, Einsle F, Martini J. Maternal anxiety versus depressive disorders: specific relations to infants' crying, feeding and sleeping problems. *Child Care Health Dev.* 2016;42:231-245. Available at: https://doi.org/10.1111/cch.12292.
9. Bayer JK, Hiscock H, Hampton A, Wake M. Sleep problems in young infants and maternal mental and physical health. *J Paediatr Child Health.* 2007;43:66-73. Available at: https://doi.org/10.1111/j.1440-1754.2007.01005.x.
10. Mindell JA, Kuhn B, Lewin DS, Meltzer LJ, Sadeh A. Behavioral treatment of bedtime problems and night wakings in infants and young children. *Sleep.* 2006;29:1263-1276. Available at: https://doi.org/10.1093/sleep/29.10.1263.
11. Morgenthaler TI, Owens J, Alessi C, et al. Practice parameters for behavioral treatment of bedtime problems and night wakings in infants and young children. *Sleep.* 2006;29:1277-1281. Available at: https://doi.org/10.1093/sleep/29.10.1277.
12. Meltzer LJ, Mindell JA. Systematic review and meta-analysis of behavioral interventions for pediatric insomnia. *J Pediatr Psychol.* 2014;39:932-948. Available at: https://doi.org/10.1093/jpepsy/jsu041.
13. Meltzer LJ, Wainer A, Engstrom E, Pepa L, Mindell JA. A scoping review of behavioral treatments for pediatric insomnia. *Sleep Med Rev.* 2020;56:101410. Available at: https://doi.org/10.1016/j.smrv.2020.101410.
14. Whittall H, Kahn M, Pillion M, Gradisar M. Parents matter: barriers and solutions when implementing behavioural sleep interventions for infant sleep problems. *Sleep Med.* 2021;84:244-252. Available at: https://doi.org/10.1016/j.sleep.2021.05.042.
15. Kahn M, Juda-Hanael M, Livne-Karp E, Tikotzky L, Anders TF, Sadeh A. Behavioral interventions for pediatric insomnia: one treatment may not fit all. *Sleep.* 2020;43(4):zsz268. Available at: https://doi.org/10.1093/sleep/zsz268.

16. Adams LA, Rickert VI. Reducing bedtime tantrums: comparison between positive routines and graduated extinction. *Pediatrics*. 1989;84:756-761. Available at: https://doi.org/10.1542/peds.84.5.756.
17. Esposito S, Laino D, D'Alonzo R, et al. Pediatric sleep disturbances and treatment with melatonin.
J Transl Med. 2019;17:77. Available at: https://doi.org/10.1186/s12967-019-1835-1.
18. Bryanton J, Beck CT, Montelpare W. Postnatal parental education for optimizing infant general health
and parent-infant relationships. *Cochrane Database Syst Rev*. 2013;(11):CD004068. Available at: https://
doi.org/10.1002/14651858.CD004068.pub4.
19. Gradisar M, Jackson K, Spurrier NJ, et al. Behavioral interventions for infant sleep problems: a randomized
controlled trial. *Pediatrics*. 2016;137(6):e20151486. Available at: https://doi.org/10.1542/peds.2015-1486.
20. Edinger JD. Is it time to step up to stepped care with our cognitive-behavioral insomnia therapies? *Sleep*.
2009;32:1539-1541. Available at: https://doi.org/10.1093/sleep/32.12.1539.
21. Kempler L, Sharpe L, Miller CB, Bartlett DJ. Do psychosocial sleep interventions improve infant sleep or
maternal mood in the postnatal period? A systematic review and meta-analysis of randomised controlled
trials. *Sleep Med Rev*. 2016;29:15-22. Available at: https://doi.org/10.1016/j.smrv.2015.08.002.
22. Galland BC, Sayers RM, Cameron SL, et al. Anticipatory guidance to prevent infant sleep problems
within a randomised controlled trial: infant, maternal and partner outcomes at 6 months of age. *BMJ
Open*. 2017;7:e014908. Available at: http://dx.doi.org/10.1136/bmjopen-2016-014908.
23. Santos IS, Del-Ponte B, Tovo-Rodrigues L, et al. Effect of parental counseling on infants' healthy sleep
habits in Brazil: a randomized clinical trial. *JAMA Netw Open*. 2019;2:e1918062. Available at: http://ja-
manetwork.com/article.aspx?doi=10.1001/jamanetworkopen.2019.18062.
24. Kempler L, Sharpe LA, Marshall NS, Bartlett DJ. A brief sleep focused psychoeducation program for
sleep-related outcomes in new mothers: a randomized controlled trial. *Sleep*. 2020;43:zsaa101. Available
at: https://doi.org/10.1093/sleep/zsaa101.
25. Hiscock H. An educational intervention for improving infant sleep duration—why won't you sleep, baby?
JAMA Netw Open. 2019;2:e1918061. Available at: http://jamanetwork.com/article.aspx?doi=10.1001/
jamanetworkopen.2019.18061.
26. Adachi Y, Sato C, Nishino N, Ohryoji F, Hayama J, Yamagami T. A brief parental education for shaping
sleep habits in 4-month-old infants. *Clin Med Res*. 2009;7:85-92.
27. Stremler R, Hodnett E, Kenton L, et al. Effect of behavioural-educational intervention on sleep for
primiparous women and their infants in early postpartum: multisite randomised controlled trial. *BMJ*.
2013;346:f1164. Available at: https://doi.org/10.1136/bmj.f1164.
28. Kerr SM, Jowett SA, Smith LN. Preventing sleep problems in infants: a randomized controlled trial.
J Adv Nurs. 1996;24:938-942. Available at: https://doi.org/10.1111/j.1365-2648.1996.tb02929.x.
29. Mindell JA, Williamson AA. Benefits of a bedtime routine in young children: sleep, development, and
beyond. *Sleep Med Rev*. 2018;40:93-108. Available at: https://doi.org/10.1016/j.smrv.2017.10.007.
30. Bootzin RR. Stimulus control treatment for insomnia. *Proc Am Psychol Assoc*. 1972;7:395-396.
31. Mindell JA, Li AM, Sadeh A, Kwon R, Goh DY. Bedtime routines for young children: a dose-dependent
association with sleep outcomes. *Sleep*. 2015;38:717-722. Available at: https://doi.org/10.5665/sleep.4662.
32. Fiese BH, Cai T, Sutter C, Bost KK. Bedtimes, bedtime routines, and children's sleep across the first
2 years of life. *Sleep*. 2021;44(8):zsab045. Available at: https://doi.org/10.1093/sleep/zsab045.
33. Allen SL, Howlett MD, Coulombe JA, Corkum PV. ABCs of SLEEPING: a review of the evidence
behind pediatric sleep practice recommendations. *Sleep Med Rev*. 2016;29:1-14. Available at: https://doi.
org/10.1016/j.smrv.2015.08.006.
34. Tsai SY, Lee CC, Tsai HY, Tung YC. Bedtime routines and objectively assessed sleep in infants. *J Adv
Nurs*. 2022;78:154-164. Available at: https://doi.org/10.1111/jan.14968.
35. Hale L, Berger LM, Lebourgeois MK, Brooks-Gunn J. A longitudinal study of preschoolers' language-
based bedtime routines, sleep duration, and well-being. *J Fam Psychol*. 2011;25:423. Available at: https://
dx.doi.org/10.1037%2Fa0023564.
36. Zajicek-Farber ML, Mayer LM, Daughtery LG, Rodkey E. The buffering effect of childhood routines: Longitudinal connections between early parenting and prekindergarten learning readiness of children in low-
income families. *J Soc Serv Res*. 2014;40:699-720. Available at: https://doi.org/10.1080/01488376.2014.930946.
37. Mindell JA, Lee C, Sadeh A. Young child and maternal sleep in the Middle East. *Sleep Med*. 2017;32:
75-82. Available at: https://doi.org/10.1016/j.sleep.2016.11.011.
38. Mindell JA, Telofski LS, Wiegand B, Kurtz ES. A nightly bedtime routine: impact on sleep in young
children and maternal mood. *Sleep*. 2009;32:599-606. Available at: https://doi.org/10.1093/sleep/32.5.599.
39. Galbraith L, Hewitt K. Behavioural treatment for sleep disturbance. *Health Visit*. 1993;66:169-171.

40. Field T, Hernandez-Reif M. Sleep problems in infants decrease following massage therapy. *Early Child Dev Care*. 2001;168:95-104. Available at: https://doi.org/10.1080/0300443011680106.

41. Field T, Gonzalez G, Diego M, Mindell J. Mothers massaging their newborns with lotion versus no lotion enhances mothers' and newborns' sleep. *Infant Behav Dev*. 2016;45:31-37. Available at: https://doi.org/10.1016/j.infbeh.2016.08.004.

42. Ferber SG, Laudon M, Kuint J, Weller A, Zisapel N. Massage therapy by mothers enhances the adjustment of circadian rhythms to the nocturnal period in full-term infants. *J Dev Behav Pediatr*. 2002;23:410-415.

43. Spielman AJ, Saskin P, Thorpy MJ. Treatment of chronic insomnia by restriction of time in bed. *Sleep*. 1987;10:45-56. Available at: https://doi.org/10.1093/sleep/10.1.45.

44. Maurer LF, Espie CA, Kyle SD. How does sleep restriction therapy for insomnia work? A systematic review of mechanistic evidence and the introduction of the Triple-R model. *Sleep Med Rev*. 2018;42: 127-138. Available at: https://doi.org/10.1016/j.smrv.2018.07.005.

45. Piazza CC, Fisher WW. Bedtime fading in the treatment of pediatric insomnia. *J Behav Ther Exp Psychiatry*. 1991;22:53-56. Available at: https://doi.org/10.1016/0005-7916(91)90034-3.

46. Christodulu KV, Durand VM. Reducing bedtime disturbance and night waking using positive bedtime routines and sleep restriction. *Focus Autism Dev Disabil*. 2004;19:130-139. Available at: https://doi.org/10.1177%2F10883576040190030101.

47. Ashbaugh R, Peck SM. Treatment of sleep problems in a toddler: a replication of the faded bedtime with response cost protocol. *J Appl Behav Anal*. 1998;31:127-129. Available at: https://doi.org/10.1901/jaba.1998.31-127.

48. Deleon IG, Fisher WW, Marhefka JM. Decreasing self-injurious behavior associated with awakening in a child with autism and developmental delays. *Behav Interv*. 2004;19:111-119. Available at: https://doi.org/10.1002/bin.154.

49. Maurer LF, Schneider J, Miller CB, Espie CA, Kyle SD. The clinical effects of sleep restriction therapy for insomnia: a meta-analysis of randomised controlled trials. *Sleep Med Rev*. 2021;58:101493. Available at: https://doi.org/10.1016/j.smrv.2021.101493.

50. Cooney MR, Short MA, Gradisar M. An open trial of bedtime fading for sleep disturbances in preschool children: a parent group education approach. *Sleep Med*. 2018;46:98-106. Available at: https://doi.org/10.1016/j.sleep.2018.03.003.

51. Mcgarr RJ, Hovell MF. In search of the sand man: shaping an infant to sleep. *Educ Treat Children*. 1980;3:173-182.

52. Johnson C, Bradley-Johnson S, Stack J. Decreasing the frequency of infants' nocturnal crying with the use of scheduled awakenings. *Fam Pract Res J*. 1981;1:98-104.

53. Johnson CM, Lerner M. Amelioration of infant sleep disturbances: II. Effects of scheduled awakenings by compliant parents. *Infant Ment Health J*. 1985;6:21-30. Available at: https://doi.org/10.1002/1097-0355(198521)6:1%3C21::AID-IMHJ2280060105%3E3.0.CO;2-Q.

54. Rickert VI, Johnson CM. Reducing nocturnal awakening and crying episodes in infants and young children: a comparison between scheduled awakenings and systematic ignoring. *Pediatrics*. 1988;81:203-212. Available at: https://doi.org/10.1542/peds.81.2.203.

55. Honaker SM, Meltzer LJ. Bedtime problems and night wakings in young children: an update of the evidence. *Paediatr Respir Rev*. 2014;15:333-339. Available at: https://doi.org/10.1016/j.prrv.2014.04.011.

56. Hogg T, Blau M. *The Baby Whisperer Solves All Your Problems: Sleeping, Feeding, and Behavior— Beyond the Basics from Infancy Through Toddlerhood*. Simon and Schuster; 2006.

57. Freedman J, Karol S, Aicardi E, Symon B. *The Dream Feed Method: How We Got Our Babies Sleeping from Dusk till Dawn. Without Crying-It-Out*. BookBaby; 2018.

58. Dewar G. *Dream Feeding: An Evidence-Based Guide to Helping Babies Sleep Longer*. 2018. Available at: https://parentingscience.com/dream-feeding/. Accessed November 22, 2021.

59. Paul IM, Savage JS, Anzman-Frasca S, Marini ME, Mindell JA, Birch LL. INSIGHT responsive parenting intervention and infant sleep. *Pediatrics*. 2016;138. Available at: https://dx.doi.org/10.1542%2Fpeds.2016-0762.

60. Pinilla T, Birch LL. Help me make it through the night: behavioral entrainment breast-fed infants' sleep patterns. *Pediatrics*. 1993;91:436-444. Available at: https://publications.aap.org/pediatrics/article-abstract/91/2/436/58621/Help-Me-Make-It-Through-the-Night-Behavirol?redirectedFrom=fulltext.

61. Burnham MM, Goodlin-Jones BL, Gaylor EE, Anders TF. Nighttime sleep-wake patterns and self-soothing from birth to one year of age: a longitudinal intervention study. *J Child Psychol Psychiatry*. 2002;43:713-725. Available at: https://doi.org/10.1111/1469-7610.00076.

62. Mindell JA, Sadeh A, Kohyama J, How TH. Parental behaviors and sleep outcomes in infants and toddlers: a cross-cultural comparison. *Sleep Med.* 2010;11:393-399. Available at: https://doi.org/10.1016/j.
sleep.2009.11.011.
63. Tikotzky L, Sadeh A. Maternal sleep-related cognitions and infant sleep: a longitudinal study from
pregnancy through the 1st year. *Child Dev.* 2009;80:860-874. Available at: https://doi.org/10.1111/
j.1467-8624.2009.01302.x.
64. Burnham MM, Goodlin-Jones BL, Gaylor EE, Anders TF. Use of sleep aids during the first year of life.
Pediatrics. 2002;109:594-601. Available at: https://doi.org/10.1542/peds.109.4.594.
65. Ficca G, Fagioli I, Giganti F, Salzarulo P. Spontaneous awakenings from sleep in the first year of life.
Early Hum Dev. 1999;55:219-228. Available at: https://doi.org/10.1016/S0378-3782(99)00016-X.
66. Williams CD. The elimination of tantrum behavior by extinction procedures. *J Abnorm Soc Psychol.*
1959;59:269. Available at: https://psycnet.apa.org/doi/10.1037/h0046688.
67. France KG, Hudson SM. Behavior management of infant sleep disturbance. *J Appl Behav Anal.*
1990;23:91-98. Available at: https://doi.org/10.1901/jaba.1990.23-91.
68. Honaker SM, Schwichtenberg AJ, Kreps TA, Mindell JA. Real-world implementation of infant behavioral sleep interventions: results of a parental survey. *J Pediatr.* 2018;199:106-111.e2. Available at: https://
doi.org/10.1016/j.jpeds.2018.04.009.
69. Douglas PS. High level evidence does not support first wave behavioural approaches to parent-infant
sleep. *Sleep Med Rev.* 2015;30:121-122. Available at: https://doi.org/10.1016/j.smrv.2015.10.007.
70. Kempler L, Sharpe L, Bartlett DJ. Response to SMRV-D-15-564: not yet time to throw the baby out
with the bathwater, a paradigm shift is premature. *Sleep Med Rev.* 2016;100:119-120. Available at:
https://doi.org/10.1016/j.smrv.2015.11.001.
71. Sadeh A. The role and validity of actigraphy in sleep medicine: an update. *Sleep Med Rev.* 2011;15:
259-267. Available at: https://doi.org/10.1016/j.smrv.2010.10.001.
72. Blunden SL, Thompson KR, Dawson D. Behavioural sleep treatments and night time crying in infants:
challenging the status quo. *Sleep Med Rev.* 2011;15:327-334. Available at: https://doi.org/10.1016/j.
smrv.2010.11.002.
73. Rolider A, van Houten R. Training parents to use extinction to eliminate nighttime crying by gradually
increasing the criteria for ignoring crying. *Educ Treat Children.* 1984;119-124.
74. Ferber R. *Solve Your Child's Sleep Problems.* New York: Simon & Schuster; 1985.
75. Eckerberg B. Treatment of sleep problems in families with young children: effects of treatment on family
well-being. *Acta Paediatr.* 2004;93:126-134. Available at: https://doi.org/10.1111/j.1651-2227.2004.
tb00686.x.
76. Hall WA, Hutton E, Brant RF, et al. A randomized controlled trial of an intervention for infants' behavioral
sleep problems. *BMC Pediatr.* 2015;15:181. Available at: https://doi.org/10.1186/s12887-015-0492-7.
77. Hiscock H, Bayer J, Gold L, Hampton A, Ukoumunne OC, Wake M. Improving infant sleep and
maternal mental health: a cluster randomised trial. *Arch Dis Child.* 2007;92:952-958. Available at: http://
dx.doi.org/10.1136/adc.2006.099812.
78. Hiscock H, Bayer JK, Hampton A, Ukoumunne OC, Wake M. Long-term mother and child mental
health effects of a population-based infant sleep intervention: cluster-randomized, controlled trial.
Pediatrics. 2008;122:e621-e627. Available at: https://doi.org/10.1542/peds.2007-3783.
79. Sadeh A. Assessment of interventions for infant night waking- parental reports and activity-based home
monitoring. *J Consult Clin Psychol.* 1994;62:63-68. Available at: https://psycnet.apa.org/doi/10.1037/
0022-006X.62.1.63.
80. Skuladottir A, Thome M. Changes in infant sleep problems after a family-centered intervention. *Pediatr
Nurs.* 2003;29:375-378.
81. Matthey S, Črnčec R. Comparison of two strategies to improve infant sleep problems, and associated
impacts on maternal experience, mood and infant emotional health: a single case replication design study.
Early Hum Dev. 2012;88:437-442. Available at: https://doi.org/10.1016/j.earlhumdev.2011.10.010.
82. Kahn M, Livne-Karp E, Juda-Hanael M, et al. Behavioral interventions for infant sleep problems: the
role of parental cry tolerance and sleep-related cognitions. *J Clin Sleep Med.* 2020;16:1275-1283. Available at: https://doi.org/10.5664/jcsm.8488.
83. Kahn M, Gradisar M. Sleeping through COVID-19: a longitudinal comparison of 2019 and 2020
infant auto-videosomnography metrics. *J Child Psychol Psychiatry.* 2022;63(6):693-700. Available at:
https://doi.org/10.1111/jcpp.13509.

84. Norris LA, Kendall PC. Moderators of outcome for youth anxiety treatments: current findings and future directions. *J Clin Child Adolesc Psychol.* 2021;50:450-463. Available at: https://doi.org/10.1080/1 5374416.2020.1833337.
85. Danzi BA, La Greca AM. Treating children and adolescents with posttraumatic stress disorder: moderators of treatment response. *J Clin Child Adolesc Psychol.* 2021;50:510-516. Available at: https://doi.or g/10.1080/15374416.2020.1823849.
86. Jenni OG, Borbély AA, Achermann P. Development of the nocturnal sleep electroencephalogram in human infants. *Am J Physiol Regul Integr Comp Physiol.* 2004;286:R528-R538. Available at: https://doi. org/10.1152/ajpregu.00503.2003.
87. Jenni OG, Deboer T, Achermann P. Development of the 24-h rest-activity pattern in human infants. *Infant Behav Dev.* 2006;29:143-152. Available at: https://doi.org/10.1016/j.infbeh.2005.11.001.
88. Douglas PS, Hill PS. Behavioral sleep interventions in the first six months of life do not improve outcomes for mothers or infants: a systematic review. *J Dev Behav Pediatr.* 2013;34:497-507. Available at: https://doi.org/10.1097/DBP.0b013e31829cafa6.
89. Middlemiss W, Granger DA, Goldberg WA, Nathans L. Asynchrony of mother–infant hypothalamic–pituitary–adrenal axis activity following extinction of infant crying responses induced during the transition to sleep. *Early Hum Dev.* 2012;88:227-232. Available at: https://doi.org/10.1016/j.earlhum-dev.2011.08.010.
90. Kahn M, Bauminger Y, Volkovich E, Meiri G, Sadeh A, Tikotzky L. Links between infant sleep and parental tolerance for infant crying: longitudinal assessment from pregnancy through six months postpartum. *Sleep Med.* 2018;50:72-78. Available at: https://doi.org/10.1016/j.sleep.2018.05.014.
91. Sadeh A, Juda-Hanael M, Livne-Karp E, et al. Low parental tolerance for infant crying: an underlying factor in infant sleep problems? *J Sleep Res.* 2016;25:501-507. Available at: https://doi.org/10.1111/jsr.12401.
92. Camerota M, Propper CB, Teti DM. Intrinsic and extrinsic factors predicting infant sleep: moving beyond main effects. *Dev Rev.* 2019;53:100871. Available at: https://doi.org/10.1016/j.dr.2019.100871.
93. Sadeh A, Tikotzky L, Scher A. Parenting and infant sleep. *Sleep Med Rev.* 2010;14:89-96. Available at: https://doi.org/10.1016/j.smrv.2009.05.003.
94. Alpha P. *Sleep Training and Learned Helplessness.* Available at: https://www.thealphaparent.com/sleep-training-and-learned-helplessness/. Accessed November 30, 2021.
95. Mckay P. *When Baby Sleep Training Goes Wrong—The Risks of Controlled Crying.* Available at: https://www.pinkymckay.com/when-baby-sleep-training-goes-wrong-the-risks-of-controlled-crying/. Accessed November 29, 2021.
96. Cinelli M, Morales GDF, Galeazzi A, Quattrociocchi W, Starnini M. The echo chamber effect on social media. *Proc Natl Acad Sci.* 2021;118. Available at: https://doi.org/10.1073/pnas.2023301118.
97. Moon RY, Mathews A, Oden R, Carlin R. Mothers' perceptions of the Internet and social media as sources of parenting and health information: qualitative study. *J Med Internet Res.* 2019;21:e14289. Available at: https://doi.org/10.2196/14289.
98. Tangherlini TR, Roychowdhury V, Glenn B, et al. "Mommy blogs" and the vaccination exemption narrative: results from a machine-learning approach for story aggregation on parenting social media sites. *JMIR Public Health Surveill.* 2016;2:e6586. Available at: https://doi.org/10.2196/publichealth.6586.
99. Bail CA, Argyle LP, Brown TW, et al. Exposure to opposing views on social media can increase political polarization. *Proc Natl Acad Sci.* 2018;115:9216-9221.
100. Schmidt AL, Zollo F, Scala A, Betsch C, Quattrociocchi W. Polarization of the vaccination debate on Facebook. *Vaccine.* 2018;36:3606-3612. Available at: https://doi.org/10.1016/j.vaccine.2018.05.040.
101. Rosier JG, Cassels T. From "Crying Expands the Lungs" to "You're Going to Spoil That Baby": how the Cry-It-Out method became authoritative knowledge. *J Fam Issues.* 2021;42:1516-1535. Available at: https://doi.org/10.1177%2F0192513X20949891.
102. Ball HL, Tomori C, Mckenna JJ. Toward an integrated anthropology of infant sleep. *Am Anthropol.* 2019;121:595-612. Available at: https://doi.org/10.1111/aman.13284.
103. Munroe RL, Munroe RH, Whiting BB. *Handbook of Cross-Cultural Human Development.* Taylor & Francis; 1981.
104. Henderson JM, France KG, Blampied NM. The consolidation of infants' nocturnal sleep across the first year of life. *Sleep Med Rev.* 2011;15:211-220. Available at: https://doi.org/10.1016/j.smrv.2010.08.003.
105. Tikotzky L, Volkovich E. Infant nocturnal wakefulness: a longitudinal study comparing three sleep assessment methods. *Sleep.* 2018;42:zsy191. Available at: https://doi.org/10.1093/sleep/zsy191.

106. Ben-Zion H, Volkovich E, Meiri G, Tikotzky L. Mother–infant sleep and maternal emotional distress in solo-mother and two-parent families. *J Pediatr Psychol*. 2020;45:181-193. Available at: https://doi.org/10.1093/jpepsy/jsz097.

107. Davies L. Babies co-sleeping with parents. *Midwives*. 1995;108:384-386.

108. Gottlieb A. Where have all the babies gone? Toward an anthropology of infants (and their caretakers). *Anthropol Q*. 2000;73:121-132.

109. Obladen M. Lethal lullabies: a history of opium use in infants. *J Hum Lact*. 2016;32:75-85. Available at: https://doi.org/10.1177%2F0890334415594615.

110. Mathianaki K, Tzatzarakis M, Karamanou M. Poppies as a sleep aid for infants: the "Hypnos" remedy of Cretan folk medicine. *Toxicol Rep*. 2021;8:1729-1733. Available at: https://doi.org/10.1016/j.toxrep.2021.10.002.

111. Mindell JA, Moline ML, Zendell SM, Brown LW, Fry JM. Pediatricians and sleep disorders: training and practice. *Pediatr Neonatol*. 1994;94:194-200. Available at: https://doi.org/10.1542/peds.94.2.194.

112. Liew SC, Aung T. Sleep deprivation and its association with diseases-a review. *Sleep Med*. 2021;77: 192-204. Available at: https://doi.org/10.1016/j.sleep.2020.07.048.

113. King LS, Rangel E, Simpson N, Tikotzky L, Manber R. Mothers' postpartum sleep disturbance is associated with the ability to sustain sensitivity toward infants. *Sleep Med*. 2020;65:74-83. Available at: https://doi.org/10.1016/j.sleep.2019.07.017.

114. McQuillan ME, Bates JE, Staples AD, Deater-Deckard K. Maternal stress, sleep, and parenting. *J Fam Psychol*. 2019;33:349. Available at: https://psycnet.apa.org/doi/10.1037/fam0000516.

115. Tikotzky L. Postpartum maternal sleep, maternal depressive symptoms and self-perceived mother–infant emotional relationship. *Behav Sleep Med*. 2016;14:5-22. Available at: https://doi.org/10.1080/15402002.2014.940111.

116. Tikotzky L, Chambers AS, Kent J, Gaylor E, Manber R. Postpartum maternal sleep and mothers' perceptions of their attachment relationship with the infant among women with a history of depression during pregnancy. *Int J Behav Dev*. 2012;36:440-448. Available at: https://doi.org/10.1177%2F0165025412450528.

117. Bartels L, Easteal P. Mothers who kill: the forensic use and judicial reception of evidence of postnatal depression and other psychiatric disorders in Australian filicide cases. *Melb Univ Law Rev*. 2013;37:297-341.

118. Chaffin M, Kelleher K, Hollenberg J. Onset of physical abuse and neglect: Psychiatric, substance abuse, and social risk factors from prospective community data. *Child Abuse Negl*. 1996;20:191-203. Available at: https://doi.org/10.1016/S0145-2134(95)00144-1.

119. Kahn M, Fridenson S, Lerer R, Bar-Haim Y, Sadeh A. Effects of one night of induced night-wakings versus sleep restriction on sustained attention and mood: a pilot study. *Sleep Med*. 2014;15:825-832. Available at: https://doi.org/10.1016/j.sleep.2014.03.016.

120. Ben Simon E, Vallat R, Barnes CM, Walker MP. Sleep loss and the socio-emotional brain. *Trends Cogn Sci*. 2020;24:435-450. Available at: https://doi.org/10.1016/j.tics.2020.02.003.

121. Kahn M, Sheppes G, Sadeh A. Sleep and emotions: bidirectional links and underlying mechanisms. *Int J Psychophysiol*. 2013;89:218-228. Available at: https://doi.org/10.1016/j.ijpsycho.2013.05.010.

122. Sadeh A, Mindell JA, Owens J. Why care about sleep of infants and their parents? *Sleep Med Rev*. 2011;15:335-337. Available at: http://dx.doi.org/10.1016/j.smrv.2011.03.001.

123. Thunström M. Severe sleep problems in infancy associated with subsequent development of attention-deficit/hyperactivity disorder at 5.5 years of age. *Acta Paediatr*. 2002;91:584-592. Available at: https://doi.org/10.1111/j.1651-2227.2002.tb03281.x.

124. Kaar JL, Schmiege SJ, Kalkwarf HJ, Woo JG, Daniels SR, Simon SL. Longitudinal assessment of sleep trajectories during early childhood and their association with obesity. *Child Obes*. 2020;16:211-217. Available at: https://doi.org/10.1089/chi.2019.0126.

125. Bowlby J. *Attachment, Volume 1, Attachment and Loss*. New York: Basic Books; 1969.

126. Acebo C, Thoman EB. Role of infant crying in the early mother-infant dialogue. *Physiol Behav*. 1995;57:541-547. Available at: https://doi.org/10.1016/0031-9384(94)00345-6.

127. Bell SM, Ainsworth MDS. Infant crying and maternal responsiveness. *Child Dev*. 1972;43:1171-1190.

128. Feldman R. The adaptive human parental brain: implications for children's social development. *Trends Neurosci*. 2015;38:387-399. Available at: https://doi.org/10.1016/j.tins.2015.04.004.

129. Swain JE. The human parental brain: in vivo neuroimaging. *Prog Neuro-Psychopharmacol Biol Psychiatry*. 2011;35:1242-1254. Available at: https://doi.org/10.1016/j.pnpbp.2010.10.017.

130. Davis AM, Kramer RS. Commentary: does "cry it out" really have no adverse effects on attachment? Reflections on Bilgin and Wolke (2020). *J Child Psychol Psychiatry*. 2021;62:1488-1490. Available at: https://doi.org/10.1111/jcpp.13223.

131. van Ijzendoorn MH, Hubbard FO. Are infant crying and maternal responsiveness during the first year related to infant-mother attachment at 15 months? *Attach Hum Dev*. 2000;2:371-391. Available at: https://doi.org/10.1080/14616730010001596.

132. Gewirtz JL, Boyd EF. Does maternal responding imply reduced infant crying? A critique of the 1972 Bell and Ainsworth report. *Child Dev*. 1977:1200-1207. Available at: https://doi.org/10.2307/1128476.

133. Bilgin A, Wolke D. Parental use of "cry it out" in infants: no adverse effects on attachment and behavioural development at 18 months. *J Child Psychol Psychiatry*. 2020;61:1184-1193. Available at: https://doi.org/10.1111/jcpp.13223.

134. Hubbard FO, van Ijzendoorn MH. Maternal unresponsiveness and infant crying across the first 9 months: a naturalistic longitudinal study. *Infant Behav Dev*. 1991;14:299-312. Available at: https://doi.org/10.1016/0163-6383(91)90024-M.

135. Winnicott DW. Transitional objects and transitional phenomena: a study of the first not-me. *Int J Psychoanal*. 1953;34:89-97.

136. Winnicott DW. The capacity to be alone. *Int J Psychoanal*. 1958;39:416-420.

137. Kohut H. *The Analysis of the Self*. New York: International Universities; 1971.

138. Baumrind D. Child care practices anteceding three patterns of preschool behavior. *Genet Psychol Monogr*. 1967;75:43-88.

139. Baumrind D. Authoritative parenting revisited: history and current status. In: Larzelere RE, Morris AS, Harrist AW, eds. *Authoritative Parenting: Synthesizing Nurturance and Discipline for Optimal Child Development*. American Psychological Association; 2013:11-34.

140. Price A, Wake M, Ukoumunne OC, Hiscock H. Five-year follow-up of harms and benefits of behavioral infant sleep intervention: randomized trial. *Pediatrics*. 2012;130:643-651. Available at: https://doi.org/10.1542/peds.2011-3467.

141. Price A, Hiscock H, Gradisar M. Let's help parents help themselves: a letter to the editor supporting the safety of behavioural sleep techniques. *Early Hum Dev*. 2012;89:39-40. Available at: https://doi.org/10.1016/j.earlhumdev.2012.07.018.

142. Ivars K, Nelson N, Theodorsson A, Theodorsson E, Ström JO, Mörelius E. Development of salivary cortisol circadian rhythm and reference intervals in full-term infants. *PLoS One*. 2015;10:e0129502. Available at: https://doi.org/10.1371/journal.pone.0151888.

143. Mindell JA, du Mond CE, Sadeh A, Telofski LS, Kulkarni N, Gunn E. Efficacy of an internet-based intervention for infant and toddler sleep disturbances. *Sleep*. 2011;34:451-458. Available at: https://doi.org/10.1093/sleep/34.4.451.

144. Leichman ES, Gould RA, Williamson AA, Walters RM, Mindell JA. Effectiveness of an mHealth intervention for infant sleep disturbances. *Behav Ther*. 2020;51:548-558. Available at: https://doi.org/10.1016/j.beth.2019.12.011.

145. Mahler MS. Symbiosis and individuation: the psychological birth of the human infant. *Psychoanal Study Child*. 1974;29:89-106.

146. Wilson KR, Prior MR. Father involvement and child well-being. *J Paediatr Child Health*. 2011;47:405-407. Available at: https://doi.org/10.1111/j.1440-1754.2010.01770.x.

147. Tikotzky L, Sadeh A, Volkovich E, Manber R, Meiri G, Shahar G. VII. Infant sleep development from 3 to 6 months postpartum: links with maternal sleep and paternal involvement. *Monogr Soc Res Child Dev*. 2015;80:107-124. Available at: https://doi.org/10.1111/mono.12147.

148. Mindell JA, Sadeh A, Wiegand B, How TH, Goh DY. Cross-cultural differences in infant and toddler sleep. *Sleep Med Clin*. 2010;11:274-280. Available at: https://doi.org/10.1016/j.sleep.2009.04.012.

149. Honaker SM, Mindell JA, Slaven JE, Schwichtenberg A. Implementation of infant behavioral sleep intervention in a diverse sample of mothers. *Behav Sleep Med*. 2021;19(4):547-561. Available at: https://doi.org/10.1080/15402002.2020.1817745.

Infant Sleep Health Disparities and Cross-Cultural Differences

Francesca Lupini ■ Ariel A. Williamson

Infant Sleep Health Disparities and Cross-Cultural Differences

The National Institute of Minority Health and Health Disparities (NIMHD) defines a health disparity as a health difference that adversely affects disadvantaged populations, based on one or more health outcomes.[1] NIMHD identifies racial and ethnic minoritized populations, those of less privileged socioeconomic status (SES), rural populations, sexual and gender minorities, and any subpopulations that may fit two or more of these descriptions as health disparity populations. In this chapter, we review literature on disparities in infant sleep health and sleep problems, with a focus on potential mechanisms and directions for future infant sleep research. The majority of extant research focuses on racial, ethnic, and socioeconomic disparities. In addition to reviewing these sleep health disparities, we will include studies of variation in infant sleep health and sleep problems across cultures and contexts. In this chapter, sleep health refers to a multidimensional construct that includes sleep patterns, such as sleep duration and timing (bed and wake times), as well as perceived sleep quality, sleep continuity (efficiency, or night awakenings), alertness, and sleep-related behaviors, in line with the expansion of Buysse's definition[2] to pediatrics.[3] Sleep problems refer to medical sleep disorders, such as obstructive sleep apnea, as well as caregiver- and/or family-perceived behavioral child sleep problems, including difficulties initiating and/or maintaining sleep (i.e., insomnia symptoms).

In discussing infant sleep disparities by race and ethnicity, as well as potential determinants of these disparities, it is crucial to acknowledge that both race and ethnicity are sociopolitical constructs.[4,5] Observed racial and ethnic disparities are not due to biological or genetic differences and instead reflect historical and ongoing racism and discrimination at multiple social and environmental levels.[6,7] Recognition of the contextual nature of race and ethnicity is important, as it allows us to consider the systemic causes and develop multilevel solutions to eradicate health disparities, rather than accept them as inevitable differences based on the false notion of biological determinism.

CROSS-CULTURAL RESEARCH ON INFANT SLEEP HEALTH

Over the first few years of life, sleep patterns rapidly develop, with many changes in sleep timing, consolidation, naps, and total (24-hour) sleep duration.[8,9] Although sleep is often conceptualized as a physiological phenomenon driven by biological need, a large body of evidence indicates that cultural and contextual factors play a major role in pediatric sleep patterns.[10,11] Norms and expectations of infant sleep are largely based on cultural expectations; that is, culture helps to determine what constitutes "normal" infant sleep. As such, acknowledging cultural differences in infant sleep patterns is critical for understanding variation in infant sleep health across contexts.

It can be challenging to make cross-cultural comparisons of infant sleep health due to methodological differences and a limited number of countries/regions included in the sampling. However, a few studies utilizing the same measures and procedures in a large number of countries/regions have been conducted and show stark differences across cultures. A study of 29,287 caregivers of infants ages 0 to 36 months across 17 countries found that infants and toddlers from "predominantly Asian (PA)" countries/regions (e.g., China, Korea, Vietnam) had significantly later bedtimes and later wake times than infants and toddlers in "predominantly Caucasian (PC)" countries/regions (e.g., United States, Australia, New Zealand).[12] For example, bedtimes ranged from 19:27 (New Zealand) to 22:17 (Hong Kong), while wake times ranged from 5:56 (Indonesia) to 7:58 (Korea). On average, PA infants and toddlers were going to bed an hour later (21:26) than PC infants and toddlers (20:25).

Regarding other dimensions of sleep health, the same study found that PA infants and toddlers had significantly longer and more frequent night wakings than PC infants and toddlers. There was also variation within the PA group; for instance, infants and toddlers in Korea had fewer night wakings compared to infants and toddlers in other PA countries/regions, although night waking frequency was still increased relative to infants and toddlers in PC countries/regions. Infants and toddlers in PA countries also had significantly shorter sleep duration, both overnight and in a 24-hour period compared to infants and toddlers in PC countries/regions. Nighttime sleep duration ranged from 8.7 hours (Taiwan) to 10.6 hours (New Zealand) and total sleep duration ranged from 11.6 hours (Japan) to 13.3 hours (New Zealand). These differences in sleep duration have been examined longitudinally, with one study showing that young children in Singapore tend to exhibit shortened overnight and total sleep durations but a longer daytime sleep duration from ages 3 to 54 months compared to estimates of overnight sleep among "predominantly Caucasian" samples in other studies.[13]

As noted above, it is important to examine variation in infant sleep health both across and *within* countries/regions. One study utilizing the same data from the broader PA and PC infant sleep research found that infants in Korea had even shorter total sleep duration (11.89 hours) and even later bedtimes (22:08) than infants and toddlers in both PA (12.33 hours, 21:25) and PC (13.02 hours, 20:25) countries/regions overall.[14] Similarly, another study compared the sleep of infants in the broader PA sample to those from Japan, who showed fewer and shorter night awakenings and fewer and shorter naps compared to those of other Asian countries/regions.[15]

Cross-cultural research on infant sleep health behaviors has also shown variation in the consistency and activities involved in bedtime routines. In the same cross-cultural studies referenced above, infants and toddlers from PA countries/regions were less likely to implement a consistent bedtime routine (implemented 5 or more nights/week) than those in PC countries/regions.[10] Activities involved in bedtime routines, including book-reading, watching television, singing songs, and praying, also vary by country/region, and warrant further exploration both within and across contexts, given that research to date has shown a dose-response link between consistent bedtime routines and better early childhood sleep outcomes.[16] As an example of cross-cultural variation within a single country, a recent study of infants and toddlers ages 3 to 36 months in Israel compared Arab and Jewish cultural groups on infant sleep patterns and ecology.[17] Roomsharing and maternal involvement at bedtime were more prevalent among Arab families, with Arab children showing later bedtimes, longer night awakenings, and shorter nighttime sleep durations compared to Jewish children. Interestingly, whereas sleep onset latency was a strong correlate of nighttime sleep duration in Arab children, caregiver behaviors at bedtime were strong correlates of this outcome in Jewish children.[17]

These findings underscore the importance of comparing cultures within a country/regional context, and converge with broader cross-cultural research, which has highlighted that caregiver bedtime presence and family sleep arrangements, in addition to bedtime routines, are associated with variation in early childhood sleep patterns.[12] For instance, sleeping in a separate room was associated with a shorter sleep onset latency, fewer night wakings, and longer nighttime sleep duration, but these associations were stronger among infants in PC countries/regions, who were more likely to fall asleep independently, without caregiver presence, when sleeping in a separate room. By contrast, infants in PA countries/regions were more likely to fall asleep with a caregiver present, regardless of whether the infant slept in a separate or shared room.[12]

INFANT SLEEP HEALTH DISPARITIES

In addition to cross-cultural differences in infant sleep health, there is a growing body of research highlighting sleep health disparities by race, ethnicity, and SES. This research primarily examines infant sleep within instead of across countries/regions, with most studies conducted in the United States. Several studies have found that non-Hispanic/Latinx White (hereafter, "White") infants and toddlers obtain more nighttime sleep compared to infants and toddlers of African American/Black (hereafter, "Black"), Hispanic/Latinx (hereafter, "Latinx"), and Asian racial and ethnic backgrounds.[18-23] Racial and ethnic disparities in infant sleep duration have continued in the context of the coronavirus (COVID-19) pandemic, with a recent study showing shorter nighttime sleep duration in Latinx infants compared to their White counterparts during the ongoing pandemic.[20]

A longitudinal study of infants over the first 2 years of life also found that overall, Black, Latinx, and Asian children showed a consistently shorter total (24-hour) sleep duration compared to White children.[21] One study of predominantly racial and ethnic minoritized preschoolers from lower-SES backgrounds found that over 20% of caregivers reported that their child obtained insufficient total sleep duration (<10 hours), according to age-based US guidelines.[24] Similarly, a longitudinal cohort study examining caregiver-reported child sleep duration of 1288 children at ages 6 months to 2 years, 3 to 4 years, and 5 to 7 years found that Black, Latinx, and Asian children were more likely to experience insufficient sleep than White children at each age.[22] A recent study following 306 infants from age 1 month to 6 months found that Black and Latinx infants experienced smaller increases in nighttime sleep over this developmental period compared to White infants, with Asian infants experiencing more frequent night wakings relative to White infants.[25] At the same time, studies have also shown that children of racial and ethnic minoritized backgrounds tend to obtain more sleep during the day (i.e., more frequent and longer naps) than White children.[21,23] Longer daytime sleep could compensate for the observed shorter nighttime sleep duration, or vice versa.

Notably, some of the racial and ethnic differences in infant sleep described above are partially attenuated when considering SES and other social and environmental factors.[18,22,25] For instance, in the longitudinal cohort study described above, racial and ethnic differences in sleep duration between ages 6 months and 7 years were diminished when considering lower maternal education level and household income, both of which were linked to insufficient sleep.[22] Another study found that Latinx infants were three times more likely to obtain insufficient sleep based on sleep duration recommendations compared to White infants; however, these differences were attenuated when having a foreign-born mother, a lower maternal education level, and a later bedtime were included in analyses.[19] Indeed, independent of racial and ethnic disparities in infant sleep health, there is mounting evidence of socioeconomic sleep disparities. In this research, SES is often indexed using a variety of individual and contextual economic indicators. Child or family-level SES is typically measured using one or a combination of variables such as household income, household poverty level (household size, income, and US poverty guidelines), and caregiver education level or occupational status. For example, several studies in addition to those referenced above have found shortened total infant sleep duration among those living in lower-income homes and/or whose caregivers have not graduated college compared to infants living in higher-income homes and/or with more highly educated caregivers.[21,23]

Other studies have used neighborhood-level indicators of SES, drawing upon available federal data sources, such as the US Census, to identify the average neighborhood income, proportion of families living in poverty, and other metrics. One study of 14,980 caregivers in the United States found later bedtimes, longer sleep onset latencies, and shorter sleep durations for infants living in the most distressed neighborhoods, compared to those in more advantaged neighborhoods, according to a neighborhood economic index based on multiple Census-derived indicators.[26] Another study of 1226 mothers of 12-month-old infants examined infant sleep duration as a function of urbanicity, which is the proportion of urban land use.[27] In this study, average infant sleep duration was shorter in higher quintiles of urbanicity. A recent systematic review found that, overall, lower neighborhood SES was associated with poorer sleep outcomes, including shorter sleep duration and later sleep timing, in young children ages 0 to 5 years.[28] While aspects of the neighborhood social environment, such as crime and safety, were also associated with child sleep outcomes, these studies were conducted with school-aged children and adolescents.

Research on the unique contribution of neighborhood factors to infant sleep health disparities is mixed. In the cross-sectional study of infant sleep and urbanicity, living closer to major roadways and in densely populated neighborhoods were also associated with shorter infant sleep duration, but these associations were no longer significant when sociodemographic variables, such as prenatal tobacco smoke exposure and television viewing at age 1 year, were included in analyses.[27] However, a study of 80 Black infants and their caregivers found that greater neighborhood deprivation was associated with increased infant actigraphy-derived night wakings, even after controlling for family-level sociodemographic factors, including maternal education, family poverty level, and a single-mother household.[29] A Canadian study found that beyond infant ethnicity and family income, an index of neighborhood disorder, based on community-level crime reports, and maternal perceptions of an unsafe neighborhood were associated with less consolidated nighttime sleep among 12-month-old infants.[30] In addition, a Canadian Census-derived neighborhood deprivation measure was indirectly linked to infant sleep consolidation, such that neighborhood deprivation was associated with more disorder and less safety, which in turn was associated with poorer sleep consolidation. While longitudinal research is needed to better understand these associations, these studies underscore the need to examine multiple family- and neighborhood-level SES indicators, along with family race and ethnicity data, when examining infant sleep health disparities.

Overall, there are fewer studies that examine disparities in dimensions of infant sleep health beyond sleep duration, efficiency, and timing.[3] One study found that in families of lower-SES backgrounds, maternal race and ethnicity were related to child bedtime routine consistency, such that children of White mothers were the most likely (94.4%) to have a regular bedtime routine, followed by children of Latinx (89.7%) and Black (85.3%) mothers.[24] In a study examining multilevel cumulative risk factors, including caregiver education, employment, income, and neighborhood-level SES, with each increase in the number of these sociodemographic risks, there was a 10% increase in the likelihood of poor early childhood sleep health behaviors, including the absence of a bedtime routine, caffeine consumption, insufficient sleep duration, and electronics present in the child's bedroom, even when covarying for child race and ethnicity.[31] Another study examining infant sleep health outcomes among caregivers of lower-SES backgrounds found that nearly half (49.6%) of caregivers had a TV in the room where the infant slept and 26.6% of caregivers reported inconsistent infant nap and bedtimes.[32] Further, lower caregiver health literacy was associated with greater likelihood of having a TV in the infant's bedroom, as well as greater likelihood of insufficient infant sleep duration. A longitudinal study following children from 6 months to 7 years found that having a TV in the bedroom at any point during the study was more common among racial and ethnic minoritized children compared to White children.[33] Interestingly, although the effect of lifetime TV viewing on child sleep duration longitudinally did not vary by race and ethnicity, the presence of a TV in the bedroom did, such that having a TV in the bedroom was associated with a 32-minute shorter sleep duration in minoritized children, but not among White children.

CROSS-CULTURAL DIFFERENCES IN BEHAVIORAL INFANT SLEEP PROBLEMS

Broadly defined behavioral sleep problems are very common in infancy and early childhood, with studies indicating that 15% to 30% of children experience caregiver-identified sleep problems in the first few years of life.[34-38] Infant sleep problems are often assessed using a single question directed to caregivers.[39-41] For instance, the Brief Infant Sleep Questionnaire (BISQ), a widely used infant sleep assessment measure, asks caregivers to rate whether they consider their child's sleep to be a problem on a Likert scale ranging from *not a problem* to *a serious problem*.[35] Frequent night awakenings are a common correlate of caregiver-identified infant sleep problems,[37,38] although some research suggests there may be cross-cultural variation in both the prevalence and correlates of infant sleep problems.

The previously discussed cross-cultural research comparing infant sleep patterns and problems in 17 countries/regions found that caregivers in PA countries/regions were more likely to consider their infant's sleep a problem than caregivers in PC countries/regions (51.9% versus 26.3%, respectively)[12]; this was also the case when examining the prevalence of a "severe" infant sleep problem (17% in PA versus 2% in PC countries/regions).[37] PA caregivers (22.3%) were also more likely to endorse child bedtime difficulty compared to PC caregivers (14.3%).[10] A follow-up study examining sleep problem correlates in this sample found that overall frequency of night wakings and cultural context were the strongest predictors of a severe sleep problem.[37] That is, caregivers from PA countries/regions were 6.5 times more likely to report a child sleep problem than caregivers from PC countries/regions. Interestingly, in PC countries/regions child night waking frequency and sleep onset latency were the strongest correlates of a child sleep problem, whereas in PA countries/regions, sociodemographic characteristics, such as child and caregiver age, were most strongly linked to a child sleep problem. Variation in caregiver-perceived child sleep problems may reflect cultural differences in expectations for "normal" versus "problematic" sleep, as well as differences in the perceived impact of child sleep on family functioning. For instance, in 10,085 mothers of young children across 13 different countries/regions, similarly divided into PA versus PC groups, mothers' own sleep was more robustly associated with the perception of her child's sleep as being problematic in PC compared to PA countries/regions.[42]

As with research on infant sleep patterns, findings from this cross-cultural sample showed some within-country/region variation in caregiver-reported sleep problems. For instance, caregivers from Japan were less likely to endorse an infant sleep problem (19.6%) compared to the rest of the PA group (53.3%) but were more likely to report bedtime difficulties.[15] In Korea, fewer severe sleep problems (2.3%) were reported compared to other PA countries/regions (18.1%), with severe sleep problem endorsement more comparable to those in PC countries/regions.[14] In a smaller study examining infant and toddler sleep in Australia and New Zealand, close to one-third of caregivers reported a child sleep problem, which was comparable to rates in these countries drawn from the larger cross-cultural study.[43] Another study found that 49% of infants and toddlers in Spain had a caregiver-identified sleep problem, which was associated with shorter child sleep duration and more frequent and longer night wakings.[44] In a cross-cultural study of Arab and Jewish families in Israel, 14.1% of Arab mothers perceived their 3- to 18-month-old child's sleep to be a problem compared to 4.29% of Jewish mothers, with notable differences in the degree of caregiver bedtime involvement, the sleep ecology, and infant sleep patterns between these cultural groups.[17]

DISPARITIES IN BEHAVIORAL INFANT SLEEP PROBLEMS

Few studies have examined disparities in broadly defined, caregiver-perceived behavioral sleep problems and symptoms in young children, especially during infancy. This literature gap is also found in behavioral sleep treatment research, where few studies have included families of racial and ethnic minoritized and/or lower-SES backgrounds,[45] underscoring the need for additional studies of disparities in both infant behavioral sleep problem identification and treatment. In the United States, there is some initial evidence that White caregivers are more likely to report early childhood sleep problems than caregivers of racial or ethnic minoritized backgrounds.[46] White mothers of preschoolers reported significantly more concerns about their child having sleep onset difficulties (38%) compared to Black mothers (28%), but not Latinx mothers (33%).[46] A retrospective study examining pediatric sleep disorders diagnosed in well child visits found that infants and toddlers of Black and "other" racial and ethnic backgrounds were less likely to have received any (medical or behavioral) sleep disorder diagnosis compared to White infants and toddlers.[47]

A large-scale study of 14,980 caregivers found that caregivers from more socioeconomically distressed neighborhoods, defined using US Census data, were less likely to endorse an infant/toddler sleep problem (42.6%) compared to caregivers from more advantaged neighborhoods (57.9%), despite caregivers in distressed neighborhoods being more likely to report poorer child sleep outcomes, including a longer sleep onset latency and shorter sleep duration.[26] A follow-up study using the same sample demonstrated that although correlates of a caregiver-endorsed child sleep problem were similar across levels of neighborhood distress, the perceived impact of child sleep on caregiver sleep was more robustly associated with a child sleep problem in more advantaged neighborhoods.[48] Importantly, however, information about family-level SES, race, and ethnicity were not available in the dataset. In one of the few studies to examine specific symptoms of insomnia in young children, increased exposure to cumulative sociodemographic risk factors, including family and neighborhood disadvantage, was associated with greater likelihood of caregiver-reported insomnia symptoms in young children, covarying for child race and ethnicity.[31] Of note, however, overall rates of caregiver-perceived sleep problems (15.1%) were lower than anticipated based on previous research.[31]

DISPARITIES IN MEDICAL INFANT SLEEP PROBLEMS

The vast majority of research on disparities in medical sleep disorders in pediatrics has been conducted with school-aged children and adolescents, with a focus on sleep-disordered breathing (SDB). SDB reflects a continuum of breathing difficulties during sleep, from obstructive sleep apnea (OSA), which is the most severe form of SDB, to mild snoring.[49-51] Pediatric SDB is found in between 10.5% and 17.1% of children, with 1% to 3% experiencing OSA.[52] Research on older children indicates that Black youth are approximately four to six times more likely than White youth to experience SDB.[51,53] The sparse early childhood literature indicates similar racial disparities, although smaller in magnitude. A study of infants and toddlers found that Black children were significantly more likely to snore 3 or more times/week than White children (25% versus 15%, respectively).[54] Another study found that Black preschoolers were 2.5 times as likely as White preschoolers to exhibit caregiver-reported SDB symptoms, while Latinx preschoolers were 2.3 times as likely as White preschoolers to exhibit these symptoms.[55] School-aged Black children diagnosed with OSA have also shown increased disease severity (measured by apnea-hypopnea index) on polysomnogram compared to White children with OSA, controlling for other OSA risk factors such as prematurity.[56] Independent of race and ethnicity, SES has also been associated with SDB, such that children from lower-SES homes and/or neighborhoods are more likely to experience SDB than those living in more advantaged contexts.[57-59]

There are additional racial, ethnic, and socioeconomic disparities in the treatment of OSA, potentially reflecting differential access to and experiences with pediatric health care. For instance, a number of studies in older youth indicate lower rates of OSA treatment via adenotonsillectomy, the primary treatment approach, in Black and Latinx compared to White youth.[57,60-62] A study using state health care data found that in addition to lower rates of adenotonsillectomy in Black and Latinx children, there were also lower rates of adenotonsillectomy in children who were publicly insured compared to those with private insurance, suggesting income-related disparities.[60] Another study in a smaller sample found that children who were publicly insured experienced increased delays in SDB treatment, including initial polysomnogram and surgical treatment, than privately insured children.[63] Although in older children, there is also preliminary evidence that the benefits of adenotonsillectomy for treating OSA and its neurobehavioral symptoms may be diminished in Black youth compared to those of White and other racial and ethnic backgrounds.[62] However, more research is needed on disparities in the identification and treatment of SDB, as well as other medical sleep disorders, in infancy and early childhood, especially as medical symptoms and treatment approaches may differ substantially for infants and toddlers compared to youth of older ages.

MULTILEVEL CONTRIBUTORS TO INFANT SLEEP DISPARITIES

A 2020 NIMHD workshop report on sleep health disparities highlighted the need to identify and test multilevel and multifactorial interventions to address these disparities.[5] A socioecological framework[64] is well-suited for understanding the multiple and interactive factors at different social and ecological levels that contribute to sleep health disparities, and this model has been previously applied to sleep patterns, problems, and disparities across the lifespan.[3,11,65-67] Briefly, within this model there are *microsystem* factors, or individual child characteristics, that interact with factors in the *mesosystem* (e.g., family/home, school, health care, and neighborhood environments) and *macrosystem* (e.g., broader social, cultural, and political climate), which also interact within and across levels to contribute to developmental outcomes and disparities.[64] In the sections that follow, we summarize selected socioecological factors that have been associated with infant sleep patterns and problems and could contribute to or buffer against infant sleep disparities. The socioecological factors described below are not an exhaustive list of putative mechanisms, and future research is needed to understand the multifactorial and multilevel nature of sleep health disparities in infancy.

Child Factors

Individual child factors including a history of prematurity, asthma, and obesity, among others, have been linked to variation in sleep patterns (e.g., duration) and disorders[51,53] (e.g., SDB). Temperament is another individual factor thought to interact with caregiver characteristics (e.g., caregiver mood and parenting style) to influence sleep outcomes.[11,67] For instance, in a longitudinal study of 72 mother-infant dyads from ages 1 to 6 months old, child temperament moderated the association between maternal emotional availability at bedtime on infant sleep duration, such that high surgency infants showed greater increases in sleep duration over time than other infants when their mothers were emotionally available at bedtime.[68] Furthermore, child temperament has also been associated with poorer sleep health (e.g., less consistent bedtimes), which in turn has been linked to bedtime resistance.[69] As previously discussed, caregiving patterns at bedtime vary cross-culturally, and additional research is needed to identify whether infant temperament and caregiving experiences interact to predict sleep outcomes in culturally diverse samples.

Family Factors

Many studies of infant sleep health disparities examine potential contributors at the family level, including caregiver sleep health literacy and behaviors. As previously discussed, a study examining caregiver health literacy among families of lower-SES backgrounds found that lower health literacy was associated with poorer child sleep health behaviors and reduced sleep duration.[32] Similarly, greater caregiver sleep knowledge has been associated with more positive sleep health behaviors.[70] Another previously mentioned study indicated that TVs in the bedroom were more common among children of racial and ethnic minoritized backgrounds, and importantly, the impact of the presence of TVs in the bedroom was more robust for these children compared to their White counterparts.[33] Some pilot data indicate that sleep education interventions can increase caregiver knowledge about child sleep health,[71] with one study showing that both bed provision and sleep health education in families living in poverty and without an individual child bed resulted in improved sleep.[72] However, more efforts are needed to test the longitudinal impacts of sleep education in larger, sociodemographically diverse samples.

Maternal mood and cognitions about infant sleep also may impact infant and child sleep outcomes. For instance, a longitudinal study found that mothers whose cognitions indicated difficulty limiting their involvement in their child's sleep at age 12 months were associated with more actigraphy-derived sleep fragmentation and caregiver involvement in child sleep at age 4 years.[73] Another study examining caregiver cognitions and child sleep found that caregivers whose infant had sleep problems also had more difficulty with limit setting or resisting an infant's demands.[74] Caregiver difficulty with limit setting was also associated with increased infant nocturnal wakefulness. Another study found that greater maternal depressive symptoms and dysfunctional cognitions (i.e., worries about infants' night needs) were associated with increased infant night wakings.[75] Furthermore, maternal depressive symptoms and dysfunctional cognitions were also associated with maternal behaviors, including overnight presence, which mediated the linkages between depressive symptoms, dysfunctional cognitions, and infant night wakings. Contrary to these findings, a study of 388 mother-infant dyads at infants 6 and 12 months of age found no associations between maternal depressive symptoms and infant sleep consolidation (6 or 8 hours of uninterrupted sleep),[76] highlighting the need for additional research.

Sleep arrangement, which varies both across and within cultures and contexts, may also contribute to infant sleep disparities and cross-cultural differences. A clinical review of over 600 studies found that generally, African and Asian countries/regions have higher prevalence rates of bedsharing compared to Europe and North and South America.[77] These results are corroborated by the previously discussed large-scale study comparing infant sleep and sleep health behaviors spanning 17 countries/regions, which found infants and toddlers in PA countries/regions were more likely to both roomshare and bedshare with their caregivers than those in PC countries/regions.[10] In addition to variation across countries/regions, there is also evidence of variation in bedsharing by race and ethnicity within contexts. For instance, one US study of families from low-income backgrounds found that Black and Latinx mothers were more likely to bed-share than their White counterparts.[78] In addition, a longitudinal study in the Netherlands comparing bedsharing over the first 2 years of life in a sample of Dutch, Turkish or Moroccan, and Caribbean children found that while rates of bedsharing decreased over time for Dutch infants, the other ethnic groups showed higher rates of bedsharing at baseline and increases in bedsharing over time.[79] Additionally, bedsharing in Dutch families was related to family and child characteristics, such as temperament and maternal depression, but not in other ethnic groups, underscoring the role of cultural factors in family sleep arrangements.

Bedsharing is a common point of debate in sleep medicine, especially in infancy when this can increase risk for sudden unexplained infant death syndrome.[77] While some advocate against bedsharing due to this increased risk and additional negative sleep outcomes, others endorse bedsharing, citing potential coregulatory and sleep benefits for infants and their mothers.[77] There are many reasons that families may decide to bedshare, from cultural norms to reactive bedsharing, or bedsharing that occurs in response to a child sleep disturbance.[80] Bedsharing may occur due to fewer available beds or sleep spaces, which could be the case for families of lower SES, who are more likely to bedshare.[81] A qualitative study in Korea found that mothers generally perceived bed- and roomsharing to promote better, less disrupted infant sleep, although many also noted their own sleep disruption due to hearing their infant's overnight sounds and movements.[82] In another study, mothers who perceived greater toddler sleep problems also reported shorter maternal sleep duration by nearly an hour when cosleeping.[83] Interestingly, a recent study found that bedsharing in the first 6 months of life was not associated with any negative or positive infant behavior or mother-infant attachment outcomes at 18 months of age.[84] Given that family sleep arrangements may vary by culture, context, and child age, more research in this regard is needed to identify how these arrangements could contribute to infant and maternal sleep outcomes.

External family stressors, such as family organization and work schedules, could also contribute to sleep health disparities. For instance, a study of toddlers and preschoolers from racial and ethnic minoritized backgrounds found that household chaos may mediate linkages between positive parenting and better child sleep health, including sufficient sleep duration.[85] Another study examining household chaos in children entering kindergarten found that household chaos also mediates the relationship between family resources and child sleep duration.[86] Caregivers in one qualitative study indicated that their family's work and school schedules, as well as household responsibilities, and the sleep patterns of other family members are barriers to a good night's sleep.[87] Future research should explore modifiable family factors, such as parenting style and household chaos, in relation to disparities in infant sleep health and sleep disorders.

In addition to these external stressors, maternal experiences of racism and discrimination may impact racial disparities in infant sleep. Racism is a social determinant of both physical and mental health throughout the lifespan.[7,88] In particular, caregiver experiences of personally mediated racism (i.e., implicit and explicit bias and discrimination)[6,88] can affect the entire family context, including infant sleep and development. For instance, caregiver experiences of racism have been associated with poorer caregiver mental health, including depression and anxiety,[7,89] and poorer caregiver sleep.[90] In addition, a recent study found that increased caregiver experiences of racial discrimination were associated with shorter child sleep duration longitudinally, from 6 months to 2 years of age.[91]

Health Care Factors

Discrimination and bias in the health care system may also account for disparities by race, ethnicity, and SES in access to pediatric sleep and other related health care services.[92,93] For instance, research has demonstrated that physicians and other health care professionals tend to have implicit (unconscious) pro-White and anti-Black biases toward both adults and children, which could contribute to variation in patient-provider interactions and treatment decision-making.[94-96] Explicit biases may also influence disparities in access to care by SES or insurance status. In a California study of otolaryngologists, while 97% indicated they would offer an appointment to children with commercial insurance, only 27% indicated the same appointment offer to children with government-funded insurance.[97] Administrative burdens (e.g., excessive paperwork) and low monetary reimbursement were commonly cited as reasons that appointments were not offered to those with government-funded insurance. Research that specifically examines discrimination and bias in health care systems in relation to pediatric sleep disorder diagnosis, treatment, and management is needed, as this work could identify points of clinician- and systems-level intervention in these contexts.

Neighborhood Factors

Characteristics of neighborhoods themselves may contribute to disparities in pediatric sleep health as well. A recent systematic review found that poorer neighborhood characteristics, both social (e.g., perception of safety) and physical (e.g., noise, air quality, urban land use, etc.), were related to poorer child sleep outcomes, including increased SDB symptoms, insufficient sleep, and self-reported sleep problems.[28] The presence of environmental allergens could contribute to airway inflammation and risk for SDB symptoms.[58,59] Furthermore, exposure to toxins within the home, such as lead in poor-quality housing, is associated with adverse development, especially in infants and young children, resulting in poor neurobehavioral and socioemotional outcomes.[98-100] However, very little research has been conducted examining environmental toxins in relation to pediatric sleep disparities.

FUTURE DIRECTIONS

There are a number of directions for future research on infant sleep health disparities and cross-cultural differences. Most of the research to date on infant sleep disparities focuses on Black-White differences or SES, with fewer studies focusing on other health disparity populations, such as Asian and Latinx infants or families living in rural contexts. In addition to the limited knowledge of other health disparity populations, there is also a lack of research on the intersecting nature of these disparities. Intersectionality, a term coined by legal scholar Kimberlé Crenshaw, refers to a framework that considers the multilayered and overlapping identities that inform an individual's experience in society.[101] To apply intersectionality theory to pediatric sleep health research, one might examine sleep outcomes in young children of racial and ethnic minoritized backgrounds who also experience neurodevelopmental differences and are living in lower-SES homes. There is a need for more pediatric sleep research using this intersectional lens, as all individuals have overlapping identities that inform health outcomes and focusing on only one aspect of an individual's identity likely overlooks critical nuances. Another important but often excluded population is fathers. The majority of infant sleep research focuses on mothers and infants, with few studies examining the role of fathers in relation to infant sleep outcomes. There is some evidence that paternal involvement positively impacts infant sleep outcomes, but more research involving fathers, especially in treatment studies, is necessary.[102]

There are also methodological limitations in infant sleep health disparities research. Longitudinal studies examining determinants of infant medical and behavioral sleep disorders and disparities are needed, given that sleep patterns change drastically and rapidly over the first few years of life. Most of the available research is cross-sectional, which limits the identification and evaluation of potential causal mechanisms of infant sleep health disparities. Mechanistic research is additionally needed to better understand how determinants of infant sleep health disparities unfold, interact, and evolve over time. Such research can inform the much-needed multilevel treatment strategies for sleep health equity promotion, particularly when modifiable factors are identified.

There is also limited qualitative and mixed methods research considering family perspectives on cultural norms around infant sleep, as well as treatment for medical and behavioral sleep disorders. In a recent qualitative study, caregivers and primary care clinicians identified a lack of knowledge of early childhood sleep-related recommendations, which may inform expectations of normative versus problematic sleep across different populations.[103] Another qualitative study found that mothers from lower-SES backgrounds reported applying the bedtime routine and other sleep strategies they had learned from their own families to their young children's sleep, indicating a legacy of cultural sleep beliefs.[104] Caregiver perspectives from each of these studies also suggested that adaptations to address social and contextual factors (e.g., caregiver work schedules, family sleep beliefs) are needed in behavioral sleep interventions. In a rare qualitative study of family decision-making in treatment for pediatric SDB, caregivers expressed the importance of trust in their physician when identifying the best course of treatment.[105] Collectively, these studies underscore the value of soliciting family perspectives in pediatric sleep research, as these qualitative data can provide insights into sleep intervention foci and adaptations for health disparity populations.

Much of the infant sleep health disparities studies to date have focused on describing the nature and extent of these disparities. Although additional research on determinants of these disparities is needed, there is also a paucity of interventional research for behavioral sleep problems in health disparity populations. A recent systematic review of behavioral sleep interventions found that less than half of intervention studies reported family race and ethnicity, and of those studies, 78% of participants were White.[45] Furthermore, most caregivers included had moderate to high levels of education. Without more diverse participants included in these studies, results of interventions may lack generalizability. Recently, however, a secondary analysis of randomized clinical trial with Black mothers and infants found evidence of longer total infant sleep duration and fewer nighttime awakenings at 16 weeks of age among dyads that received a responsive parenting intervention compared to those who received a safety control condition.[106] Future research should also focus on designing and/or adapting early childhood behavioral sleep treatment strategies as well as broad sleep health promotion efforts in collaboration with families from health disparity populations. Community-engaged research strategies may be especially beneficial in this regard. Initial research on an early childhood behavioral sleep treatment adapted for families from lower-SES and/or racial and ethnic minoritized backgrounds has demonstrated that a community-engaged approach to intervention adaptation is feasible, with families endorsing high levels of intervention acceptability and cultural humility.[107]

CONCLUSION

There are salient cross-cultural differences in infant sleep patterns and problems as well as important racial, ethnic, and socioeconomic sleep health disparities. The evidence of cross-cultural variation in sleep patterns and perceptions of infant sleep problems highlights the notion that infant sleep is determined by multiple factors, including biological needs, cultural norms and expectations of child sleep, and the family context. Considering these and additional factors at multiple socioecological levels is necessary to understand and effectively address infant sleep health disparities. To promote sleep health equity, future research should include an intersectional framework, longitudinal and qualitative designs, as well as a focus on intervention design, adaptation, and evaluation with sociodemographically diverse and health disparity populations.

References

1. *Minority Health and Health Disparities: Definitions and Parameters*. NIMHD; n.d. Available at: https://www.nimhd.nih.gov/about/strategic-plan/nih-strategic-plan-definitions-and-parameters.html.
2. Buysse DJ. Sleep health: can we define it? Does it matter? *Sleep*. 2014;37(1):9-17. Available at: https://doi.org/10.5665/sleep.3298.
3. Meltzer LJ, Williamson AA, Mindell JA. Pediatric sleep health: it matters, and so does how we define it. *Sleep Med Rev*. 2021;57:101425. Available at: https://doi.org/10.1016/j.smrv.2021.101425.
4. Boyd RW, Lindo EG, Weeks LD, McLemore MR. *On Racism: A New Standard for Publishing on Racial Health Inequities*. Health Affairs Blog; July 2, 2020. Available at: https://www-healthaffairs-org.ezproxy.sju.edu/do/10.1377/hblog20200630.939347/full/.
5. Jackson CL, Walker JR, Brown MK, Das R, Jones NL. A workshop report on the causes and consequences of sleep health disparities. *Sleep*. 2020;43(8):zsaa037. Available at: https://doi.org/10.1093/sleep/zsaa037.
6. Jones CP. Invited commentary: "Race," racism, and the practice of epidemiology. *Am J Epidemiol*. 2001;154(4):299-304. Available at: https://doi.org/10.1093/aje/154.4.299.
7. Paradies Y, Ben J, Denson N, et al. Racism as a determinant of health: a systematic review and meta-analysis. *PLoS One*. 2015;10(9):e0138511. Available at: https://doi.org/10.1371/journal.pone.0138511.
8. Galland BC, Taylor BJ, Elder DE, Herbison P. Normal sleep patterns in infants and children: a systematic review of observational studies. *Sleep Med Rev*. 2012;16(3):213-222. Available at: https://doi.org/10.1016/j.smrv.2011.06.001.

9. Mindell JA, Leichman ES, Composto J, Lee C, Bhullar B, Walters RM. Development of infant and toddler sleep patterns: Real-world data from a mobile application. *J Sleep Res.* 2016;25(5):508-516. Available at: https://doi.org/10.1111/jsr.12414.

10. Mindell JA, Sadeh A, Kohyama J, How TH. Parental behaviors and sleep outcomes in infants and toddlers: a cross-cultural comparison. *Sleep Med.* 2010;11(4):393-399. Available at: https://doi.org/10.1016/j.sleep.2009.11.011.

11. Sadeh A, Tikotzky L, Scher A. Parenting and infant sleep. *Sleep Med Rev.* 2010;14(2):89-96. Available at: https://doi.org/10.1016/j.smrv.2009.05.003.

12. Mindell JA, Sadeh A, Wiegand B, How TH, Goh DY. Cross-cultural differences in infant and toddler sleep. *Sleep Med.* 2010;11(3):274-280. Available at: https://doi.org/10.1016/j.sleep.2009.04.012.

13. Tham EK, Xu HY, Fu X, et al. Variations in longitudinal sleep duration trajectories from infancy to early childhood. *Sleep Health.* 2021;7(1):56-64. Available at: https://doi.org/10.1016/j.sleh.2020.06.007.

14. Ahn Y, Williamson AA, Seo HJ, Sadeh A, Mindell JA. Sleep patterns among South Korean infants and toddlers: global comparison. *J Korean Med Sci.* 2016;31(2):261-269. Available at: https://doi.org/10.3346/jkms.2016.31.2.261.

15. Kohyama J, Mindell JA, Sadeh A. Sleep characteristics of young children in Japan: Internet study and comparison with other Asian countries. *Pediatr Int.* 2011;53(5):649-655. Available at: https://doi.org/10.1111/j.1442-200X.2010.03318.x.

16. Mindell JA, Williamson AA. Benefits of a bedtime routine in young children: sleep, development, and beyond. *Sleep Med Rev.* 2018;40:93-108. Available at: https://doi.org/10.1016/j.smrv.2017.10.007.

17. Zreik G, Asraf K, Tikotzky L, Haimov I. Sleep Ecology and sleep patterns among infants and toddlers: a cross-cultural comparison between the Arab and Jewish societies in Israel. *Sleep Med.* 2020;75:117-127. Available at: https://doi.org/10.1016/j.sleep.2020.07.017.

18. Ash T, Davison KK, Haneuse S, et al. Emergence of racial/ethnic differences in infant sleep duration in the first six months of life. *Sleep Med X.* 2019;1:100003. Available at: https://doi.org/10.1016/j.sleepx.2019.100003.

19. Ash T, Taveras EM, Redline S, Haneuse S, Quante M, Davison K. Contextual and parenting factors contribute to shorter sleep among Hispanic/Latinx compared to Non-Hispanic White infants. *Ann Behav Med.* 2021;55(5):424-435. Available at: https://doi.org/10.1093/abm/kaaa062.

20. Lucchini M, Kyle M, Pini N, et al. Racial/ethnic disparities in sleep in mothers and infants during the Covid-19 pandemic. *MedRxiv.* 2021. Available at: https://doi.org/10.1101/2021.03.22.21254093.

21. Nevarez MD, Rifas-Shiman SL, Kleinman KP, Gillman MW, Taveras EM. Associations of early life risk factors with infant sleep duration. *Acad Pediatr.* 2010;10(3):187-193.

22. Peña MM, Rifas-Shiman SL, Gillman MW, Redline S, Taveras EM. Racial/ethnic and socio-contextual correlates of chronic sleep curtailment in childhood. *Sleep.* 2016;39(9):1653-1661. Available at: https://doi.org/10.5665/sleep.6086.

23. Zhang Z, Adamo KB, Ogden N, et al. Longitudinal correlates of sleep duration in young children. *Sleep Med.* 2021;78:128-134. Available at: https://doi.org/10.1016/j.sleep.2020.12.023.

24. Schlieber M, Han J. The sleeping patterns of Head Start children and the influence on developmental outcomes. *Child Care Health Dev.* 2018;44(3):462-469. Available at: https://doi.org/10.1111/cch.12522.

25. Yu X, Quante M, Rueschman M, et al. Emergence of racial/ethnic and socioeconomic differences in objectively measured sleep–wake patterns in early infancy: Results of the Rise & SHINE study. *Sleep.* 2021;44:zsaa193. Available at: https://doi.org/10.1093/sleep/zsaa193.

26. Williamson AA, Gould R, Leichman ES, Walters RM, Mindell JA. Socioeconomic disadvantage and sleep in early childhood: Real-world data from a mobile health application. *Sleep Health.* 2021. Available at: https://doi.org/10.1016/j.sleh.2021.01.002.

27. Bottino CJ, Rifas-Shiman SL, Kleinman KP, et al. The association of urbanicity with infant sleep duration. *Health Place.* 2012;18(5):1000-1005. Available at: https://doi.org/10.1016/j.healthplace.2012.06.007.

28. Mayne SL, Mitchell JA, Virudachalam S, Fiks AG, Williamson AA. Neighborhood environments and sleep among children and adolescents: a systematic review. *Sleep Med Rev.* 2021;57:101465. Available at: https://doi.org/10.1016/j.smrv.2021.101465.

29. Grimes M, Camerota M, Propper CB. Neighborhood deprivation predicts infant sleep quality. *Sleep Health.* 2019;5(2):148-151. Available at: https://doi.org/10.1016/j.sleh.2018.11.001.

30. MacKinnon AL, Tomfohr-Madsen L, Tough S. Neighborhood socio-economic factors and associations with infant sleep health. *Behav Sleep Med.* 2021;19(4):458-470. Available at: https://doi.org/10.1080/15402002.2020.1778478.

31. Williamson AA, Mindell JA. Cumulative socio-demographic risk factors and sleep outcomes in early childhood. *Sleep.* 2020;43(3):zsz233. Available at: https://doi.org/10.1093/sleep/zsz233.

32. Bathory E, Tomopoulos S, Rothman R, et al. Infant sleep and parent health literacy. *Acad Pediatr.* 2016;16(6):550-557. Available at: https://doi.org/10.1016/j.acap.2016.03.004.

33. Cespedes EM, Gillman MW, Kleinman K, Rifas-Shiman SL, Redline S, Taveras EM. Television viewing, bedroom television, and sleep duration from infancy to mid-childhood. *Pediatrics.* 2014;133(5):e1163-e1171. Available at: https://doi.org/10.1542/peds.2013-3998.

34. Blunden SL. Behavioural sleep disorders across the developmental age span: An overview of causes, consequences and treatment modalities. *Psychology.* 2012;3(3):249-256. Available at: https://doi.org/10.4236/psych.2012.33035.

35. Sadeh A. A brief screening questionnaire for infant sleep problems: validation and findings for an Internet sample. *Pediatrics.* 2004;113(6):e570-e577. Available at: https://doi.org/10.1542/peds.113.6.e570.

36. Sadeh A, Mindell JA, Luedtke K, Wiegand B. Sleep and sleep ecology in the first 3 years: a web-based study. *J Sleep Res.* 2009;18(1):60-73. Available at: https://doi.org/10.1111/j.1365-2869.2008.00699.x.

37. Sadeh A, Mindell J, Rivera L. "My child has a sleep problem": a cross-cultural comparison of parental definitions. *Sleep Med.* 2011;12(5):478-482. Available at: https://doi.org/10.1016/j.sleep.2010.10.008.

38. Williamson AA, Mindell JA, Hiscock H, Quach J. Child sleep behaviors and sleep problems from infancy to school-age. *Sleep Med.* 2019;63:5-8. Available at: https://doi.org/10.1016/j.sleep.2019.05.003.

39. Mindell JA, Du Mond CE, Sadeh A, Telofski LS, Kulkarni N, Gunn E. Efficacy of an internet-based intervention for infant and toddler sleep disturbances. *Sleep.* 2011;34(4):451-458.

40. Owens JA. The practice of pediatric sleep medicine: Results of a community survey. *Pediatrics.* 2001;108(3):e51. Available at: https://doi.org/10.1542/peds.108.3.e51.

41. Quach J, Hiscock H, Ukoumunne OC, Wake M. A brief sleep intervention improves outcomes in the school entry year: a randomized controlled trial. *Pediatrics.* 2011;128(4):692-701. Available at: https://doi.org/10.1542/peds.2011-0409.

42. Mindell JA, Sadeh A, Kwon R, Goh DY. Relationship between child and maternal sleep: a developmental and cross-cultural comparison. *J Pediatr Psychol.* 2015;40(7):689-696. Available at: https://doi.org/10.1093/jpepsy/jsv008.

43. Teng A, Bartle A, Sadeh A, Mindell J. Infant and toddler sleep in Australia and New Zealand. *J Paediatr Child Health.* 2012;48(3):268-273. Available at: https://doi.org/10.1111/j.1440-1754.2011.02251.x.

44. Cassanello P, Ruiz-Botia I, Díez-Izquierdo A, Cartanyà-Hueso À, Martínez-Sanchez JM, Balaguer A. How do infants and toddlers sleep in Spain? A cross-sectional study. *Eur J Pediatr.* 2021;180(3):775-782. Available at: https://doi.org/10.1007/s00431-020-03786-2.

45. Schwichtenberg AJ, Abel EA, Keys E, Honaker SM. Diversity in pediatric behavioral sleep intervention studies. *Sleep Med Rev.* 2019;47:103-111. Available at: https://doi.org/10.1016/j.smrv.2019.07.004.

46. Milan S, Snow S, Belay S. The context of preschool children's sleep: racial/ethnic differences in sleep locations, routines, and concerns. *J Fam Psychol.* 2007;21(1):20-28. Available at: https://doi.org/10.1037/0893-3200.21.1.20.

47. Meltzer LJ, Johnson C, Crosette J, Ramos M, Mindell JA. Prevalence of diagnosed sleep disorders in pediatric primary care practices. *Pediatrics.* 2010;125(6):e1410-e1418. Available at: https://doi.org/10.1542/peds.2009-2725.

48. Lupini F, Leichman ES, Gould R, Walters RM, Mindell JA, Williamson AA. Correlates of a caregiver-reported child sleep problem and variation by community disadvantage. *Sleep Med.* 2022;90:83-90. Available at: https://doi.org/10.1016/j.sleep.2022.01.009.

49. Bixler EO, Vgontzas AN, Lin HM, et al. Sleep disordered breathing in children in a general population sample: prevalence and risk factors. *Sleep.* 2009;32(6):731-736.

50. Bonuck KA, Chervin RD, Cole TJ, et al. Prevalence and persistence of sleep disordered breathing symptoms in young children: a 6-year population-based cohort study. *Sleep.* 2011;34(7):875-884. Available at: https://doi.org/10.5665/SLEEP.1118.

51. Rosen CL, Larkin EK, Kirchner HL, et al. Prevalence and risk factors for sleep-disordered breathing in 8- to 11-year-old children: Association with race and prematurity. *J Pediatr.* 2003;142(4):383-389. Available at: https://doi.org/10.1067/mpd.2003.28.

52. Marcus CL, Brooks LJ, Draper KA, et al. Diagnosis and management of childhood obstructive sleep apnea syndrome. *Pediatrics.* 2012;130(3):576-584. Available at: https://doi.org/10.1542/peds.2012-1671.

53. Redline S, Tishler PV, Schluchter M, Aylor J, Clark K, Graham G. Risk factors for sleep-disordered breathing in children. *Am J Respir Crit Care Med.* 1999;159(5):1527-1532. Available at: https://doi.org/10.1164/ajrccm.159.5.9809079.

54. Montgomery-Downs HE, Gozal D. Sleep habits and risk factors for sleep-disordered breathing in infants and young toddlers in Louisville, Kentucky. *Sleep Med.* 2006;7(3):211-219. Available at: https://doi.org/10.1016/j.sleep.2005.11.003.

55. Goldstein NA, Abramowitz T, Weedon J, Koliskor B, Turner S, Taioli E. Racial/ethnic differences in the prevalence of snoring and sleep disordered breathing in young children. *J Clin Sleep Med.* 2011;7(2):163-171.

56. Weinstock TG, Rosen CL, Marcus CL, et al. Predictors of obstructive sleep apnea severity in adenotonsillectomy candidates. *Sleep.* 2014;37(2):261-269. Available at: https://doi.org/10.5665/sleep.3394.

57. Boss EF, Smith DF, Ishman SL. Racial/ethnic and socioeconomic disparities in the diagnosis and treatment of sleep-disordered breathing in children. *Int J Pediatr Otorhinolaryngol.* 2011;75(3):299-307. Available at: https://doi.org/10.1016/j.ijporl.2010.11.006.

58. Spilsbury JC, Storfer-Isser A, Kirchner HL, et al. Neighborhood disadvantage as a risk factor for pediatric obstructive sleep apnea. *J Pediatr.* 2006;149(3):342-347. Available at: https://doi.org/10.1016/j.jpeds.2006.04.061.

59. Wang R, Dong Y, Weng J, et al. Associations among neighborhood, race, and sleep apnea severity in children. A six-city analysis. *Ann Am Thorac Soc.* 2017;14(1):76-84. Available at: https://doi.org/10.1513/AnnalsATS.201609-662OC.

60. Cooper JN, Koppera S, Boss EF, Lind MN. Differences in tonsillectomy utilization by race/ethnicity, type of health insurance, and rurality. *Acad Pediatr.* 2021;21(6):1031-1036. Available at: https://doi.org/10.1016/j.acap.2020.11.007.

61. Kum-Nji P, Mangrem C, Wells P, Klesges L, Herrod H. Black/white differential use of health services by young children in a rural Mississippi community. *South Med J.* 2006. Available at: https://doi.org/10.1097/01.smj.0000232966.81950.a4.

62. Marcus CL, Moore RH, Rosen CL, et al. A randomized trial of adenotonsillectomy for childhood sleep apnea. *N Engl J Med.* 2013;368(25):2366-2376. Available at: https://doi.org/10.1056/NEJMoa1215881.

63. Boss EF, Benke JR, Tunkel DE, Ishman SL, Bridges JFP, Kim JM. Public insurance and timing of polysomnography and surgical care for children with sleep-disordered breathing. *JAMA Otolaryngol Head Neck Surg.* 2015;141(2):106-111. Available at: https://doi.org/10.1001/jamaoto.2014.3085.

64. Bronfenbrenner U. Ecological systems theory. In: Vasta R, ed. *Six Theories of Child Development: Revised Formulations and Current Issues.* Jessica Kingsley Publishers; 1992:187-249.

65. Billings ME, Cohen RT, Baldwin CM, et al. Disparities in sleep health and potential intervention models: a focused review. *Chest.* 2021;159(3):1232-1240. Available at: https://doi.org/10.1016/j.chest.2020.09.249.

66. Grandner MA, Hale L, Moore M, Patel NP. Mortality associated with short sleep duration: the evidence, the possible mechanisms, and the future. *Sleep Med Rev.* 2010;14(3):191-203. Available at: https://doi.org/10.1016/j.smrv.2009.07.006.

67. Sadeh A, Anders TF. Infant sleep problems: origins, assessment, interventions. *Infant Ment Health J.* 1993;14(1):17-34. Available at: https://doi.org/10.1002/1097-0355(199321)14:1<17::AID-IMHJ2280140103>3.0.CO;2-Q.

68. Jian N, Teti DM. Emotional availability at bedtime, infant temperament, and infant sleep development from 1 to 6 months. *Sleep Med.* 2016;23:49-58. Available at: https://doi.org/10.1016/j.sleep.2016.07.001.

69. Wilson KE, Lumeng JC, Kaciroti N, et al. Sleep hygiene practices and bedtime resistance in low-income preschoolers: does temperament matter? *Behav Sleep Med.* 2015;13(5):412-423. Available at: https://doi.org/10.1080/15402002.2014.940104.

70. Owens JA, Jones C. Parental knowledge of healthy sleep in young children: results of a primary care clinic survey. *J Dev Behav Pediatr.* 2011;32(6):447-453. Available at: https://doi.org/10.1097/DBP.0b013e31821bd20b.

71. Jones CH, Owens JA, Pham B. Can a brief educational intervention improve parents' knowledge of healthy children's sleep? A pilot-test. *Health Educ J.* 2013;72(5):601-610. Available at: https://doi.org/10.1177/0017896912464606.

72. Mindell JA, Sedmak R, Boyle JT, Butler R, Williamson AA. Sleep Well!: A pilot study of an education campaign to improve sleep of socioeconomically disadvantaged children. *J Clin Sleep Med.* 2016;12(12):1593-1599. Available at: https://doi.org/10.5664/jcsm.6338.

73. Tikotzky L, Shaashua L. Infant sleep and early parental sleep-related cognitions predict sleep in pre-school children. *Sleep Med.* 2012;13(2):185-192. Available at: https://doi.org/10.1016/j.sleep.2011.07.013.

74. Sadeh A, Flint-Ofir E, Tirosh T, Tikotzky L. Infant sleep and parental sleep-related cognitions. *J Fam Psychol.* 2007;21(1):74-87. Available at: https://doi.org/10.1037/0893-3200.21.1.74.

75. Teti DM, Crosby B. Maternal depressive symptoms, dysfunctional cognitions, and infant night waking: the role of maternal nighttime behavior. *Child Dev.* 2012;83(3):939-953. Available at: https://doi.org/10.1111/j.1467-8624.2012.01760.x.

76. Pennestri MH, Laganière C, Bouvette-Turcot AA, et al. Uninterrupted infant sleep, development, and maternal mood. *Pediatrics.* 2018;142(6):e20174330. Available at: https://doi.org/10.1542/peds.2017-4330.

77. Mileva-Seitz VR, Bakermans-Kranenburg MJ, Battaini C, Luijk MP. Parent-child bed-sharing: the good, the bad, and the burden of evidence. *Sleep Med Rev.* 2017;32:4-27. Available at: https://doi.org/10.1016/j.smrv.2016.03.003.

78. Barajas RG, Martin A, Brooks-Gunn J, Hale L. Mother-child bed-sharing in toddlerhood and cognitive and behavioral outcomes. *Pediatrics.* 2011;128(2):e339-e347. Available at: https://doi.org/10.1542/peds.2010-3300.

79. Luijk MP, Mileva-Seitz VR, Jansen PW, et al. Ethnic differences in prevalence and determinants of mother–child bed-sharing in early childhood. *Sleep Med.* 2013;14(11):1092-1099. Available at: https://doi.org/10.1016/j.sleep.2013.04.019.

80. Covington LB, Armstrong B, Black MM. Bed sharing in toddlerhood: choice versus necessity and provider guidelines. *Glob Pediatr Health.* 2019;6:2333794X19843929. Available at: https://doi.org/10.1177/2333794X19843929.

81. Colson ER, Willinger M, Rybin D, et al. Trends and factors associated with infant bed sharing, 1993-2010: The National Infant Sleep Position Study. *JAMA Pediatr.* 2013;167(11):1032-1037. Available at: https://doi.org/10.1001/jamapediatrics.2013.2560.

82. Chae SM, Yeo JY, Chung N. A qualitative study of the sleep ecology of infants under 2 years old and their mothers in South Korea. *Sleep Health.* 2022;8(1):101-106. Available at: https://doi.org/10.1016/j.sleh.2021.10.013.

83. Covington LB, Armstrong B, Black MM. Perceived toddler sleep problems, co-sleeping, and maternal sleep and mental health. *J Dev Behav Pediatr.* 2018;39(3):238-245. Available at: https://doi.org/10.1097/DBP.0000000000000535.

84. Bilgin A, Wolke D. Bed-sharing in the first 6 months: associations with infant-mother attachment, infant attention, maternal bonding, and sensitivity at 18 months. *J Dev Behav Pediatr.* 2022;43(1):e9-e19. Available at: https://doi.org/10.1097/DBP.0000000000000966.

85. Daniel LC, Childress JL, Flannery JL, et al. Identifying modifiable factors linking parenting skills and sleep outcomes in racial/ethnic minority children. *J Pediatr Psychol.* 2020;45(8):867-876. doi:10.1093/jpepsy/jsaa034.

86. Fronberg KM, Bai S, Teti DM. Household chaos mediates the link between family resources and child sleep. *Sleep Health.* 2022;8(1):121-129. Available at: https://doi.org/10.1016/j.sleh.2021.10.005.

87. Zambrano DN, Mindell JA, Reyes NR, Hart CN, Herring SJ. "It's not all about my baby's sleep": a qualitative study of factors influencing low-income African American mothers' sleep quality. *Behav Sleep Med.* 2016;14(5):489-500. Available at: https://doi.org/10.1080/15402002.2015.1028063.

88. Trent M, Dooley DG, Dougé J, et al. The impact of racism on child and adolescent health. *Pediatrics.* 2019;144(2):e20191765. Available at: https://doi.org/10.1542/peds.2019-1765.

89. Pieterse AL, Todd NR, Neville HA, Carter RT. Perceived racism and mental health among Black American adults: a meta-analytic review. *J Couns Psychol.* 2012;59(1):1-9. Available at: https://doi.org/10.1037/a0026208.

90. Slopen N, Lewis TT, Williams DR. Discrimination and sleep: a systematic review. *Sleep Med.* 2016;18:88-95. Available at: https://doi.org/10.1016/j.sleep.2015.01.012.

91. Powell CA, Rifas-Shiman SL, Oken E, et al. Maternal experiences of racial discrimination and offspring sleep in the first 2 years of life: Project Viva cohort, Massachusetts, USA (1999-2002). *Sleep Health.* 2020;6(4):463-468. Available at: https://doi.org/10.1016/j.sleh.2020.02.002.

92. Johnson TJ. Intersection of bias, structural racism, and social determinants with health care inequities. *Pediatrics.* 2020;146(2):e2020003657. Available at: https://doi.org/10.1542/peds.2020-003657.

93. van Ryn M. Research on the provider contribution to race/ethnicity disparities in medical care. *Med Care.* 2002;40(1):I140-I151.

94. Johnson TJ, Winger DG, Hickey RW, et al. A comparison of physician implicit racial bias towards adults versus children. *Acad Pediatr.* 2017;17(2):120-126. Available at: https://doi.org/10.1016/j.acap.2016.08.010.

95. Maina IW, Belton TD, Ginzberg S, Singh A, Johnson TJ. A decade of studying implicit racial/ethnic bias in healthcare providers using the implicit association test. *Soc Sci Med.* 2018;199:219-229. Available at: https://doi.org/10.1016/j.socscimed.2017.05.009.

96. Sabin JA, Greenwald AG. The influence of implicit bias on treatment recommendations for 4 common pediatric conditions: pain, urinary tract infection, attention deficit hyperactivity disorder, and asthma. *Am J Publ Health.* 2012;102(5):988-995. Available at: https://doi.org/10.2105/AJPH.2011.300621.

97. Wang E, Choe M, Meara J, Koempel J. Inequality of access to surgical specialty health care: why children with government-funded insurance have less access than those with private insurance in Southern California. *Pediatrics.* 2004;114:e584-e590. Available at: https://doi.org/10.1542/peds.2004-0210.

98. Mattison DR. Environmental exposures and development. *Curr Opin Pediatr.* 2010;22(2):208-218. Available at: https://doi.org/10.1097/MOP.0b013e32833779bf.

99. Rauh VA, Margolis A. Research Review: Environmental exposures, neurodevelopment and child mental health—new paradigms for the study of brain and behavioral effects. *J Child Psychol Psychiatry.* 2016;57(7):775-793. Available at: https://doi.org/10.1111/jcpp.12537.

100. Sanders T, Liu Y, Buchner V, Tchounwou PB. Neurotoxic effects and biomarkers of lead exposure: a review. *Rev Environ Health.* 2009;24(1):15-45.

101. Crenshaw K. Demarginalizing the intersection of race and sex: a Black feminist critique of antidiscrimination doctrine, feminist theory and antiracist politics. *Univ Chic Leg Forum.* 1989;1989(1). Available at: https://chicagounbound.uchicago.edu/uclf/vol1989/iss1/8.

102. Ragni B, De Stasio S, Barni D. Fathers and sleep: a systematic literature review of bidirectional links between paternal factors and children's sleep in the first three years of life. *Clin Neuropsychiatry.* 2020;17(6):349-360. Available at: https://doi.org/10.36131/cnfioritieditore20200604.

103. Williamson AA, Milaniak I, Watson B, et al. Early childhood sleep intervention in urban primary care: caregiver and clinician perspectives. *J Pediatr Psychol.* 2020;45(8):933-945. Available at: https://doi.org/10.1093/jpepsy/jsaa024.

104. Caldwell BA, Ordway MR, Sadler LS, Redeker NS. Parent perspectives on sleep and sleep habits among young children living with economic adversity. *J Pediatr Health Care.* 2020;34(1):10-22. Available at: https://doi.org/10.1016/j.pedhc.2019.06.006.

105. Boss EF, Links AR, Saxton R, Cheng TL, Beach MC. Parent experience of care and decision making for children who snore. *JAMA Otolaryngol Head Neck Surg.* 2017;143(3):218-225. Available at: https://doi.org/10.1001/jamaoto.2016.2400.

106. Lavner JA, Hohman EE, Beach SRH, Stansfield BK, Savage JS. Effects of a responsive parenting intervention among black families on infant sleep: a secondary analysis of the sleep SAAF randomized clinical trial. *JAMA Netw Open.* 2023;6(3):e236276. doi:10.1001/jamanetworkopen.2023.6276.

107. Williamson AA, Okoroji C, Cicalese O, et al. *Sleep Well!* An adapted behavioral sleep intervention implemented in urban primary care. *J Clin Sleep Med.* 2022;18(4):1153-1166. doi:10.5664/jcsm.9822.

Note: page numbers followed by "*f*" indicate figures, by "*t*" indicate tables.